STEM CELLS:
SCIENTIFIC PROGRESS
AND FUTURE
RESEARCH DIRECTIONS

June 2001

TABLE OF CONTENTS

OPPORTUNITIES AND CHALLENGES:
A FOCUS ON FUTURE STEM CELL APPLICATIONS

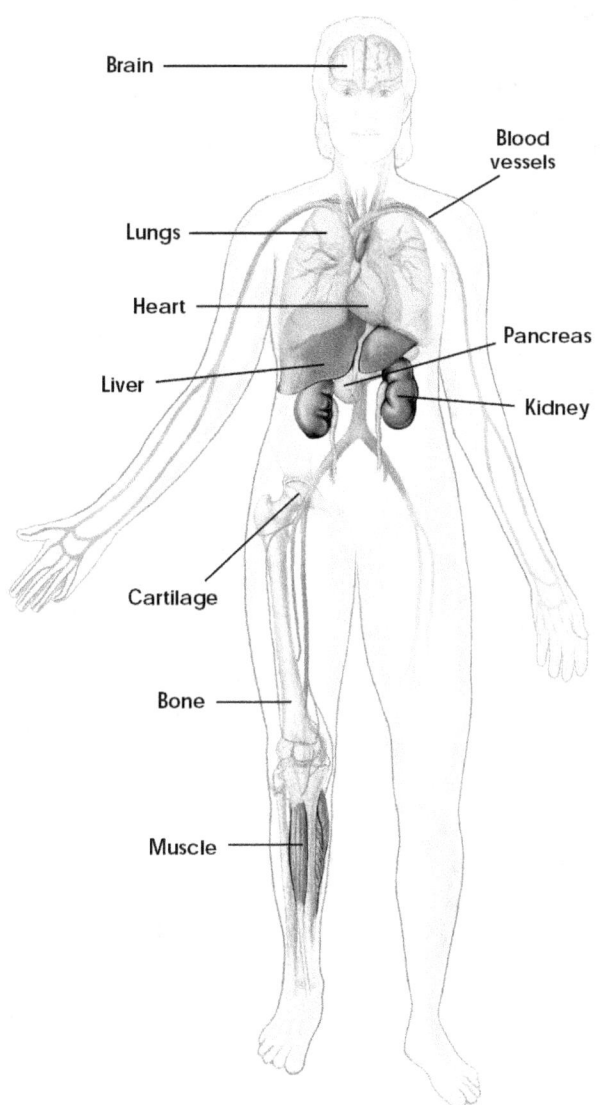

Brain

Blood
vessels

Lungs

Heart

Pancreas

Liver

Kidney

Cartilage

Bone

Muscle

The makings of future news headlines about tomorrow's life saving therapies starts in the biomedical research laboratory. Ideas abound; early successes and later failures and knowledge gained from both; the rare lightning bolt of an unexpected breakthrough discovery — this is a glimpse of the behind the scenes action of some of the world's most acclaimed stem cell scientists' quest to solve some of the human body's most challenging mysteries.

Stem cells — what lies ahead? The following chapters explore some of the cutting edge research featuring stem cells. Disease and disorders with no therapies or at best, partially effective ones, are the lure of the pursuit of stem cell research. Described here are examples of significant progress that is a prologue to an era of medical discovery of cell-based therapies that will one day restore function to those whose lives are now challenged every day — but perhaps in the future, no longer.

REPORT PREPARED BY THE NATIONAL INSTITUTES OF HEALTH

Ruth Kirschstein, M.D.
Acting Director

Office of Science Policy
Lana R. Skirboll, Ph.D.
Director

PREFACE

On February 28, 2001, Tommy G. Thompson, Secretary of Health and Human Services, requested that the National Institutes of Health prepare a summary report on the state of the science on stem cells. This report was developed in response to his request. It provides the current information about the biology of stem cells derived from all sources—embryo, fetal tissue, and adult.

Since 1998, when human pluripotent stem cells were first isolated, research on stem cells has received much public attention, both because of its extraordinary promise and because of relevant legal and ethical issues. Underlying this recent public scrutiny is decades of painstaking work by scientists in many fields, who have been deciphering some of the most fundamental questions about life with the goal of improving health.

In the last several decades, investments in basic research have yielded extensive knowledge about the many and complex processes involved in the development of an organism, including the control of cellular development. But many questions remain. How does a single cell—the fertilized egg—give rise to a complex, multi-cellular organism? The question represents a fundamental challenge in developmental biology. Researchers are now seeking to understand in greater detail the genetic factors that regulate cell differentiation in early development.

Put simply, stem cells are self-renewing, unspecialized cells that can give rise to multiple types all of specialized cells of the body. The process by which dividing, unspecialized cells are equipped to perform specific functions—muscle contraction or nerve cell communication, for example—is called differentiation, and is fundamental to the development of the mature organism. It is now known that stem cells, in various forms, can be obtained from the embryo, the fetus, and the adult.

How and whether stem cells derived from any of these sources can be manipulated to replace cells in diseased tissues, used to screen drugs and toxins, or studied to better understand normal development depends on knowing more about their basic properties. In this respect, stem cell research is in many ways no different than many other areas of modern biology; it is advancing because new tools and new knowledge are providing the opportunities for new insights. Like all fields of scientific inquiry, research on stem cells raises as many questions as it answers. This report describes the state of the science of stem cell biology and gives some clues as to the many and varied questions that remain to be answered.

WHAT IS THE SCOPE OF THE REPORT?

The report is a review of the state of the science of stem cell research as of June 17, 2001. Included in this report is subject matter addressing stem cells from adult, fetal tissue, and embryonic sources. Because so much of the progress made to date was dependent on animal models, a significant emphasis is placed on understandings gained from mouse models of development and mouse stem cell research. The report also devotes substantial attention to scientific publications on the characterization of specialized cells developed from embryonic stem cells and the plasticity of adult stem cells. A general overview of early development is provided in the Appendix to assist the reader in understanding the key events in formation of cells, tissues, and the whole organism.

Both scientific and lay publications use a variety of terms to describe stem cells and their properties. For this reason, this report adopts a lexicon of terms and it is used consistently throughout. To aid the reader, a glossary and terms section is provided. In several places in the report, discovery timelines are provided. The various sources of stem cells are described, as are the techniques used to isolate and develop them. A comprehensive listing of various stem cell isolation and characterizations is also included.

In order to ensure the reader is provided information both about the basic biology of stem cells, and their therapeutic potential, the report contains several chapters focused on particular diseases which might benefit from stem cell research. These chapters on the use of hematopoietic stem cells, followed by focus features on specific nervous system diseases, diabetes, heart disease, and autoimmune diseases serve merely as examples of the many applications of stem cells that are being pursued. Also included are features that review aspects of stem cells as therapeutic delivery tools for gene therapy and, importantly, the safety considerations for developing stem cell-based therapies.

WHAT IS NOT IN THE SCOPE OF THE REPORT?

NIH recognizes the compelling ethical and legal issues surrounding human pluripotent stem cell research. Because extensive discussions regarding these issues have been presented in various forums elsewhere, they are not part of this review of the state of the science. Also, the report does not make recommendations pertaining to the policies governing Federal funding of such research.

HOW WAS THE REPORT DEVELOPED?

The report was prepared under the auspices of the Office of Science Policy, Office of the Director, NIH. Several approaches were taken to obtain relevant scientific information for the report. A thorough review of the extant literature, including more than 1200 scientific publications was conducted. Scientific experts (both domestic and international) from all areas of relevant biomedical research in stem cells were interviewed in depth. While the majority of the work presented in this report emanates from investigators in academic laboratories, extensive discussions were held with scientists in the private pharmaceutical and biotechnology sectors. Thus, the report makes every effort to encompass what is known and not known about stem cell biology and is, therefore, not limited to research that is or has been funded by the NIH.

In recent months, there have been many reports in the lay press regarding scientific discoveries on various types of stem cells. The science represented in this report focuses exclusively on scientific publications or public presentations. In cases where technical or logistical information key to the understanding of the details of science was needed, personal communications with the information sources were cited.

EXECUTIVE SUMMARY

INTRODUCTION

A stem cell is a special kind of cell that has a unique capacity to renew itself and to give rise to specialized cell types. Although most cells of the body, such as heart cells or skin cells, are committed to conduct a specific function, a stem cell is uncommitted and remains uncommitted, until it receives a signal to develop into a specialized cell. Their proliferative capacity combined with the ability to become specialized makes stem cells unique. Researchers have for years looked for ways to use stem cells to replace cells and tissues that are damaged or diseased. Recently, stem cells have received much attention. What is "new" and what has brought stem cell biology to the forefront of science and public policy?

Scientists interested in human development have been studying animal development for many years. This research yielded our first glimpse at a class of stem cells that can develop into any cell type in the body. This class of stem cells is called pluripotent, meaning the cells have the potential to develop almost all of the more than 200 different known cell types. Stem cells with this unique property come from embryos and fetal tissue.

In 1998, for the first time, investigators were able to isolate this class of pluripotent stem cell from early human embryos and grow them in culture. In the few years since this discovery, evidence has emerged that these stem cells are, indeed, capable of becoming almost all of the specialized cells of the body and, thus, may have the potential to generate replacement cells for a broad array of tissues and organs, such as the heart, the pancreas, and the nervous system. Thus, this class of human stem cell holds the promise of being able to repair or replace cells or tissues that are damaged or destroyed by many of our most devastating diseases and disabilities.

At about the same time as scientists were beginning to explore human pluripotent stem cells from embryos and fetal tissue, a flurry of new information was emerging about a class of stem cells that have been in clinical use for years—so-called adult stem cells. An adult stem cell is an undifferentiated cell that is found in a differentiated (specialized) tissue in the adult, such as blood. It can yield the specialized cell types of the tissue from which it originated. In the body, it too, can renew itself. During the past decade, scientists discovered adult stem cells in tissues that were previously not thought to contain them, such as the brain. More recently, they reported that adult stem cells from one tissue appear to be capable of developing into cell types that are characteristic of other tissues. For example, although adult hematopoietic stem cells from bone marrow have long been recognized as capable of developing into blood and immune cells, recently scientists reported that, under certain conditions, the same stem cells could also develop into cells that have many of the characteristics of neurons. So, a new concept and a new term emerged-adult stem cell plasticity.

Are human adult and embryonic stem cells equivalent in their potential for generating replacement cells and tissues? Current science indicates that, although both of these cell types hold enormous promise, adult and embryonic stem cells differ in important ways. What is not known is the extent to which these different cell types will be useful for the development of cell-based therapies to treat disease.

Some considerations are noteworthy regarding this report. First, in recent months, there have been many discussions in the lay press about the anticipated abilities of stem cells from various sources and projected benefits to be realized from them in replacing cells and tissues in patients with various diseases. The terminology used to describe stem cells in the lay literature is often confusing or misapplied. Second, even among biomedical researchers, there is a lack of consistency in common terms to describe what stem cells are and how they behave in the research laboratory. Third, the field of stem cell biology is advancing at an incredible pace with new discoveries being reported in the scientific literature on a weekly basis.

This summary begins with common definitions and explanations of key concepts about stem cells. It ends with an assessment of how adult, embryonic and fetal stem cells are similar and how they are different. In between lie important details that describe what researchers have discovered about stem cells and how they are being used in the laboratory.

DEFINITIONS AND GENERAL CONCEPTS ABOUT STEM CELLS

In developing this report, some conventions were established to describe consistently what stem cells are, what characteristics they have, and how they are used in biomedical research. Here are some of the key definitions that are used throughout this report.

Stem cell. A stem cell is a cell from the embryo, fetus, or adult that has, under certain conditions, the ability to reproduce itself for long periods or, in the case of adult stem cells, throughout the life of the organism. It also can give rise to specialized cells that make up the tissues and organs of the body. Much basic understanding about embryonic stem cells has come from animal research. In the laboratory, this type of stem cell can proliferate indefinitely, a property that is not shared by adult stem cells.

Pluripotent stem cell. A single pluripotent stem cell has the ability to give rise to types of cells that develop from the three germ layers (mesoderm, endoderm, and ectoderm) from which all the cells of the body arise. The only known sources of human pluripotent stem cells are those isolated and cultured from early human embryos and from fetal tissue that was destined to be part of the gonads.

Embryonic stem cell. An embryonic stem cell is derived from a group of cells called the inner cell mass, which is part of the early (4- to 5-day) embryo called the blastocyst. Once removed from the blastocyst, the cells of the inner cell mass can be cultured into embryonic stem cells. These embryonic stem cells are not themselves embryos. In fact, evidence is emerging that these cells do not behave in the laboratory as they would in the developing embryo—that is, the conditions in which these cells develop in culture are likely to differ from those in the developing embryo.

Embryonic germ cell. An embryonic germ cell is derived from fetal tissue. Specifically, they are isolated from the primordial germ cells of the gonadal ridge of the 5- to 10-week fetus. Later in development, the gonadal ridge develops into the testes or ovaries and the primordial germ cells give rise to eggs or sperm. Embryonic stem cells and embryonic germ cells are pluripotent, but they are not identical in their properties and characteristics.

Differentiation. Differentiation is the process by which an unspecialized cell (such as a stem cell) becomes specialized into one of the many cells that make up the body. During differentiation, certain genes become activated and other genes become inactivated in an intricately regulated fashion. As a result, a differentiated cell develops specific structures and performs certain functions. For example, a mature, differentiated nerve cell has thin, fiber-like projections that send and receive the electrochemical signals that permit the nerve cell to communicate with other nerve cells. In the laboratory, a stem cell can be manipulated to become specialized or partially specialized cell types (e.g., heart muscle, nerve, or pancreatic cells) and this is known as directed differentiation.

Adult stem cell. An adult stem cell is an undifferentiated (unspecialized) cell that occurs in a differentiated (specialized) tissue, renews itself, and becomes specialized to yield all of the specialized cell types of the tissue from which it originated. Adult stem cells are capable of making identical copies of themselves for the lifetime of the organism. This property is referred to as "self-renewal." Adult stem cells usually divide to generate progenitor or precursor cells, which then differentiate or develop into "mature" cell types that have characteristic shapes and specialized functions, e.g., muscle cell contraction or nerve cell signaling. Sources of adult stem cells include bone marrow, blood, the cornea and the retina of the eye, brain, skeletal muscle, dental pulp, liver, skin, the lining of the gastrointestinal tract, and pancreas. The most abundant information about adult human stem cells comes from studies of hematopoietic (blood-forming) stem cells isolated from the bone marrow and blood. These adult stem cells have been extensively studied and applied therapeutically for various diseases. At this point, there is no isolated population of adult stem cells that is capable of forming all the kinds of cells of the body. Adult stem cells are rare. Often they are difficult to identify, isolate, and purify. There are insufficient numbers of cells available for transplantation and adult stem cells do not replicate indefinitely in culture.

Plasticity. Plasticity is the ability of an adult stem cell from one tissue to generate the specialized cell type(s) of another tissue. A recently reported example of plasticity is that, under specific experimental conditions, adult stem cells from bone marrow generated cells that resemble neurons and other cell types that are commonly found in the brain. The concept of adult stem cell plasticity is new, and the phenomenon is not thoroughly understood. Evidence suggests that, given the right environment, some adult stem cells are capable of being "genetically reprogrammed" to generate specialized cells that are characteristic of different tissues.

Clonality or clonally derived stem cell. A cell is said to be clonally derived or to exhibit clonality if it was generated by the division of a single cell and is genetically identical to that cell. In stem cell research, the concept of clonality is important for several reasons. For researchers to fully understand and harness the ability of stem cells to generate replacement cells and tissues, the exact identity of those cells' genetic capabilities and functional qualities must be known. Human pluripotent stem cells from embryos and fetal tissue are by their nature clonally derived. However, very few studies have shown clonal properties of the cells that are developed from adult stem cells. It is crucial to know whether a single cell is capable of developing an array of cell types, or whether multiple stem cell types, that when grown together, are capable of forming multiple cell types. For instance, recent research has shown that a mixture of cells removed from fat tissue or umbilical cord blood are capable of developing into blood cells, bone cells, and perhaps others. Researchers have not shown that a single cell is responsible for giving rise to other cell types or, if so, what kind of cell it is. These results may well be attributable to multiple types of precursor cells

in the starting tissue; such results from fat cells may, in fact, be due to the presence of hematopoietic stem cells in the fat tissue. The importance of showing that one cell type can reproducibly become another and self-replicate cannot be overemphasized.

Progenitor or precursor cell. A progenitor or precursor cell occurs in fetal or adult tissues and is partially specialized; it divides and gives rise to differentiated cells. Researchers often distinguish precursor/progenitor cells from adult stem cells in the following way: when a stem cell divides, one of the two new cells is often a stem cell capable of replicating itself again. In contrast, when a progenitor/precursor cell divides, it can form more progenitor/precursor cells or it can form two specialized cells, neither of which is capable of replicating itself. Progenitor/precursor cells can replace cells that are damaged or dead, thus maintaining the integrity and functions of a tissue such as liver or brain. Progenitor/precursor cells give rise to related types of cells-lymphocytes such as T cells, B cells, and natural killer cells, for example—but in their normal state do not generate a wide variety of cell types.

CHALLENGES IN STEM CELL RESEARCH

It is important to understand some of the difficulties that researchers have had in isolating various types of stem cells, working with the cells in the laboratory, and proving experimentally that the cells are true stem cells. Most of the basic research discoveries on embryonic and adult stem cells come from research using animal models, particularly mice.

In 1981, researchers reported methods for growing mouse embryonic stem cells in the laboratory, and it took nearly 20 years before similar achievements could be made with human embryonic stem cells. Much of the knowledge about embryonic stem cells has emerged from two fields of research: applied reproductive biology, i.e., in vitro fertilization technologies, and basic research on mouse embryology.

There have been many technical challenges that have been overcome in adult stem cell research as well. Some of the barriers include: the rare occurrence of adult stem cells among other, differentiated cells, difficulties in isolating and identifying the cells (researchers often use molecular "markers" to identify adult stem cells), and in many cases, difficulties in growing adult stem cells in tissue culture. Much of the research demonstrating the plasticity of adult stem cells comes from studies of animal models in which a mixture of adult stem cells from a donor animal is injected into another animal, and the development of new, specialized cells is traced.

In 1998, James Thomson at the University of Wisconsin-Madison isolated cells from the inner cell mass of the early embryo, called the blastocyst, and developed the first human embryonic stem cell lines. At the same time, John Gearhart at Johns Hopkins University reported the first derivation of human embryonic germ cells from an isolated population of cells in fetal gonadal tissue, known as the primordial germ cells, which are destined to become the eggs and sperm. From both of these sources, the researchers developed pluripotent stem cell "lines," which are capable of renewing themselves for long periods and giving rise to many types of human cells or tissues. Human embryonic stem cells and embryonic germ cells differ in some characteristics, however, and do not appear to be equivalent.

Why are the long-term proliferation ability and pluripotency of embryonic stem cells and embryonic germ cells so important? First, for basic research purposes, it is important to understand the genetic and molecular basis by which these cells continue to make many copies of themselves overlong periods of time. Second, if the cells are to be manipulated and used for transplantation, it is important to have sufficient quantities of cells that can be directed to differentiate into the desired cell type(s) and used to treat the many patients that may be suffering from a particular disease.

In recent months, other investigators have been successful in using somewhat different approaches to deriving human pluripotent stem cells. At least 5 other laboratories have been successful in deriving pluripotent stem cells from human embryos and one additional laboratory has created cell lines from fetal tissue. In each case, the methods for deriving pluripotent stem cells from human embryos and embryonic germ cells from fetal tissue are similar, yet they differ in the isolation and culture conditions as initially described by Thomson and Gearhart, respectively. It is not known to what extent U.S.-based researchers are using these additional sources of embryonic stem and germ cells.

At present, there have been multiple human adult stem cell lines that have been created through a combination of public and private resources (e.g., hematopoietic stem cells). Substantial adult stem cell research has been underway for many years, and in recent years this has included basic studies on the "plasticity" of such cells.

WHAT KINDS OF RESEARCH MIGHT BE CONDUCTED WITH STEM CELLS?

There has been much written about the new discoveries of various stem cell types and their properties. Importantly, these cells are research tools and they open many doors of opportunity for bio-medical research.

Transplantation Research—Restoring Vital Body Functions

Stem cells may hold the key to replacing cells lost in many devastating diseases. There is little doubt that this potential benefit underpins the vast interest about stem cell research. What are some of these diseases? Parkinson's disease, diabetes, chronic heart disease, end-stage kidney disease, liver failure, and cancer are just a few for which stem cells have thera-peutic potential. For many diseases that shorten lives, there are no effective treatments but the goal is to find a way to replace what natural processes have taken away. For example, today, science has brought us to a point where the immune response can be subdued, so that organs from one person can be used to replace the diseased organs and tissues of another. But, despite recent advances in transplanta-tion sciences, there is a shortage of donor organs that makes it unlikely that the growing demand for lifesaving organ replacements will be fully met through organ donation strategies.

The use of stem cells to generate replacement tissues for treating neurological diseases is a major focus of research. Spinal cord injury, multiple sclerosis, Parkin-son's disease, and Alzheimer's disease are among those diseases for which the concept of replacing destroyed or dysfunctional cells in the brain or spinal cord is a practical goal. This report features several recent advances that demonstrate the regenerative properties of adult and embryonic stem cells.

Another major discovery frontier for research on adult and embryonic stem cells is the development of transplantable pancreatic tissues that can be used to treat diabetes. Scientists in academic and industrial research are vigorously pursuing all possible avenues of research, including ways to direct the specialization of adult and embryonic stem cells to become pancreatic islet-like cells that produce insulin and can be used to control blood glucose levels. Researchers have recently shown that human embryonic stem cells to be directly differentiated into cells that produce insulin.

There are common misconceptions about both adult and human embryonic stem cells. First, the lines of unaltered human embryonic stem cells that exist will not be suitable for direct use in patients. These cells will need to be differentiated or otherwise modified before they can be used clinically. Current challenges are to direct the differentiation of embryonic stem cells into specialized cell populations, and also to devise ways to control their development or proliferation once placed in patients.

A second misconception is that adult stem cells are ready to use as therapies. With the exception of the clinical application of hematopoietic stem cells to restore the blood and immune system, this is not the case. The therapeutic use of this mixture of cells has proven safe because the mixture is place back into the environment from which it was taken, e.g., the bone marrow. In fact, many of the adult stem cell preparations currently being developed in the laboratory represent multiple cell types that are not fully characterized. In order to safely use stem cells or cells differentiated from them in tissues other than the tissue from which they were isolated, researchers will need purified populations (clonal lines) of adult stem cells.

In addition, the potential for the recipient of a stem cell transplant to reject these tissues as foreign is very high. Modifications to the cells, to the immune system, or both will be a major requirement for their use. In sum, with the exception of the current practice of hematopoietic stem cell transplantation, much basic research lies ahead before direct patient application of stem cell therapies is realized.

Basic Research Applications

Embryonic stem cells will undoubtedly be key research tools for understanding fundamental events in embryonic development that one day may explain the causes of birth defects and approaches to correct or prevent them. Another important area of

research that links developmental biology and stem cell biology is understanding the genes and molecules, such as growth factors and nutrients, that function during the development of the embryo so that they can be used to grow stem cells in the laboratory and direct their development into specialized cell types.

Therapeutic Delivery Systems

Stem cells are already being explored as a vehicle for delivering genes to specific tissues in the body. Stem cell-based therapies are a major area of investigation in cancer research. For many years, restoration of blood and immune system function has been used as a component in the care of cancer patients who have been treated with chemotherapeutic agents. Now, researchers are trying to devise more ways to use specialized cells derived from stem cells to target specific cancerous cells and directly deliver treatments that will destroy or modify them.

Other Applications of Stem Cells

Future uses of human pluripotent cell lines might include the exploration of the effects of chromosomal abnormalities in early development. This might include the ability to monitor the development of early childhood tumors, many of which are embryonic in origin. Another future use of human stem cells and their derivatives include the testing of candidate therapeutic drugs. Although animal model testing is a mainstay of pharmaceutical research, it cannot always predict the effects that a developmental drug may have on human cells. Stem cells will likely be used to develop specialized liver cells to evaluate drug detoxifying capabilities and represents a new type of early warning system to prevent adverse reactions in patients. The coupling of stem cells with the information learned from the human genome project will also likely have many unanticipated benefits in the future.

Critical Evidence and Questions about Stem Cell Research

What is the evidence that specialized cells generated from human stem cells can replace damaged or diseased cells and tissues? Currently, there are more questions than answers.

Most of the evidence that stem cells can be directed to differentiate into specific types of cells suitable for transplantation—for example, neurons, heart muscle cells, or pancreatic islet cells—comes from experiments with stem cells from mice. And although more is known about mouse stem cells, not all of that information can be translated to the understanding of human stem cells. Mouse and human cells differ in significant ways, such as the laboratory conditions that favor the growth and specialization of specific cell types.

Another important aspect of developing therapies based on stem cells will be devising ways to prevent the immune system of recipients from rejecting the donated cells and tissues that are derived from human pluripotent stem cells. Modifying or evading the immune rejection of cells or tissues developed from embryonic stem cells will not be able to be done exclusively using mouse models and human adult stem cells.

As with any new research tool, it will also be important to compare the techniques and approaches that various laboratories are using to differentiate and use human embryonic stem cells. Such research will provide a more complete understanding of the cells' characteristics. One key finding about the directed differentiation of pluripotent stem cells learned thus far is that relatively subtle changes in culture conditions can have dramatic influences on the types of cells that develop.

What Is Known About Adult Stem Cells?

- To date, published scientific papers indicate that adult stem cells have been identified in brain, bone marrow, peripheral blood, blood vessels, skeletal muscle, epithelia of the skin and digestive system, cornea, dental pulp of the tooth, retina, liver, and pancreas. Thus, adult stem cells have been found in tissues that develop from all three embryonic germ layers.

- There is no evidence of an adult stem cell that is pluripotent. It has not been demonstrated that one adult stem cell can be directed to develop into any cell type of the body. That is, no adult stem cell has been shown to be capable of developing into cells from all three embryonic germ layers.

- In the body, adult stem cells can proliferate without differentiating for a long period (the characteristic referred to as long-term self-renewal),

and they can give rise to mature cell types that have characteristic shapes and specialized functions of a particular tissue.

- Adult stem cells are rare. Often they are difficult to identify, isolate, and purify.

- One important, limiting factor for the use of adult stem cells in future cell-replacement strategies is that there are insufficient numbers of cells available for transplantation. This is because most adult stem cell lines when grown in a culture dish are unable to proliferate in an unspecialized state for long periods of time. In cases where they can be grown under these conditions, researchers have not been able to direct them to become specialized as functionally useful cells.

- Stem cells from the bone marrow are the most-studied type of adult stem cells. Currently, they are used clinically to restore various blood and immune components to the bone marrow via transplantation. There are two major types of stem cells found in bone: hematopoietic stem cells which form blood and immune cells, and stromal (mesenchymal) stem cells that normally form bone, cartilage, and fat. The restricted capacity of hematopoietic stem cells to grow in large numbers and remain undifferentiated in the culture dish is a major limitation to their broader use for research and transplantation studies. Researchers have reported that at least two other populations of adult stem cells occur in bone marrow and blood, but these cells are not well characterized.

- Evidence to date indicates that umbilical cord blood is an abundant source of hematopoietic stem cells. There do not appear to be any qualitative differences between the stem cells obtained from umbilical cord blood and those obtained from bone marrow or peripheral blood.

- Several populations of adult stem cells have been identified in the brain, particularly in a region important in memory, known as the hippocampus. Their function in the brain is unknown. When the cells are removed from the brain of mice and grown in tissue culture, their proliferation and differentiation can be influenced by various growth factors.

- Current methods for characterizing adult stem cells depend on determining cell-surface markers and making observations about their differentiation patterns in culture dishes.

- Some adult stem cells appear to have the capability to differentiate into tissues other than the ones from which they originated; this is referred to as plasticity. Reports of human or mouse adult stem cells that demonstrate plasticity and the cells they differentiate or specialize into include: 1) blood and bone marrow (unpurified hematopoietic) stem cells differentiate into the 3 major types of brain cells (neurons, oligodendrocytes, and astrocytes), skeletal muscle cells, cardiac muscle cells, and liver cells; 2) bone marrow (stromal) cells differentiates into cardiac muscle cells, skeletal muscle cells, fat, bone, and cartilage; and 3) brain stem cells differentiate into blood cells and skeletal muscle cells.

- Very few published research reports on the plasticity of adult stem cells shown that a single, identified adult stem cell can give rise to a differentiated cell type of another tissue. That is, there is limited evidence that a single adult stem cell or genetically identical line of adult stem cells demonstrates plasticity. Researchers believe that it is most likely that a variety of populations of stem cells may be responsible for the phenomena of developing multiple cell types.

- A few experiments have shown plasticity of adult stem cells by demonstrating the development of mature, fully functional cells in tissues other than which they were derived and the restoration of lost or diminished function in an animal model.

What is Known About Human Pluripotent Stem Cells?

- Since 1998, research teams have refined the techniques for growing human pluripotent cells in culture systems. Collectively, the studies indicate that it is now possible to grow these cells for up to two years in a chemically defined medium.

- The cell lines have been shown to have a normal number of chromosomes and they generate cell types that originate from all three primary germ layers.

- Cultures of human pluripotent stem cells have active telomerase, which is an enzyme that maintains the length of telomeres and is important for cells to maintain their capacity to replicate. Human pluripotent stem cells appear to maintain relatively long telomeres, indicating that they have the ability to replicate for many, many generations.

- Evidence of structural, genetic, and functional cells characteristic of specialized cells developed from cultured human and mouse embryonic stem cells has been shown for: 1) Pancreatic islet-cell like cells that secrete insulin (mouse and human); 2) cardiac muscle cells with contractile activity (mouse and human); 3) blood cells (human and mouse); 4) nerve cells that produce certain brain chemicals (mouse).

- At the time of this report, there are approximately 30 cell lines of human pluripotent stem cells that have been derived from human blastocysts or fetal tissue.

- Overall, it appears human embryonic cells and embryonic germ cells are not equivalent in their potential to proliferate or differentiate.

What are Some of the Questions that Need to be Answered about Stem Cells?

- What are the mechanisms that allow human embryonic stem cells and embryonic germ cells to proliferate *in vitro* without differentiating?

- What are the intrinsic controls that keep stem cells from differentiating?

- Is there a universal stem cell? That is, could a kind of stem cell exist (possibly circulating in the blood) that can generate the cells of any organ or tissue?

- Do adult stem cells exhibit plasticity as a normal event in the body or is it an artifact of the culture conditions? If plasticity occurs normally, is it a characteristic of all adult stem cells? What are the signals that regulate the proliferation and differentiation of stem cells that demonstrate plasticity?

- What are the factors responsible for stem cells to "home" to sites of injury or damage?

- What are the intrinsic controls that direct stem cells along a particular differentiation pathway to form one specialized cell over another? How are such intrinsic regulators, in turn, influenced by the microenvironment, or niche, where stem cells normally reside?

- Will the knowledge about the genetic mechanisms regulating the specialization of embryonic cells into cells from all embryonic germ layers during development enable the scientists to engineer adult stem cells to do the same?

- What are the sources of adult stem cells in the body? Are they "leftover" embryonic stem cells, or do they arise in some other way? And if the latter is true—which seems to be the case—exactly how do adult stem cells arise, and why do they remain in an undifferentiated state when all the cells around them have differentiated?

- How many kinds of adult stem cells exist, and in which tissues do they exist?

- Is it possible to manipulate adult stem cells to increase their ability to proliferate in a culture dish so that adult stem cells can be used as a sufficient source of tissue for transplants?

- Does the genetic programming status of stem cells play a significant role in maintaining the cells, directing their differentiation, or determining their suitability for transplant?

- Are the human embryonic stem and germ cells that appear to be homogeneous and undifferentiated in culture, in fact, homogeneous and undifferentiated? Or are they heterogeneous and/or "partially" differentiated?

- What are the cellular and molecular signals that are important in activating a human pluripotent stem cell to begin differentiating into a specialized cell type?

- Will analysis of genes from human pluripotent stem cells reveal a common mechanism that maintains cells in an undifferentiated state?

- Do all pluripotent stem cells pass through a progenitor/precursor cell stage while becoming specialized? If so, can a precursor or progenitor cell stage be maintained as optimal cells for therapeutic transplantation?

- What stage of differentiation of stem cells will be best for transplantation? Would the same stage be optimal for all transplantation applications, or will it differ on a case-by-case basis?

- What differentiation stages of stem cells would be best for screening drugs or toxins, or for delivering potentially therapeutic drugs?

COMPARISONS OF ADULT STEM CELLS AND EMBRYONIC STEM CELLS

Biomedical research on stem cells is at an early stage, but is advancing rapidly. After many years of isolating and characterizing these cells, researchers are just now beginning to employ stem cells as discovery tools and a basis for potential therapies. This new era of research affords an opportunity to use what has already been learned to explore the similarities and differences of adult and embryonic stem cells. (In this discussion, comments about embryonic stem cells derived from human embryos, and embryonic germ cells derived from fetal tissue, will be referred to equally as embryonic stem cells, unless otherwise distinguished.)

How are Adult and Embryonic Stem Cells Similar?

By definition, stem cells have in common the ability to self-replicate and to give rise to specialized cells and tissues (such as cells of the heart, brain, bone, etc.) that have specific functions. In most cases, stem cells can be isolated and maintained in an unspecialized state. Scientists use similar techniques (i.e., cell-surface markers and monitoring the expression of certain genes) to identify or characterize stem cells as being unspecialized. Scientists then use different genetic or molecular markers to determine that the cells have differentiated—a process that might be compared to distinguishing a particular cell type by reading its cellular barcode.

Stem cells from both adult and embryonic sources can proliferate and specialize when transplanted into an animal with a compromised immune system. (Immune-deficient animals are less likely to reject the transplanted tissue). Scientists also have evidence that differentiated cells generated from either stem cell type, when injected or transplanted into an animal model of disease or injury, undergo "homing," a process whereby the transplanted cells are attracted by and travel to the injured site. Similarly, researchers are finding that the cellular and non-cellular "environment" into which stem cell-derived tissues are placed (e.g., whether they are grown in a culture dish or transplanted into an animal) prominently influences how the cells differentiate.

Another important area that requires substantially more research concerns the immunologic characteristics of human adult and embryonic stem cells. If any of these stem cells are to be used as the basis for therapy, it is critical understand how the body's immune system will respond to the transplantation of tissue derived from these cells. At this time, there is no clear advantage of one stem cell source over the other in this regard.

How are Adult and Embryonic Stem Cells Different?

Perhaps the most distinguishing feature of embryonic stem cells and adult stem cells is their source. Most scientists now agree that adult stem cells exist in many tissues of the human body (*in vivo*), although the cells are quite rare. In contrast, it is less certain that embryonic stem cells exist as such in the embryo. Instead, embryonic stem cells and embryonic germ cells develop in tissue culture after they are derived from the inner cell mass of the early embryo or from the gonadal ridge tissue of the fetus, respectively.

Depending on the culture conditions, embryonic stem cells may form clumps of cells that can differentiate spontaneously to generate many cell types. This property has not been observed in cultures of adult stem cells. Also, if undifferentiated embryonic stem cells are removed from the culture dish and injected into a mouse with a compromised immune system, a benign tumor called a teratoma can develop. A teratoma typically contains a mixture of partially differentiated cell types. For this reason, scientists do not anticipate that undifferentiated embryonic stem cells will be used for transplants or other therapeutic applications. It is not known whether similar results are observed with adult stem cells.

Stem cells in adult tissues do not appear to have the same capacity to differentiate as do embryonic stem cells or embryonic germ cells. Embryonic stem and germ cells are clearly pluripotent; they can differentiate into any tissues derived from all three germ layers of the embryo (ectoderm, mesoderm, and endoderm). But are adult stem cells also pluripotent? When they reside in their normal tissue compartments—the brain, the bone marrow, the epithelial lining of the gut, etc.—they produce the cells that are specific to that kind of tissue and they have been found in tissues derived from all three embryonic layers. But can adult stem cells be taken out of their normal environment and be manipulated or otherwise induced to have the same differentiation

potential as embryonic stem and germ cells? To date, there are no definitive answers to these questions, and the answers that do exist are sometimes conflicting.

These sources of stem cells do not seem to have the same ability to proliferate in culture and at the same time retain the capacity to differentiate into functionally useful cells. Human embryonic stem cells can be generated in abundant quantities in the laboratory and can be grown (allowed to proliferate) in their undifferentiated (or unspecialized) state for many, many generations. From a practical perspective in basic research or eventual clinical application, it is significant that millions of cells can be generated from one embryonic stem cell in the laboratory. In many cases, however, researchers have had difficulty finding laboratory conditions under which some adult stem cells can proliferate without becoming specialized. This problem is most pronounced with hematopoietic stem cells isolated from blood or bone marrow. These cells when cultured in the laboratory either fail to proliferate or do so to a limited extent, although they do proliferate if transplanted into an animal or human. This technical barrier to proliferation has limited the ability of researchers to explore the capacity of certain types of adult stem cells to generate sufficient numbers of specialized cells for transplantation purposes.

These differences in culturing conditions contribute to the contrasts in the experimental systems used to evaluate the ability to become specialized under particular laboratory conditions. Much of the information on the directed differentiation of embryonic stem cells into cells with specialized function comes from studying mouse or human embryonic cell lines grown in laboratory culture dishes. In contrast, most knowledge about the differentiation of adult stem cells differentiation are from observations of cells and tissues in animal models in which mixtures of cells have been implanted.

Stem cells also differ in their capacity to specialize into various cell and tissue types. Current evidence indicates that the capability of adult stem cells to give rise to many different specialized cell types is more limited than that of embryonic stem cells. A single embryonic stem cell has been shown to give rise to specialized cells from all three embryonic layers. However, it has not yet been shown that a single adult stem cell can give rise to specialized cells derived from all three embryonic germ cell layers. Therefore, a single adult stem cell has not been shown to have the same degree of pluripotency as embryonic stem cells.

CONCLUSIONS

Two important points about embryonic and adult stem cells have emerged so far: the cells are different and present immense research opportunities for potential therapy. As research goes forward, scientists will undoubtedly find other similarities and differences between adult and embryonic stem cells. During the next several years, it will be important to compare embryonic stem cells and adult stem cells in terms of their ability to proliferate, differentiate, survive and function after transplant, and avoid immune rejection. Investigators have shown that differentiated cells generated from both adult and embryonic stem cells can repair or replace damaged cells and tissues in animal studies.

Scientists upon making new discoveries often verify reported results in different laboratories and under different conditions. Similarly, they will often conduct experiments with different animal models or, in this case, different cell lines. However, there have been very few studies that compare various stem cell lines with each other. It may be that one source proves better for certain applications, and a different cell source proves better for others.

For researchers and patients, there are many practical questions about stem cells that cannot yet be answered. How long will it take to develop therapies for Parkinson's Disease and diabetes with and without human pluripotent stem cells? Can the full range of new therapeutic approaches be developed using only adult stem cells? How many different sources of stem cells will be needed to generate the best treatments in the shortest period of time?

Predicting the future of stem cell applications is impossible, particularly given the very early stage of the science of stem cell biology. To date, it is impossible to predict which stem cells—those derived from the embryo, the fetus, or the adult—or which methods for manipulating the cells, will best meet the needs of basic research and clinical applications. The answers clearly lie in conducting more research.

1. THE STEM CELL

WHAT IS A STEM CELL?

A stem cell is a cell that has the ability to divide (self replicate) for indefinite periods—often throughout the life of the organism. Under the right conditions, or given the right signals, stem cells can give rise (differentiate) to the many different cell types that make up the organism. That is, stem cells have the potential to develop into mature cells that have characteristic shapes and specialized functions, such as heart cells, skin cells, or nerve cells.

THE DIFFERENTIATION POTENTIAL OF STEM CELLS: BASIC CONCEPTS AND DEFINITIONS

Many of the terms used to define stem cells depend on the behavior of the cells in the intact organism (in vivo), under specific laboratory conditions (in vitro), or after transplantation in vivo, often to a tissue that is different from the one from which the stem cells were derived.

For example, the fertilized egg is said to be totipotent—from the Latin totus, meaning entire—because it has the potential to generate all the cells and tissues that make up an embryo and that support its development in utero. The fertilized egg divides and differentiates until it produces a mature organism. Adult mammals, including humans, consist of more than 200 kinds of cells. These include nerve cells (neurons), muscle cells (myocytes), skin (epithelial) cells, blood cells (erythrocytes, monocytes, lymphocytes, etc.), bone cells (osteocytes), and cartilage cells (chondrocytes). Other cells, which are essential for embryonic development but are not incorporated into the body of the embryo, include the extra-embryonic tissues, placenta, and umbilical cord. All of these cells are generated from a single, totipotent cell—the zygote, or fertilized egg.

Most scientists use the term pluripotent to describe stem cells that can give rise to cells derived from all three embryonic germ layers—mesoderm, endoderm, and ectoderm. These three germ layers are the embryonic source of all cells of the body (see Figure 1.1. Differentiation of Human Tissues). All of the many different kinds of specialized cells that make up the body are derived from one of these germ layers (see Table 1.1. Embryonic Germ Layers From Which Differentiated Tissues Develop). "Pluri"—derived from the Latin plures—means several or many. Thus, pluripotent cells have the potential to give rise to any type of cell, a property observed in the natural course of embryonic development and under certain laboratory conditions.

Unipotent stem cell, a term that is usually applied to a cell in adult organisms, means that the cells in question are capable of differentiating along only one lineage. "Uni" is derived from the Latin word unus, which means one. Also, it may be that the adult stem cells in many differentiated, undamaged tissues are typically unipotent and give rise to just one cell type under normal conditions. This process would allow for a steady state of self-renewal for the tissue. However, if the tissue becomes damaged and the replacement of multiple cell types is required, pluripotent stem cells may become activated to repair the damage [2].

The embryonic stem cell is defined by its origin—that is from one of the earliest stages of the development of the embryo, called the blastocyst. Specifically, embryonic stem cells are derived from the inner cell mass of the blastocyst at a stage before it would implant in the uterine wall. The embryonic stem cell can self-replicate and is pluripotent—it can give rise to cells derived from all three germ layers.

The adult stem cell is an undifferentiated (unspecialized) cell that is found in a differentiated (specialized)

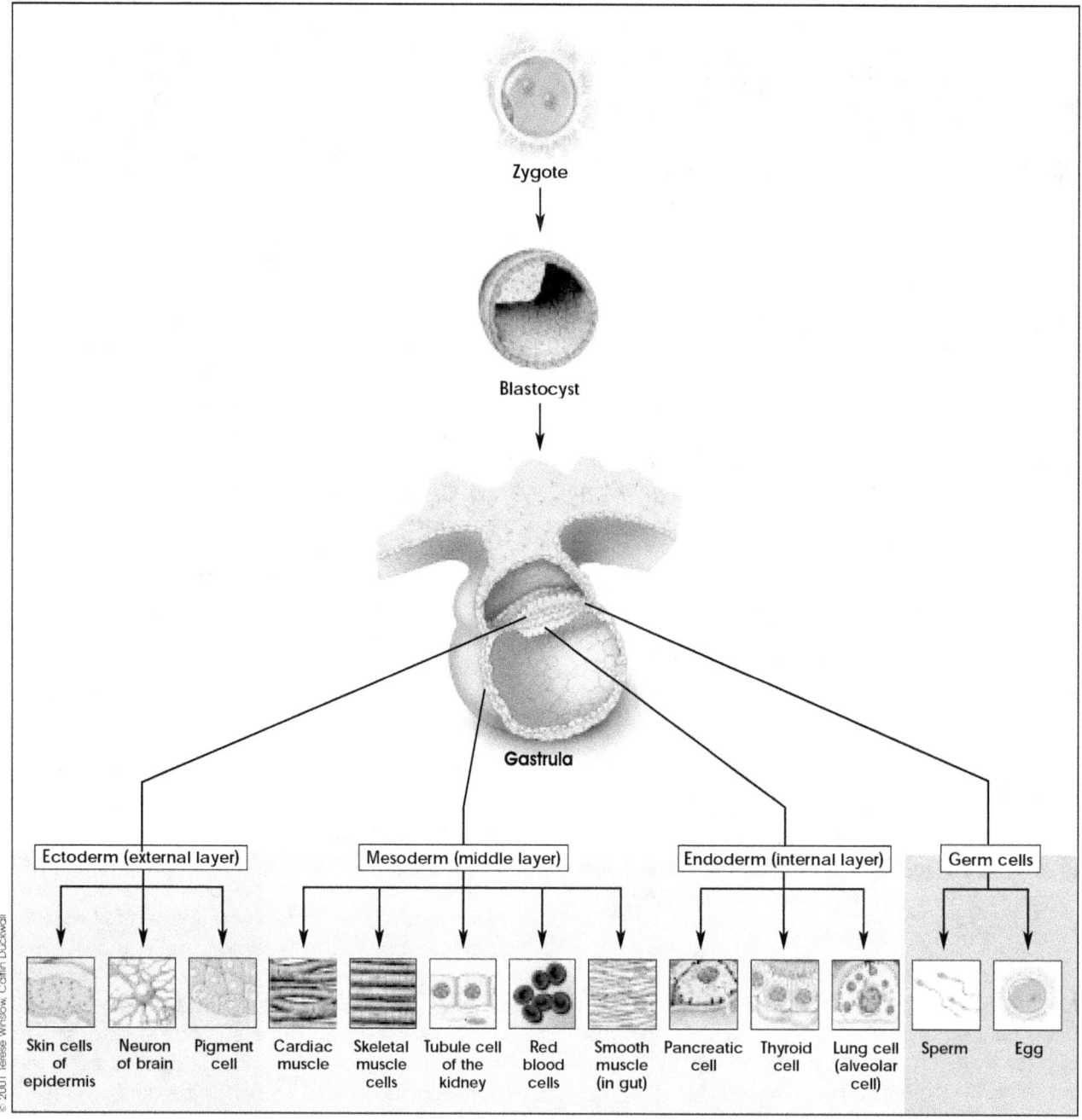

Figure 1.1. Differentiation of Human Tissues.

tissue; it can renew itself and become specialized to yield all of the specialized cell types of the tissue from which it originated. Adult stem cells are capable of self-renewal for the lifetime of the organism. Sources of adult stem cells have been found in the bone marrow, blood stream, cornea and retina of the eye, the dental pulp of the tooth, liver, skin, gastrointestinal tract, and pancreas. Unlike embryonic stem cells, at this point in time, there are no isolated adult stem cells that are capable of forming all cells of the body. That is, there is no evidence, at this time, of an adult stem cell that is pluripotent.

Table 1.1. Embryonic Germ Layers From Which Differentiated Tissues Develop

Embryonic Germ Layer	Differentiated Tissue
Endoderm	Thymus
	Thyroid, parathyroid glands
	Larynx, trachea, lung
	Urinary bladder, vagina, urethra
	Gastrointestinal (GI) organs (liver, pancreas)
	Lining of the GI tract
	Lining of the respiratory tract
Mesoderm	Bone marrow (blood)
	Adrenal cortex
	Lymphatic tissue
	Skeletal, smooth, and cardiac muscle
	Connective tissues (including bone, cartilage)
	Urogenital system
	Heart and blood vessels (vascular system)
Ectoderm	Skin
	Neural tissue (neuroectoderm)
	Adrenal medulla
	Pituitary gland
	Connective tissue of the head and face
	Eyes, ears

[1]

REFERENCES

1. Chandross, K.J. and Mezey, E. (2001). Plasticity of adult bone marrow stem cells. Mattson, M.P. and Van Zant, G. eds. (Greenwich, CT: JAI Press).

2. Slack, J.M. (2000). Stem cells in epithelial tissues. Science. 287, 1431-1433.

This page intentionally left blank

2. THE EMBRYONIC STEM CELL

As stated in the first chapter, an embryonic stem cell (ES cell) is defined by its origin. It is derived from the blastocyst stage of the embryo. The blastocyst is the stage of embryonic development prior to implantation in the uterine wall. At this stage, the preimplantation embryo of the mouse is made up of 150 cells and consists of a sphere made up of an outer layer of cells (the trophectoderm), a fluid-filled cavity (the blastocoel), and a cluster of cells on the interior (the inner cell mass).

Studies of ES cells derived from mouse blastocysts became possible 20 years ago with the discovery of techniques that allowed the cells to be grown in the laboratory. Embryonic–like stem cells, called embryonic germ (EG) cells, can also be derived from primordial germ (PG) cells (the cells of the developing fetus from which eggs and sperm are formed) of the mouse [20] and human fetus [30].

In this chapter the discussion will be limited to mouse embryonic stem cells. Chapter 3 describes the human embryonic stem cell.

DO EMBRYONIC STEM CELLS ACTUALLY OCCUR IN THE EMBRYO?

Some scientists argue that ES cells do not occur *in* the embryo as such. ES cells closely resemble the cells of the preimplantation embryo [3], but are not in fact the same [32]. An alternative perspective is that the embryos of many animal species contain stem cells. These cells proliferate extensively in the embryo, are capable of differentiating into all the types of cells that occur in the adult, and can be isolated and grown *ex vivo* (outside the organism), where they continue to replicate and show the potential to differentiate [18].

For research purposes, the definition of an ES cell is more than a self-replicating stem cell derived from the embryo that can differentiate into almost all of the cells of the body. Scientists have found it necessary to develop specific criteria that help them better define the ES cell. Austin Smith, whose studies of mouse ES cells have contributed significantly to the field, has offered a list of essential characteristics that define ES cells [18, 32].

DEFINING PROPERTIES OF AN EMBRYONIC STEM CELL

- [a]Derived from the inner cell mass/epiblast of the blastocyst.
- [a]Capable of undergoing an unlimited number of symmetrical divisions without differentiating (long-term self-renewal).
- Exhibit and maintain a stable, full (diploid), normal complement of chromosomes (karyotype).
- Pluripotent ES cells can give rise to differentiated cell types that are derived from all three primary germ layers of the embryo (endoderm, mesoderm, and ectoderm).
- [a,b]Capable of integrating into all fetal tissues during development. (Mouse ES cells maintained in culture for long periods can still generate any tissue when they are reintroduced into an embryo to generate a chimeric animal.)
- [a,b]Capable of colonizing the germ line and giving rise to egg or sperm cells.
- [a]Clonogenic, that is a single ES cell can give rise to a colony of genetically identical cells, or clones, which have the same properties as the original cell.

- Expresses the transcription factor Oct-4, which then activates or inhibits a host of target genes and maintains ES cells in a proliferative, non-differentiating state.

- Can be induced to continue proliferating or to differentiate.

- Lacks the G1 checkpoint in the cell cycle. ES cells spend most of their time in the S phase of the cell cycle, during which they synthesize DNA. Unlike differentiated somatic cells, ES cells do not require any external stimulus to initiate DNA replication.

- Do not show X inactivation. In every somatic cell of a female mammal, one of the two X chromosomes becomes permanently inactivated. X inactivation does not occur in undifferentiated ES cells.

[a Not shown in human EG cells. b Not shown in human ES cells. All of the criteria have been met by mouse ES cells.]

ARE EMBRYONIC STEM CELLS TRULY PLURIPOTENT?

Pluripotency—that is the ability to give rise to differentiated cell types that are derived from all three primary germ layers of the embryo, endoderm, mesoderm, and ectoderm—is what makes ES cells unique. How do we know that these cells are, indeed, pluripotent? Laboratory-based criteria for testing the pluripotent nature of ES cells derived from mice include three kinds of experiments [19]. One test is conducted by injecting ES cells derived from the inner cell mass of one blastocyst into the cavity of another blastocyst. The "combination" embryos are then transferred to the uterus of a pseudopregnant female mouse, and the progeny that result are chimeras. Chimeras are a mixture of tissues and organs of cells derived from both donor ES cells and the recipient blastocyst.

This test has been extended in studies designed to test whether cultured ES cells can be used to replace the inner cell mass of a mouse blastocyst and produce a normal embryo. They can, but the process is far less efficient than that of using cells taken directly from the inner cell mass. Apparently, the ability of ES cells to generate a complete embryo depends on the number of times they have been passaged *in vitro* [21, 22]. A passage is the process of removing

cells from one culture dish and replating them into fresh culture dishes. Whether the number of passages affects the differentiation potential of human ES cells remains to be determined. (For a detailed discussion of the techniques for maintaining mouse ES cells in culture, see Appendix B. Mouse Embryonic Stem Cells.)

A second method for determining the pluripotency of mouse ES cells is to inject the cells into adult mice (under the skin or the kidney capsule) that are either genetically identical or are immune-deficient, so the tissue will not be rejected. In the host animal, the injected ES cells develop into benign tumors called teratomas. When examined under a microscope, it was noted that these tumors contain cell types derived from all three primary germ layers of the embryo—endoderm, mesoderm, and ectoderm. Teratomas typically contain gut-like structures such as layers of epithelial cells and smooth muscle; skeletal or cardiac muscle (which may contract spontaneously); neural tissue; cartilage or bone; and sometimes hair. Thus, ES cells that have been maintained for a long period *in vitro* can behave as pluripotent cells *in vivo*. They can participate in normal embryogenesis by differentiating into any cell type in the body, and they can also differentiate into a wide range of cell types in an adult animal. However, normal mouse ES cells do not generate trophoblast tissues *in vivo* [32].

A third technique for demonstrating pluripotency is to allow mouse ES cells *in vitro* to differentiate spontaneously or to direct their differentiation along specific pathways. The former is usually accomplished by removing feeder layers and adding leukemia inhibitory factor (LIF) to the growth medium. Within a few days after changing the culture conditions, ES cells aggregate and may form embryoid bodies (EBs). In many ways, EBs in the culture dish resemble teratomas that are observed in the animal. EBs consist of a disorganized array of differentiated or partially differentiated cell types that are derived from the three primary germ layers of the embryo—the endoderm, mesoderm, and ectoderm [32].

The techniques for culturing mouse ES cells from the inner cell mass of the preimplantation blastocyst were first reported 20 years ago [9, 19], and versions of these standard procedures are used today in laboratories throughout the world. It is striking that, to date, only three species of mammals have yielded long-term cultures of self-renewing ES cells: mice, monkeys, and humans [27, 34, 35, 36] (see Appendix B. Mouse Embryonic Stem Cells).

HOW DOES A MOUSE EMBRYONIC STEM CELL STAY UNDIFFERENTIATED?

As stated earlier, a true stem cell is capable of maintaining itself in a self-renewing, undifferentiated state indefinitely. The undifferentiated state of the embryonic stem cell is characterized by specific cell markers that have helped scientists better understand how embryonic stem cells—under the right culture conditions—replicate for hundreds of population doublings and do not differentiate. To date, two major areas of investigation have provided some clues. One includes attempts to understand the effects of secreted factors such as the cytokine leukemia inhibitory factor on mouse ES cells *in vitro*. The second area of study involves transcription factors such as Oct-4. Oct-4 is a protein expressed by mouse and human ES cells *in vitro*, and also by mouse inner cell mass cells *in vivo*. The cell cycle of the ES also seems to play a role in preventing differentiation. From studies of these various signaling pathways, it is clear that many factors must be balanced in a particular way for ES cells to remain in a self-renewing state. If the balance shifts, ES cells begin to differentiate [18, 31]. (For a detailed discussion of how embryonic stem cells maintain their pluripotency, see Appendix B. Mouse Embryonic Stem Cells.)

CAN A MOUSE EMBRYONIC STEM CELL BE DIRECTED TO DIFFERENTIATE INTO A PARTICULAR CELL TYPE IN VITRO?

One goal for embryonic stem cell research is the development of specialized cells such as neurons, heart muscle cells, endothelial cells of blood vessels, and insulin secreting cells similar to those found in the pancreas. The directed derivation of embryonic stem cells is then vital to the ultimate use of such cells in the development of new therapies.

By far the most common approach to directing differentiation is to change the growth conditions of the ES cells in specific ways, such as by adding growth factors to the culture medium or changing the chemical composition of the surface on which the ES cells are growing. For example, the plastic culture dishes used to grow both mouse and human ES cells can be treated with a variety of substances that allow the cells either to adhere to the surface of the dish or to avoid adhering and instead float in the culture medium. In general, an adherent substrate helps prevent them from interacting and differentiating. In contrast, a nonadherent substrate allows the ES cells to aggregate and thereby interact with each other. Cell-cell interactions are critical to normal embryonic development, so allowing some of these "natural" *in vivo* interactions to occur in the culture dish is a fundamental strategy for inducing mouse or human ES cell differentiation *in vitro*. In addition, adding specific growth factors to the culture medium triggers the activation (or inactivation) of specific genes in ES cells. This initiates a series of molecular events that induces the cells to differentiate along a particular pathway.

Another way to direct differentiation of ES cells is to introduce foreign genes into the cells via transfection or other methods [6, 39]. The result of these strategies is to add an active gene to the ES cell genome, which then triggers the cells to differentiate along a particular pathway. The approach appears to be a precise way of regulating ES cell differentiation, but it will work only if it is possible to identify which gene must be active at which particular stage of differentiation. Then, the gene must be activated at the right time—meaning during the correct stage of differentiation—and it must be inserted into the genome at the proper location.

Another approach to generate mouse ES cells uses cloning technology. In theory, the nucleus of a differentiated mouse somatic cell might be reprogrammed by injecting it into an oocyte. The resultant pluripotent cell would be immunologically compatible because it would be genetically identical to the donor cell [25].

All of the techniques just described are still highly experimental. Nevertheless, within the past several years, it has become possible to generate specific, differentiated, functional cell types by manipulating the growth conditions of mouse ES cells *in vitro*. It is not possible to explain *how* the directed differentiation occurs, however. No one knows how or when gene expression is changed, what signal-transduction systems are triggered, or what cell-cell interactions must occur to convert undifferentiated ES cells into precursor cells and, finally, into differentiated cells that look and function like their *in vivo* counterparts.

Embryonic stem cells have been shown to differentiate into a variety of cell types. For example, mouse ES cells can be directed *in vitro* to yield vascular structures [40], neurons that release dopamine and serotonin [14], and endocrine pancreatic islet cells [16]. In all three cases, proliferating, undifferentiated mouse ES cells provide the starting material and functional, differentiated cells were the result. Also, the onset of mouse ES cell differentiation can be triggered by withdrawing the cytokine LIF, which promotes the division of undifferentiated mouse ES cells. In addition, when directed to differentiate, ES cells aggregate, a change in their three-dimensional environment that presumably allowed some of the cell-cell interactions to occur *in vitro* that would occur *in vivo* during normal embryonic development. Collectively, these three studies provide some of the best examples of directed differentiation of ES cells. Two of them showed that a single precursor cell can give rise to multiple, differentiated cell types [16, 40], and all three studies demonstrated that the resulting differentiated cells function as their *in vivo* counterparts do. These two criteria—demonstrating that a single cell can give rise to multiple cells types and the functional properties of the differentiated cells—form the basis of an acid test for all claims of directed differentiation of either ES cells or adult stem cells. Unfortunately, very few experiments meet these criteria, which too often makes it impossible to assess whether a differentiated cell type resulted from the experimental manipulation that was reported. (For a detailed discussion of the methods used to differentiate mouse embryonic stem cells, see Appendix B. Mouse Embryonic Stem Cells.)

Table 2.1 provides a summary of what is known today about the types of cells that can be differentiated from mouse embryonic stem cells.

REFERENCES

1. Bagutti, C., Wobus, A.M., Fassler, R., and Watt, F.M. (1996). Differentiation of embryonal stem cells into keratinocytes: comparison of wild-type and β(1) integrin-deficient cells. Dev. Biol. *179*, 184-196.

2. Bain, G., Kitchens, D., Yao, M., Huettner, J.E., and Gottlieb, D.I. (1995). Embryonic stem cells express neuronal properties *in vitro*. Dev. Biol. *168*, 342-357.

Table 2.1. Reported differentiated cell types from mouse embryonic stem cells *in vitro**

Cell Type	Reference
Adipocyte	[7]
Astrocyte	[11]
Cardiomyocyte	[8, 17]
Chondrocyte	[13]
Definitive hematopoietic	[23, 24, 38]
Dendritic cell	[10]
Endothelial cell	[28, 40]
Keratinocyte	[1, 40]
Lymphoid precursor	[26]
Mast cell	[37]
Neuron	[2, 33]
Oligodendrocyte	[4, 15]
Osteoblast	[5]
Pancreatic islets	[16]
Primitive haematopoietic	[8, 23]
Smooth muscle	[40]
Striated muscle	[29]
Yolk sac endoderm	[8]
Yolk sac mesoderm	[8]

*Adapted with permission from reference [32].

3. Brook, F.A. and Gardner, R.L. (1997). The origin and efficient derivation of embryonic stem cells in the mouse. Proc. Natl. Acad. Sci. U. S. A. *94*, 5709-5712.

4. Brustle, O., Jones, K.N., Learish, R.D., Karram, K., Choudhary, K., Wiestler, O.D., Duncan, I.D., and McKay, R.D. (1999). Embryonic stem cell-derived glial precursors: a source of myelinating transplants. Science. *285*, 754-756.

5. Buttery, L.D., Bourne, S., Xynos, J.D., Wood, H., Hughes, F.J., Hughes, S.P., Episkopou, V., and Polak, J.M. (2001). Differentiation of osteoblasts and *in vitro* bone formation from murine embryonic stem cells. Tissue Eng. *7*, 89-99.

6. Call, L.M., Moore, C.S., Stetten, G., and Gearhart, J.D. (2000). A cre-lox recombination system for the targeted integration of circular yeast artificial chromosomes into embryonic stem cells. Hum. Mol. Genet. *9*, 1745-1751.

7. Dani, C., Smith, A.G., Dessolin, S., Leroy, P., Staccini, L., Villageois, P., Darimont, C., and Ailhaud, G. (1997). Differentiation of embryonic stem cells into adipocytes *in vitro*. J. Cel. Sci. *110*, 1279-1285.

8. Doetschman, T., Eistetter, H., Katz, M., Schmit, W., and Kemler, R. (1985). The in vitro development of blastocyst-derived embryonic stem cell lines: formation of visceral yolk sac, blood islands and myocardium. J. Embryol. Exp. Morph. 87, 27-45.

9. Evans, M.J. and Kaufman, M.H. (1981). Establishment in culture of pluripotential cells from mouse embryos. Nature. 292, 154-156.

10. Fairchild, P.J., Brook, F.A., Gardner, R.L., Graca, L., Strong, V., Tone, Y., Tone, M., Nolan, K.F., and Waldmann, H. (2000). Directed differentiation of dendritic cells from mouse embryonic stem cells. Curr. Biol. 10, 1515-1518.

11. Fraichard, A., Chassande, O., Bilbaut, G., Dehay, C., Savatier, P., and Samarut, J. (1995). In vitro differentiation of embryonic stem cells into glial cells and functional neurons. J. Cell Sci. 108, 3181-3188.

12. Itskovitz-Eldor, J., Schuldiner, M., Karsenti, D., Eden, A., Yanuka, O., Amit, M., Soreq, H., and Benvenisty, N. (2000). Differentiation of human embryonic stem cells into embryoid bodies comprising the three embryonic germ layers. Mol. Med. 6, 88-95.

13. Kramer, J., Hegert, C., Guan, K., Wobus, A.M., Muller, P.K., and Rohwedel, J. (2000). Embryonic stem cell-derived chondrogenic differentiation in vitro: activation by BMP-2 and BMP-4. Mech. Dev. 92, 193-205.

14. Lee, S.H., Lumelsky, N., Studer, L., Auerbach, J.M., and McKay, R.D. (2000). Efficient generation of midbrain and hindbrain neurons from mouse embryonic stem cells. Nat. Biotechnol. 18, 675-679.

15. Liu, S., Qu, Y., Stewart, T.J., Howard, M.J., Chakrabortty, S., Holekamp, T.F., and McDonald, J.W. (2000). Embryonic stem cells differentiate into oligodendrocytes and myelinate in culture and after spinal cord transplantation. Proc. Natl. Acad. Sci. U. S. A. 97, 6126-6131.

16. Lumelsky, N., Blondel, O., Laeng, P., Velasco, I., Ravin, R., and McKay, R. (2001). Differentiation of Embryonic Stem Cells to Insulin-Secreting Structures Similiar to Pancreatic Islets. Science. 292, 1389-1394.

17. Maltsev, V.A., Rohwedel, J., Hescheler, J., and Wobus, A.M. (1993). Embryonic stem cells differentiate in vitro into cardiomyocytes representing sinusnodal, atrial and ventricular cell types. Mech. Dev. 44, 41-50.

18. Marshak, D.R., Gottlieb, D., Kiger, A.A., Fuller, M.T., Kunath, T., Hogan, B., Gardner, R.L., Smith, A., Klar, A.J.S., Henrique, D., D'Urso, G., Datta, S., Holliday, R., Astle, C.M., Chen, J., Harrison, D.E., Xie, T., Spradling, A., Andrews, P.W., Przyborski, S.A., Thomson, J.A., Kunath, T., Strumpf, D., Rossant, J., Tanaka, S., Orkin, S.H., Melchers, F., Rolink, A., Keller, G., Pittenger, M.F., Marshak, D.R., Flake, A.W., Panicker, M.M., Rao, M., Watt, F.M., Grompe, M., Finegold, M.J., Kritzik, M.R., Sarvetnick, N., and Winton, D.J. (2001). Stem cell biology, Marshak, D.R., Gardner, R.L., and Gottlieb, D. eds. (Cold Spring Harbor, New York: Cold Spring Harbor Laboratory Press).

19. Martin, G.R. (1981). Isolation of a pluripotent cell line from early mouse embryos cultured in medium conditioned by teratocarcinoma stem cells. Proc. Natl. Acad. Sci. U. S. A. 78, 7634-7638.

20. Matsui, Y., Zsebo, K., and Hogan, B.L. (1992). Derivation of pluripotential embryonic stem cells from murine primordial germ cells in culture. Cell. 70, 841-847.

21. Nagy, A., Gocza, E., Diaz, E.M., Prideaux, V.R., Ivanyi, E., Markkula, M., and Rossant, J. (1990). Embryonic stem cells alone are able to support fetal development in the mouse. Development. 110, 815-821.

22. Nagy, A., Rossant, J., Nagy, R., Abramow-Newerly, W., and Roder, J.C. (1993). Derivation of completely cell culture-derived mice from early-passage embryonic stem cells. Proc. Natl. Acad. Sci. U. S. A. 90, 8424-8428.

23. Nakano, T., Kodama, H., and Honjo, T. (1996). In vitro development of primitive and definitive erythrocytes from different precursors. Science. 272, 722-724.

24. Nishikawa, S.I., Nishikawa, S., Hirashima, M., Matsuyoshi, N., and Kodama, H. (1998). Progressive lineage analysis by cell sorting and culture identifies FLK1(+)VE-cadherin(+) cells at a diverging point of endothelial and hemopoietic lineages. Development. 125, 1747-1757.

25. Odorico, J.S., Kaufman, D.S., and Thomson, J.A. (2001). Multilineage differentiation from human embryonic stem cell lines. Stem Cells. 19, 193-204.

26. Potocnik, A.J., Nielsen, P.J., and Eichmann, K. (1994). In vitro generation of lymphoid precursors from embryonic stem cells. EMBO. J. 13, 5274-5283.

27. Reubinoff, B.E., Pera, M.F., Fong, C.Y., Trounson, A., and Bongso, A. (2000). Embryonic stem cell lines from human blastocysts: somatic differentiation in vitro. Nat. Biotechnol. 18, 399-404.

28. Risau, W., Sariola, H., Zerwes, H.G., Sasse, J., Ekblom, P., Kemler, R., and Doetschman, T. (1988). Vasculogenesis and angiogenesis in embryonic-stem-cell-derived embryoid bodies. Development. 102, 471-478.

29. Rohwedel, J., Maltsev, V., Bober, E., Arnold, H.H., Hescheler, J., and Wobus, A.M. (1994). Muscle cell differentiation of embryonic stem cells reflects myogenesis in vivo: developmentally regulated expression of myogenic determination genes and functional expression of ionic currents. Dev. Biol. 164, 87-101.

30. Shamblott, M.J., Axelman, J., Wang, S., Bugg, E.M., Littlefield, J.W., Donovan, P.J., Blumenthal, P.D., Huggins, G.R., and Gearhart, J.D. (1998). Derivation of pluripotent stem cells from cultured human primordial germ cells. Proc. Natl. Acad. Sci. U. S. A. 95, 13726-13731.

31. Smith, A., personal communication.

32. Smith, A.G. (2001). Origins and properties of mouse embryonic stem cells. Annu. Rev. Cell. Dev. Biol.

33. Strubing, C., Ahnert-Hilger, G., Shan, J., Wiedenmann, B., Hescheler, J., and Wobus, A.M. (1995). Differentiation of pluripotent embryonic stem cells into the neuronal lineage *in vitro* gives rise to mature inhibitory and excitatory neurons. Mech. Dev. *53*, 275-287.

34. Thomson, J.A., Kalishman, J., Golos, T.G., Durning, M., Harris, C.P., Becker, R.A., and Hearn, J.P. (1995). Isolation of a primate embryonic stem cell line. Proc. Natl. Acad. Sci. U. S. A. *92*, 7844-7848.

35. Thomson, J.A. and Marshall, V.S. (1998). Primate embryonic stem cells. Curr. Top. Dev. Biol. *38*, 133-165.

36. Thomson, J.A., Itskovitz-Eldor, J., Shapiro, S.S., Waknitz, M.A., Swiergiel, J.J., Marshall, V.S., and Jones, J.M. (1998). Embryonic stem cell lines derived from human blastocysts. Science. *282*, 1145-1147.

37. Tsai, M., Wedemeyer, J., Ganiatsas, S., Tam, S.Y., Zon, L.I., and Galli, S.J. (2000). *In vivo* immunological function of mast cells derived from embryonic stem cells: an approach for the rapid analysis of even embryonic lethal mutations in adult mice *in vivo*. Proc. Natl. Acad. Sci. U. S. A. *97*, 9186-9190.

38. Wiles, M.V. and Keller, G. (1991). Multiple hematopoietic lineages develop from embryonic stem (ES) cells in culture. Development. *111*, 259-267.

39. Wiles, M.V., Vauti, F., Otte, J., Fuchtbauer, E.M., Ruiz, P., Fuchtbauer, A., Arnold, H.H., Lehrach, H., Metz, T., von Melchner, H., and Wurst, W. (2000). Establishment of a gene-trap sequence tag library to generate mutant mice from embryonic stem cells. Nat. Genet. *24*, 13-14.

40. Yamashita, J., Itoh, H., Hirashima, M., Ogawa, M., Nishikawa, S., Yurugi, T., Naito, M., Nakao, K., and Nishikawa, S. (2000). Flk1-positive cells derived from embryonic stem cells serve as vascular progenitors. Nature. *408*, 92-96.

3. THE HUMAN EMBRYONIC STEM CELL AND THE HUMAN EMBRYONIC GERM CELL

A new era in stem cell biology began in 1998 with the derivation of cells from human blastocysts and fetal tissue with the unique ability of differentiating into cells of all tissues in the body, i.e., the cells are pluripotent. Since then, several research teams have characterized many of the molecular characteristics of these cells and improved the methods for culturing them. In addition, scientists are just beginning to direct the differentiation of the human pluripotent stem cells and to identify the functional capabilities of the resulting specialized cells. Although in its earliest phases, research with these cells is proving to be important to developing innovative cell replacement strategies to rebuild tissues and restore critical functions of the diseased or damaged human body.

OVERVIEW

In 1998, James Thomson and his colleagues reported methods for deriving and maintaining human embryonic stem (ES) cells from the inner cell mass of human blastocysts that were produced through *in vitro* fertilization (IVF) and donated for research purposes [46]. At the same time, another group, led by John Gearhart, reported the derivation of cells that they identified as embryonic germ (EG) cells. The cells were cultured from primordial germ cells obtained from the gonadal ridge and mesenchyma of 5- to 9-week fetal tissue that resulted from elective abortions [41].

The two research teams developed their methods for culturing human ES and EG cells by drawing on a host of animal studies, some of which date back almost 40 years: derivations of pluripotent mouse ES cells from blastocysts [13, 15], reports of the derivation of EG cells [27, 36], experiments with stem cells derived from mouse teratocarcinomas [24] and human embryonal carcinomas and teratocarcinomas [4, 17, 24], the derivation and

culture of ES cells from the blastocysts of rhesus monkeys [46] and marmosets [47], and methods used by IVF clinics to prepare human embryos for transplanting into the uterus to produce a live birth [11, 49].

TIMELINE OF HUMAN EMBRYONIC STEM CELL RESEARCH

- **1878:** First reported attempts to fertilize mammalian eggs outside the body [49].

- **1959:** First report of animals (rabbits) produced through IVF in the United States [49].

- **1960s:** Studies of teratocarcinomas in the testes of several inbred strains of mice indicates they originated from embryonic germ cells. The work establishes embryonal carcinoma (EC) cells as a kind of stem cell [17, 24]. For a more detailed discussion of human embryonal carcinoma cells, see Appendix C.

- **1968:** Edwards and Bavister fertilize the first human egg *in vitro* [49].

- **1970s:** EC cells injected into mouse blastocysts produce chimeric mice. Cultured SC cells are explored as models of embryonic development, although their complement of chromosomes is abnormal [25].

- **1978:** Louise Brown, the first IVF baby, is born in England [49].

- **1980:** Australia's first IVF baby, Candace Reed, is born in Melbourne [49].

- **1981:** Evans and Kaufman, and Martin derive mouse embryonic stem (ES) cells from the inner cell mass of blastocysts. They establish culture conditions for growing pluripotent mouse ES cells *in vitro*. The ES cells yield cell lines with normal, diploid karyotyes and generate derivatives of all three primary germ layers as well as primordial germ cells. Injecting the ES cells into mice induces the formation of teratomas [15, 26]. The first IVF baby, Elizabeth Carr, is born in the United States [49].

- **1984-88:** Andrews et al., develop pluripotent, genetically identical (clonal) cells called embryonal carcinoma (EC) cells from Tera-2, a cell line of human testicular teratocarcinoma [5]. Cloned human teratoma cells exposed to retinoic acid differentiate into neuron-like cells and other cell types [3, 44].

- **1989:** Pera et al., derive a clonal line of human embryonal carcinoma cells, which yields tissues from all three primary germ layers. The cells are aneuploid (fewer or greater than the normal number of chromosomes in the cell) and their potential to differentiate spontaneously *in vitro* is typically limited. The behavior of human EC cell clones differs from that of mouse ES or EC cells [33].

- **1994:** Human blastocysts created for reproductive purposes using IVF and donated by patients for research, are generated from the 2-pronuclear stage. The inner cell mass of the blastocyst is maintained in culture and generates aggregates with trophoblast-like cells at the periphery and ES-like cells in the center. The cells retain a complete set of chromosomes (normal karyotype); most cultures retain a stem cell-like morphology, although some inner cell mass clumps differentiate into fibroblasts. The cultures are maintained for two passages [6, 7].

- **1995-96:** Non-human primate ES cells are derived and maintained *in vitro*, first from the inner cell mass of rhesus monkeys [46], and then from marmosets [47]. The primate ES cells are diploid and have normal karyotypes. They are pluripotent and differentiate into cells types derived from all three primary germ layers. The primate ES cells resemble human EC cells and indicate that it should be possible to derive and maintain human ES cells *in vitro*.

- **1998:** Thomson et al., derive human ES cells from the inner cell mass of normal human blastocysts donated by couples undergoing treatment for infertility. The cells are cultured through many passages, retain their normal karyotypes, maintain high levels of telomerase activity, and express a panel of markers typical

of human EC cells non-human primate ES cells. Several (non-clonal) cell lines are established that form teratomas when injected into immune-deficient mice. The teratomas include cell types derived from all three primary germ layers, demonstrating the pluripotency of human ES cells [48]. Gearhart and colleagues derive human embryonic germ (EG) cells from the gonadal ridge and mesenchyma of 5- to 9-week fetal tissue that resulted from elective abortions. They grow EG cells *in vitro* for approximately 20 passages, and the cells maintain normal karyotypes. The cells spontaneously form aggregates that differentiate spontaneously, and ultimately contain derivatives of all three primary germ layers. Other indications of their pluripotency include the expression of a panel of markers typical of mouse ES and EG cells. The EG cells do not form teratomas when injected into immune-deficient mice [41].

- **2000:** Scientists in Singapore and Australia led by Pera, Trounson, and Bongso derive human ES cells from the inner cell mass of blastocysts donated by couples undergoing treatment for infertility. The ES cells proliferate for extended periods *in vitro*, maintain normal karyotypes, differentiate spontaneously into somatic cell lineages derived from all three primary germ layers, and form teratomas when injected into immune-deficient mice.

- **2001:** As human ES cell lines are shared and new lines are derived, more research groups report methods to direct the differentiation of the cells *in vitro*. Many of the methods are aimed at generating human tissues for transplantation purposes, including pancreatic islet cells, neurons that release dopamine, and cardiac muscle cells.

DERIVATION OF HUMAN EMBRYONIC STEM CELLS

The first documentation of the isolation of embryonic stem cells from human blastocysts was in 1994 [7]. Since then, techniques for deriving and culturing human ES cells have been refined [38, 48]. The ability to isolate human ES cells from blastocysts and grow them in culture seems to depend in large part on the integrity and condition of the blastocyst from which the cells are derived. In general, blastocysts with a large and distinct inner cell mass tend to yield ES cultures most efficiently [11] (see Figure 3.1. Human Blastocyst Showing Inner Cell Mass and Trophectoderm).

Timeline for the Development of a Human

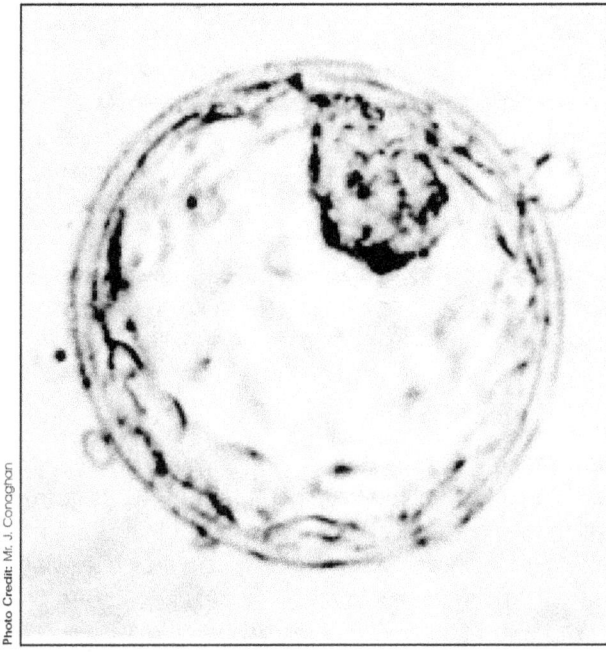

Figure 3.1. Human Blastocyst Showing Inner Cell Mass and Trophectoderm.

Blastocyst *In Vitro*

After a human oocyte is fertilized *in vitro* by a sperm cell, the following events occur according to a fairly predictable timeline [9, 12, 16]. At 18 to 24 hours after *in vitro* fertilization of the oocyte is considered day 1. By day 2 (24 to 25 hours), the zygote (fertilized egg) undergoes the first cleavage to produce a 2-cell embryo. By day 3 (72 hours), the embryo reaches the 8-cell stage called a morula. It is at this stage that the genome of the embryo begins to control its own development. This means that any maternal influences—due to the presence of mRNA and proteins in the oocyte cytoplasm—are significantly reduced. By day 4, the cells of the embryo adhere tightly to each other in a process known as compaction and by day 5, the cavity of the blastocyst is completed. The inner cell mass begins to separate from the outer cells, which become the trophectoderm that surrounds the blastocyst. This represents the first observable sign of cell differentiation in the embryo. (For a

more detailed discussion, see Appendix A. Early Development.)

Many IVF clinics now transfer day-5 embryos to the uterus for optimal implantation, a stage of development that more closely parallels the stage at which a blastocyst would implant in the wall of the uterus *in vivo*. This represents a change—and a greatly improved implantation rate—from earlier IVF procedures in which a 2-cell embryo was used for implantation.

Day-5 blastocysts are used to derive ES cell cultures. A normal day-5 human embryo *in vitro* consists of 200 to 250 cells. Most of the cells comprise the trophectoderm. For deriving ES cell cultures, the trophectoderm is removed, either by microsurgery or immunosurgery (in which antibodies against the trophectoderm help break it down, thus freeing the inner cell mass). At this stage, the inner cell mass is composed of only 30 to 34 cells [10].

The *in vitro* conditions for growing a human embryo to the blastocyst stage vary among IVF clinics and are reviewed elsewhere [6, 8, 14, 16, 18, 21, 39, 49, 50]. However, once the inner cell mass is obtained from either mouse or human blastocysts, the techniques for growing ES cells are similar. (For a detailed discussion see Appendix C. Human Embryonic Stem Cells and Human Embryonic Germ Cells.)

DERIVATION OF HUMAN EMBRYONIC GERM CELLS

As stated earlier, human embryonic germ (EG) cells share many of the characteristics of human ES cells, but differ in significant ways. Human EG cells are derived from the primordial germ cells, which occur in a specific part of the embryo/fetus called the gonadal ridge, and which normally develop into mature gametes (eggs and sperm). Gearhart and his collaborators devised methods for growing pluripotent cells derived from human EG cells. The process requires the generation of embryoid bodies from EG cells, which consists of an unpredictable mix of partially differentiated cell types [19]. The embryoid body-derived cells resulting from this process have high proliferative capacity and gene expression patterns that are representative of multiple cell lineages. This suggests that the embryoid body-derived cells are progenitor or precursor cells for a variety of differentiated cell types [19]. (For a more detailed description of the derivation of EG cells, see Appendix C. Human Embryonic Stem Cells and Human Embryonic Germ Cells.)

PLURIPOTENCY OF HUMAN EMBRYONIC STEM CELLS AND EMBRYONIC GERM CELLS

As stated earlier, a truly pluripotent stem cell is a cell that is capable of self-renewal and of differentiating into most all of the cells of the body, including cells of all three germ layers. Human ES and EG cells *in vitro* are capable of long-term self-renewal, while retaining a normal karyotype [1, 38, 41, 42, 48]. Human ES cells can proliferate for two years through 300 population doublings [29] or even 450 population doublings [30]. Cultures derived from embryoid bodies generated by human embryonic germ cells have less capacity for proliferation. Most will proliferate for 40 population doublings; the maximum reported is 70 to 80 population doublings [42].

To date, several laboratories have demonstrated that human ES cells *in vitro* are pluripotent; they can produce cell types derived from all three embryonic germ layers [1, 20, 38, 40].

Currently, the only test of the *in vivo* pluripotency of human ES cells is to inject them into immune-deficient mice where they generate differentiated cells that are derived from all three germ layers. These include gut epithelium (which, in the embryo, is derived from endoderm); smooth and striated muscle (derived from mesoderm); and neural epithelium, and stratified squamous epithelium (derived from ectoderm) [20, 38, 48].

However, two aspects of *in vivo* pluripotency typically used in animals have not been met by human ES cells: evidence that cells have the capacity to be injected into a human embryo and form an organism made up of cells from two genetic lineages; and evidence that they have the ability to generate germ cells, the precursors to eggs and sperm in a developing organism. These are theoretical considerations, however, because such tests using human ES cells have not been conducted. In any case, these two demonstrations of human ES cell pluripotency are not likely to be critical for potential therapeutic uses of the cells—in transplants or drug development, for example [43].

COMPARISONS BETWEEN HUMAN EMBRYONIC STEM CELLS AND EMBRYONIC GERM CELLS

The ES cells derived from human blastocysts by Thomson and his colleagues, and from human EG cells derived by Gearhart and his collaborators, are similar in many respects. In both cases, the cells replicate for an extended period of time, show no chromosomal abnormalities, generate both XX (female) and XY (male) cultures, and express a set of markers regarded as characteristic of pluripotent cells. When the culture conditions are adjusted to permit differentiation (see below for details), both ES and EG cells spontaneously differentiate into derivatives of all three primary germ layers— endoderm, mesoderm, and ectoderm (see Table 3.1. Comparison of Mouse, Monkey, and Human Pluripotent Stem Cells).

However, the ES cells derived from human blastocysts and EG cells differ not only in the tissue sources from which they are derived, they also vary with respect to their growth characteristics *in vitro*, and their behavior *in vivo* [34]. In addition, human ES cells have been propagated for approximately two years *in vitro*, for several hundred population doublings [1], whereas human embryoid body-derived cells from cultures of embryonic germ cells have been maintained for only 70 to 80 population doublings [42]. Also, human ES cells will generate teratomas containing differentiated cell types, if injected into immunocompromised mice colonies, while human EG cells will not [20, 37, 38, 41, 48].

Several research groups are trying to grow human ES cells without feeder layers of mouse embryo fibro-blasts (MEF), which are labor-intensive to generate. At a recent meeting, scientists from the Geron Corporation reported that they have grown human ES cell without feeder layers, in medium conditioned by MEFs and supplemented with basic FGF [51].

DIRECTED DIFFERENTIATION OF HUMAN EMBRYONIC STEM CELLS AND EMBRYONIC GERM CELLS *IN VITRO*

Currently, a major goal for embryonic stem cell research is to control the differentiation of human ES and EG cell lines into specific kinds of cells—an

Table 3.1. Comparison of Mouse, Monkey, and Human Pluripotent Stem Cells

Marker Name	Mouse EC/ ES/EG cells	Monkey ES cells	Human ES cells	Human EG cells	Human EC cells
SSEA-1	+	–	–	+	–
SSEA-3	–	+	+	+	+
SEA-4	–	+	+	+	+
TRA-1-60	–	+	+	+	+
TRA-1-81	–	+	+	+	+
Alkaline phosphatase	+	+	+	+	+
Oct-4	+	+	+	Unknown	+
Telomerase activity	+ ES, EC	Unknown	+	Unknown	+
Feeder-cell dependent	ES, EG, some EC	Yes	Yes	Yes	Some; relatively low clonal efficiency
Factors which aid in stem cell self-renewal	LIF and other factors that act through gp130 receptor and can substitute for feeder layer	Co-culture with feeder cells; other promoting factors have not been identified	Feeder cells + serum; feeder layer + serum-free medium + bFGF	LIF, bFGF, forskolin	Unknown; low proliferative capacity
Growth characteristics *in vitro*	Form tight, rounded, multi-layer clumps; can form EBs	Form flat, loose aggregates; can form EBs	Form flat, loose aggregates; can form EBs	Form rounded, multi-layer clumps; can form EBs	Form flat, loose aggregates; can form EBs
Teratoma formation *in vivo*	+	+	+	–	+
Chimera formation	+	Unknown	+	–	+

KEY

ES cell	=	Embryonic stem cell		TRA	=	Tumor rejection antigen-1
EG cell	=	Embryonic germ cell		LIF	=	Leukemia inhibitory factor
EC cell	=	Embryonal carcinoma cell		bFGF	=	Basic fibroblast growth factor
SSEA	=	Stage-specific embryonic antigen		EB	=	Embryoid bodies

objective that must be met if the cells are to be used as the basis for therapeutic transplantation, testing drugs, or screening potential toxins. The techniques now being tested to direct human ES cell differentiation are borrowed directly from techniques used to direct the differentiation of mouse ES cells *in vitro*. For more discussion on directed differentiation of human ES and EG cells see Appendix C.

POTENTIAL USES OF HUMAN EMBRYONIC STEM CELLS

Many uses have been proposed for human embryonic stem cells. The most-often discussed is their potential use in transplant therapy—i.e., to replace or restore tissue that has been damaged by disease or injury (see also Chapters 5-9).

Using Human Embryonic Stem Cells for Therapeutic Transplants

Diseases that might be treated by transplanting human ES-derived cells include Parkinson's disease, diabetes, traumatic spinal cord injury, Purkinje cell degeneration, Duchenne's muscular dystrophy, heart failure, and osteogenesis imperfecta. However, treatments for any of these diseases require that human ES cells be directed to differentiate into specific cell types prior to transplant. The research is occurring in several laboratories, but is limited because so few laboratories have access to human ES cells. Thus, at

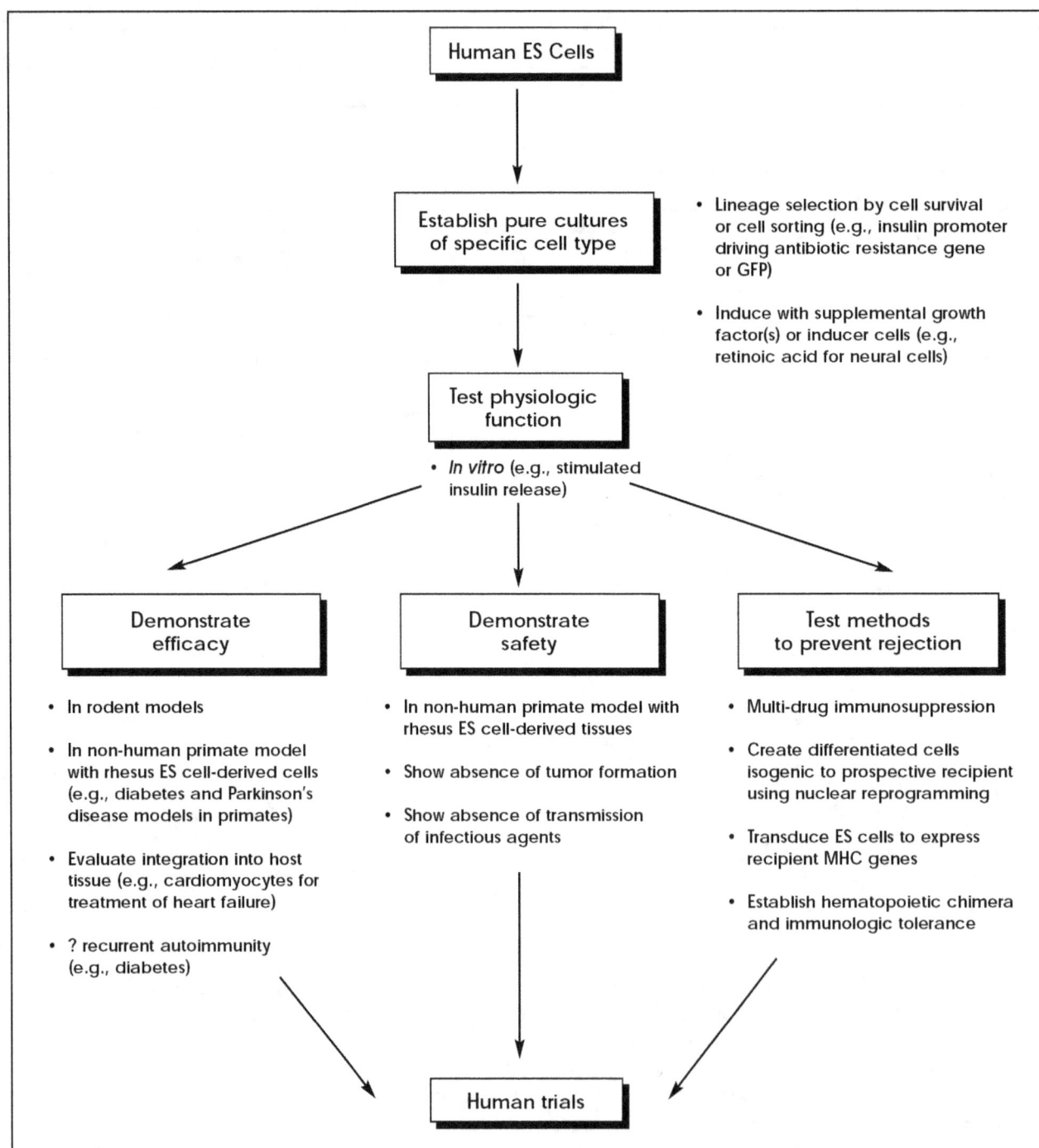

Figure 3.2. Major Goals in the Development of Transplantation Therapies from Human ES Cell Lines. (Reproduced with permission from Stem Cells, 2001)

this stage, any therapies based on the use of human ES cells are still hypothetical and highly experimental [22, 29, 31] (see Figure 3.2. Major Goals in the Development of Transplantation Therapies from Human ES Cell Lines).

One of the current advantages of using ES cells as compared to adult stem cells is that ES cells have an unlimited ability to proliferate in vitro, and are more likely to be able to generate a broad range of cell types through directed differentiation. Ultimately, it will also be necessary to both identify the optimal stage(s) of differentiation for transplant, and demonstrate that the transplanted ES-derived cells can survive, integrate, and function in the recipient.

The potential disadvantages of the use of human ES cells for transplant therapy include the propensity of undifferentiated ES cells to induce the formation of tumors (teratomas), which are typically benign. Because it is the undifferentiated cells—rather than their differentiated progeny—that have been shown to induce teratomas, tumor formation might be avoided by devising methods for removing any undifferentiated ES cells prior to transplant. Also, it should be possible to devise a fail-safe mechanism—i.e., to insert into transplanted ES-derived cells suicide genes that can trigger the death of the cells should they become tumorigenic.

Human ES derived cells would also be advantageous for transplantation purposes if they did not trigger immune rejection. The immunological status of human ES cells has not been studied in detail, and it is not known how immunogenic ES-derived cells might be. In general, the immunogenicity of a cell depends on its expression of Class I major histocompatability antigens (MHC), which allow the body to distinguish its own cells from foreign tissue, and on the presence of cells that can bind to foreign antigens and "present" them to the immune system.

The potential immunological rejection of human ES-derived cells might be avoided by genetically engineering the ES cells to express the MHC antigens of the transplant recipient, or by using nuclear transfer technology to generate ES cells that are genetically identical to the person who receives the transplant. It has been suggested that this could be accomplished by using somatic cell nuclear transfer technology (so-called therapeutic cloning) in which the nucleus is removed from one of the transplant

patient's cells, such as a skin cell, and injecting the nucleus into an oocyte. The oocyte, thus "fertilized," could be cultured in vitro to the blastocyst stage. ES cells could subsequently be derived from its inner cell mass, and directed to differentiate into the desired cell type. The result would be differentiated (or partly differentiated) ES-derived cells that match exactly the immunological profile of the person who donated the somatic cell nucleus, and who is also the intended recipient of the transplant—a labor intensive, but truly customized therapy [29].

Other Potential Uses of Human Embryonic Stem Cells

Many potential uses of human ES cells have been proposed that do not involve transplantation. For example, human ES cells could be used to study early events in human development. Still-unexplained events in early human development can result in congenital birth defects and placental abnormalities that lead to spontaneous abortion. By studying human ES cells in vitro, it may be possible to identify the genetic, molecular, and cellular events that lead to these problems and identify methods for preventing them [22, 35, 45].

Such cells could also be used to explore the effects of chromosomal abnormalities in early development. This might include the ability to monitor the development of early childhood tumors, many of which are embryonic in origin [32].

Human ES cells could also be used to test candidate therapeutic drugs. Currently, before candidate drugs are tested in human volunteers, they are subjected to a barrage of preclinical tests. These include drug screening in animal models—in vitro tests using cells derived from mice or rats, for example, or in vivo tests that involve giving the drug to an animal to assess its safety. Although animal model testing is a mainstay of pharmaceutical research, it cannot always predict the effects that a candidate drug may have on human cells. For this reason, cultures of human cells are often employed in preclinical tests. These human cell lines have usually been maintained in vitro for long periods and as such often have different characteristics than do in vivo cells. These differences can make it difficult to predict the action of a drug in vivo based on the response of human cell lines in vitro. Therefore, if human ES cells can be directed to differentiate into specific cell types that are important

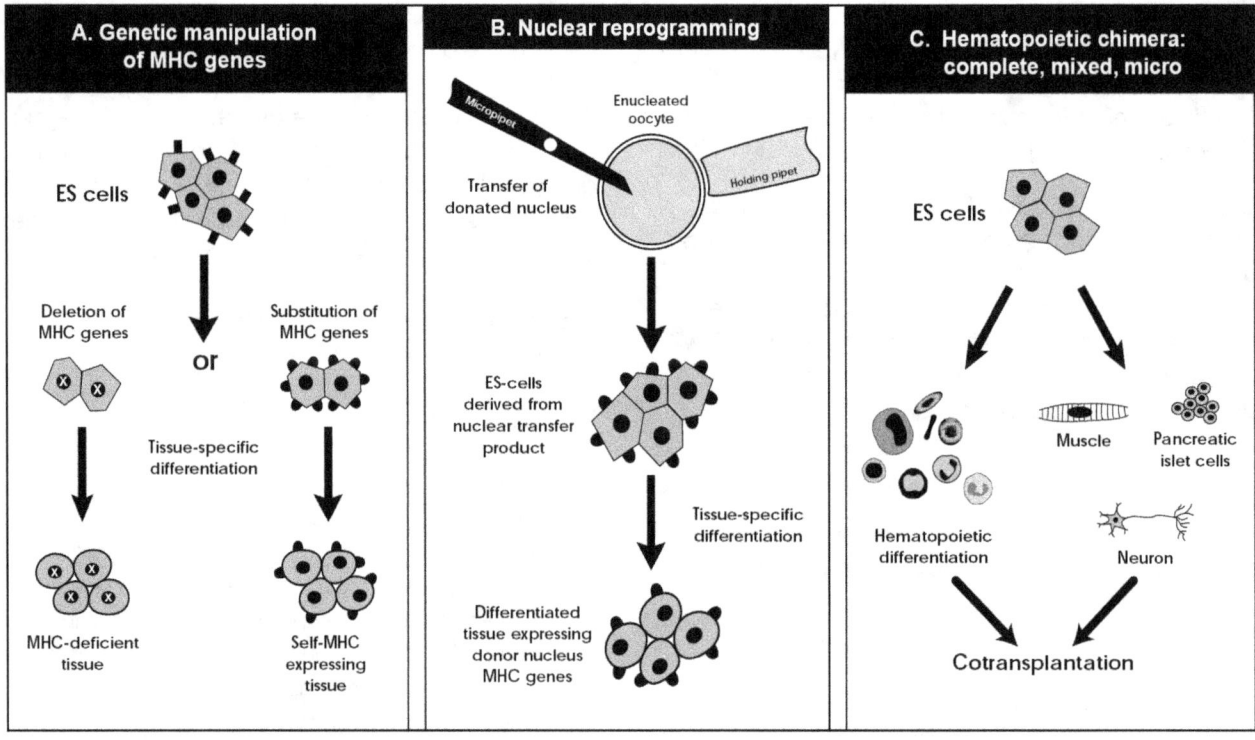

Figure 3.3. Genetic Manipulation of Human Embryonic Stem Cells. (Reproduced with permission from Stem Cells, 2001)

for drug screening, the ES-derived cells may be more likely to mimic the *in vivo* response of the cells/tissues to the drug(s) being tested and so offer safer, and potentially cheaper, models for drug screening.

Human ES cells could be employed to screen potential toxins. The reasons for using human ES cells to screen potential toxins closely resemble those for using human ES-derived cells to test drugs (above). Toxins often have different effects on different animal species, which makes it critical to have the best possible *in vitro* models for evaluating their effects on human cells.

Finally, human ES cells could be used to develop new methods for genetic engineering (see Figure 3.3. Genetic Manipulation of Human Embryonic Stem Cells). Currently, the genetic complement of mouse ES cells *in vitro* can be modified easily by techniques such as homologous recombination. This is a method for replacing or adding genes, which requires that a DNA molecule be artificially introduced into the genome and then expressed. Using this method, genes to direct differentiation to a specific cell type or genes that express a desired protein product might be introduced into the ES cell line. Ultimately, if such techniques could be developed using human ES

cells, it may be possible to devise better methods for gene therapy [35] (see Chapter 10. Assessing Human Stem Cell Safety).

SUMMARY

What Do We Know About Human Embryonic Stem Cells?

Since 1998, research teams have refined the techniques for growing human ES cells *in vitro* [1, 20, 38]. Collectively, the studies indicate that it is now possible to grow human ES cells for more than a year in serum-free medium on feeder layers. The cells have normal karyotype and are pluripotent; they generate teratomas that contain differentiated cell types derived from all three primary germ layers. The long-term cultures of human ES cells have active telomerase and maintain relatively long telomeres, another marker of proliferating cells.

Overall, the pluripotent cells that can be generated *in vitro* from human ES cells and human EG cells are apparently not equivalent in their potential to proliferate or differentiate. (ES cells are derived from the inner cell mass of the preimplantation blastocyst, approximately 5 days post-fertilization, whereas human EG cells are derived from fetal primordial germ cells, 5 to 10 weeks post-fertilization.) ES cells can proliferate for up to 300 population doublings, while cells derived from embryoid bodies that are generated from embryonic germ cells (fetal tissue) double a maximum of 70 to 80 times in vitro.

ES cells appear to have a broader ability to differentiate. Both kinds of cells spontaneously generate neural precursor-type cells (widely regarded as a default pathway for differentiation), and both generate cells that resemble cardiac myocytes [19, 45]. However, human ES and EG cells in vitro will spontaneously generate embryoid bodies that consist of cell types from all three primary germ layers [1, 20, 38, 42].

What Do We Need To Know About Human Embryonic Stem Cells?

Scientists are just beginning to understand the biology of human embryonic stem cells, and many key questions remain unanswered or only partly answered. For example, in order to refine and improve ES cell culture systems, it is important that scientists identify the mechanisms that allow human ES cells in vitro to proliferate without differentiating [29]. Once the mechanisms that regulate human ES proliferation are known, it will likely be possible to apply this knowledge to the long-standing challenge of improving the in vitro self-renewal capabilities of adult stem cells.

It will also be important to determine whether the genetic imprinting status of human ES cells plays any significant role in maintaining the cells, directing their differentiation, or determining their suitability for transplant. One of the effects of growing mouse blastocysts in culture is a change in the methylation of specific genes that control embryonic growth and development [23]. Do similar changes in gene imprinting patterns occur in human ES cells (or blastocysts)? If so, what is their effect on in vitro development and on any differentiated cell types that may be derived from cultured ES cells?

Efforts will need to be made to determine whether cultures of human ES cells that appear to be homogeneous and undifferentiated are, in fact, homogeneous and undifferentiated. Is it possible that human ES cells in vitro cycle in and out of partially differentiated states? And if that occurs, how will it affect attempts to direct their differentiation or maintain the cells in a proliferating state [28]?

Scientists will need to identify which signal transduction pathways must be activated to induce human ES cell differentiation along a particular pathway. This includes understanding ligand-receptor interaction and the intracellular components of the signaling system, as well as identifying the genes that are activated or inactivated during differentiation of specific cell types [29].

Identifying intermediate stages of human ES cell differentiation will also be important. As human ES cells differentiate in vitro, do they form distinct precursor or progenitor cells that can be identified and isolated? If ES cells do form such intermediate cell types, can the latter be maintained and expanded? Would such precursor or progenitor cells be useful for therapeutic transplantation [19]?

Finally, scientists will need to determine what differentiation stages of human ES-derived cells are optimal for other practical applications. For example, what differentiation stages of ES-derived cells would be best for screening drugs or toxins, or for delivering potentially therapeutic drugs?

REFERENCES

1. Amit, M., Carpenter, M.K., Inokuma, M.S., Chiu, C.P., Harris, C.P., Waknitz, M.A., Itskovitz-Eldor, J., and Thomson, J.A. (2000). Clonally derived human embryonic stem cell lines maintain pluripotency and proliferative potential for prolonged periods of culture. Dev. Biol. 227, 271-278.

2. Andrews, P.W., Damjanov, I., Simon, D., Banting, G.S., Carlin, C., Dracopoli, N.C., and Fogh, J. (1984). Pluripotent embryonal carcinoma clones derived from the human teratocarcinoma cell line Tera-2. Differentiation in vivo and in vitro. Lab. Invest. 50, 147-162.

3. Andrews, P.W. (1988). Human teratocarcinomas. Biochim. Biophys. Acta. 948, 17-36.

4. Andrews, P.W. (1998). Teratocarcinomas and human embryology: pluripotent human EC cell lines. Review article. APMIS 106, 158-167.

5. Andrews, P. W., personal communication.

6. Bongso, A., Fong, C.Y., Ng, S.C., and Ratnam, S.S. (1994). Blastocyst transfer in human in vitro; fertilization; the use of embryo co-culture. Cell Biol. Int. 18, 1181-1189.

7. Bongso, A., Fong, C.Y., Ng, S.C., and Ratnam, S. (1994). Isolation and culture of inner cell mass cells from human blastocysts. Hum. Reprod. 9, 2110-2117.

8. Bongso, A., Fong, C.Y., Ng, S.C., and Ratnam, S.S. (1995). Co-culture techniques for blastocyst transfer and embryonic stem cell production. Asst. Reprod. Rev. 5, 106-114.

9. Bongso, A. (1996). Behaviour of human embryos in vitro in the first 14 days: blastocyst transfer and embryonic stem cell production. Clin. Sci. (Colch.) 91, 248-249.

10. Bongso, A., Fong, C.Y., Mathew, J., Ng, L.C., Kumar, J., and Ng, S.C. (1999). The benefits to human IVF by transferring embryos after the in vitro embryonic block: alternatives to day 2 transfers. Asst. Reprod. Rev.

11. Bongso, A. (1999). Handbook on blastocyst culture, (Singapore: Sydney Press Indusprint).

12. Bongso, A., personal communication.

13. Bradley, A., Evans, M., Kaufman, M.H., and Robertson, E. (1984). Formation of germ-line chimaeras from embryo-derived teratocarcinoma cell lines. Nature. 309, 255-256.

14. De Vos, A. and Van Steirteghem, A. (2000). Zona hardening, zona drilling and assisted hatching: new achievements in assisted reproduction. Cells Tissues Organs. 166, 220-227.

15. Evans, M.J. and Kaufman, M.H. (1981). Establishment in culture of pluripotential cells from mouse embryos. Nature. 292, 154-156.

16. Fong, C.Y., Bongso, A., Ng, S.C., Kumar, J., Trounson, A., and Ratnam, S. (1998). Blastocyst transfer after enzymatic treatment of the zona pellucida: improving in-vitro fertilization and understanding implantation. Hum. Reprod. 13, 2926-2932.

17. Friedrich, T.D., Regenass, U., and Stevens, L.C. (1983). Mouse genital ridges in organ culture: the effects of temperature on maturation and experimental induction of teratocarcinogenesis. Differentiation. 24, 60-64.

18. Gardner, D.K. and Schoolcraft, W.B. (1999). Culture and transfer of human blastocysts. Curr. Opin. Obstet. Gynecol. 11, 307-311.

19. Gearhart, J., personal communication.

20. Itskovitz-Eldor, J., Schuldiner, M., Karsenti, D., Eden, A., Yanuka, O., Amit, M., Soreq, H., and Benvenisty, N. (2000). Differentiation of human embryonic stem cells into embryoid bodies comprising the three embryonic germ layers. Mol. Med. 6, 88-95.

21. Jones, G.M., Trounson, A.O., Lolatgis, N., and Wood, C. (1998). Factors affecting the success of human blastocyst development and pregnancy following in vitro fertilization and embryo transfer. Fertil. Steril. 70, 1022-1029.

22. Jones, J.M. and Thomson, J.A. (2000). Human embryonic stem cell technology. Semin. Reprod. Med. 18, 219-223.

23. Khosla, S., Dean, W., Brown, D., Reik, W., and Feil, R. (2001). Culture of preimplantation mouse embryos affects fetal development and the expression of imprinted genes. Biol. Reprod. 64, 918-926.

24. Kleinsmith, L.J. and Pierce Jr, G.B. (1964). Multipotentiality of single embryonal carcinoma cells. Cancer Res. 24, 1544-1551.

25. Martin, G.R. (1980). Teratocarcinomas and mammalian embryogenesis. Science. 209, 768-776.

26. Martin, G.R. (1981). Isolation of a pluripotent cell line from early mouse embryos cultured in medium conditioned by teratocarcinoma stem cells. Proc. Natl. Acad. Sci. U. S. A. 78, 7634-7638.

27. Matsui, Y., Toksoz, D., Nishikawa, S., Nishikawa, S., Williams, D., Zsebo, K., and Hogan, B.L. (1991). Effect of steel factor and leukaemia inhibitory factor on murine primordial germ cells in culture. Nature. 353, 750-752.

28. McKay, R., personal communication.

29. Odorico, J.S., Kaufman, D.S., and Thomson, J.A. (2001). Multilineage Differentiation from Human Embryonic Stem Cell Lines. Stem Cells. 19, 193-204.

30. Okarma, T., personal communication.

31. Pedersen, R.A. (1999). Embryonic stem cells for medicine. Sci. Am. 280, 68-73.

32. Pera, M., personal communication.

33. Pera, M.F., Cooper, S., Mills, J., and Parrington, J.M. (1989). Isolation and characterization of a multipotent clone of human embryonal carcinoma cells. Differentiation. 42, 10-23.

34. Pera, M.F., Reubinoff, B., and Trounson, A. (2000). Human embryonic stem cells. J. Cell Sci. 113 (Pt 1), 5-10.

35. Rathjen, P.D., Lake, J., Whyatt, L.M., Bettess, M.D., and Rathjen, J. (1998). Properties and uses of embryonic stem cells: prospects for application to human biology and gene therapy. Reprod. Fertil. Dev. 10, 31-47.

36. Resnick, J.L., Bixler, L.S., Cheng, L., and Donovan, P.J. (1992). Long-term proliferation of mouse primordial germ cells in culture. Nature. 359, 550-551.

37. Reubinoff BE, Pera, M., Fong, C.Y., and Trounson, A. and Bongso, A. (2000). Research Errata. Nat. Biotechnol. 18, 559.

38. Reubinoff, B.E., Pera, M.F., Fong, C.Y., Trounson, A., and Bongso, A. (2000). Embryonic stem cell lines from human blastocysts: somatic differentiation in vitro. Nat. Biotechnol. 18, 399-404.

39. Sathananthan, A.H. (1997). Ultrastructure of the human egg. Hum. Cell. 10, 21-38.

40. Schuldiner, M., Yanuka, O., Itskovitz-Eldor, J., Melton, D., and Benvenisty, N. (2000). Effects of eight growth factors on the differentiation of cells derived from human embryonic stem cells. Proc. Natl. Acad. Sci. U. S. A. 97, 11307-11312.

41. Shamblott, M.J., Axelman, J., Wang, S., Bugg, E.M., Littlefield, J.W., Donovan, P.J., Blumenthal, P.D., Huggins, G.R., and Gearhart, J.D. (1998). Derivation of pluripotent stem cells from cultured human primordial germ cells. Proc. Natl. Acad. Sci. U. S. A. 95, 13726-13731.

42. Shamblott, M.J., Axelman, J., Littlefield, J.W., Blumenthal, P.D., Huggins, G.R., Cui, Y., Cheng, L., and Gearhart, J.D. (2001). Human embryonic germ cell derivatives express a broad range of develpmentally distinct markers and proliferate extensively *in vitro*. Proc. Natl. Acad. Sci. U. S. A. *98*, 113-118.

43. Smith, A.G. (2001). Origins and properties of mouse embryonic stem cells. Annu. Rev. Cell. Dev. Biol.

44. Thompson, S., Stern, P.L., Webb, M., Walsh, F.S., Engstrom, W., Evans, E.P., Shi, W.K., Hopkins, B., and Graham, C.F. (1984). Cloned human teratoma cells differentiate into neuron-like cells and other cell types in retinoic acid. J. Cell Sci. *72*, 37-64.

45. Thomson, J., personal communication.

46. Thomson, J.A., Kalishman, J., Golos, T.G., Durning, M., Harris, C.P., Becker, R.A., and Hearn, J.P. (1995). Isolation of a primate embryonic stem cell line. Proc. Natl. Acad. Sci. U. S. A. *92*, 7844-7848.

47. Thomson, J.A., Kalishman, J., Golos, T.G., Durning, M., Harris, C.P., and Hearn, J.P. (1996). Pluripotent cell lines derived from common marmoset (Callithrix jacchus) blastocysts. Biol. Reprod. *55*, 254-259.

48. Thomson, J.A., Itskovitz-Eldor, J., Shapiro, S.S., Waknitz, M.A., Swiergiel, J.J., Marshall, V.S., and Jones, J.M. (1998). Embryonic stem cell lines derived from human blastocysts. Science. *282*, 1145-1147.

49. Trounson, A.O., Gardner, D.K., Baker, G., Barnes, F.L., Bongso, A., Bourne, H., Calderon, I., Cohen, J., Dawson, K., Eldar-Geve, T., Gardner, D.K., Graves, G., Healy, D., Lane, M., Leese, H.J., Leeton, J., Levron, J., Liu, D.Y., MacLachlan, V., Munne, S., Oranratnachai, A., Rogers, P., Rombauts, L., Sakkas, D., Sathananthan, A.H., Schimmel, T., Shaw, J., Trounson, A.O., Van Steirteghem, A., Willadsen, S., and Wood, C. (2000b). Handbook of in vitro fertilization, (Boca Raton, London, New York, Washington, D.C.: CRC Press).

50. Trounson, A.O., Anderiesz, C., and Jones, G. (2001). Maturation of human oocytes in vitro and their developmental competence. Reproduction. *121*, 51-75.

51. Xu, C., Inokuma, M.S., Denham, J., Golds, K., Kundu, P., Gold, J.D., and Carpenter, M.K. Keystone symposia. Pluripotent stem cells: biology and applications. Growth of undifferentiated human embryonic stem cells on defined matrices with conditioned medium. Poster abstract. 133.

This page intentionally left blank.

4. THE ADULT STEM CELL

For many years, researchers have been seeking to understand the body's ability to repair and replace the cells and tissues of some organs, but not others. After years of work pursuing the how and why of seemingly indiscriminant cell repair mechanisms, scientists have now focused their attention on adult stem cells. It has long been known that stem cells are capable of renewing themselves and that they can generate multiple cell types. Today, there is new evidence that stem cells are present in far more tissues and organs than once thought and that these cells are capable of developing into more kinds of cells than previously imagined. Efforts are now underway to harness stem cells and to take advantage of this new found capability, with the goal of devising new and more effective treatments for a host of diseases and disabilities. What lies ahead for the use of adult stem cells is unknown, but it is certain that there are many research questions to be answered and that these answers hold great promise for the future.

WHAT IS AN ADULT STEM CELL?

Adult stem cells, like all stem cells, share at least two characteristics. First, they can make identical copies of themselves for long periods of time; this ability to proliferate is referred to as long-term self-renewal. Second, they can give rise to mature cell types that have characteristic morphologies (shapes) and specialized functions. Typically, stem cells generate an intermediate cell type or types before they achieve their fully differentiated state. The intermediate cell is called a precursor or progenitor cell. Progenitor or precursor cells in fetal or adult tissues are partly differentiated cells that divide and give rise to differentiated cells. Such cells are usually regarded as "committed" to differentiating along a particular cellular development pathway, although this

characteristic may not be as definitive as once thought [82] (see Figure 4.1. Distinguishing Features of Progenitor/Precursor Cells and Stem Cells).

Adult stem cells are rare. Their primary functions are to maintain the steady state functioning of a cell—called homeostasis—and, with limitations, to replace cells that die because of injury or disease [44, 58]. For example, only an estimated 1 in 10,000 to 15,000 cells in the bone marrow is a hematopoietic (blood-forming) stem cell (HSC) [105]. Furthermore, adult stem cells are dispersed in tissues throughout the mature animal and behave very differently, depending on their local environment. For example, HSCs are constantly being generated in the bone marrow where they differentiate into mature types of blood cells. Indeed, the primary role of HSCs is to replace blood cells [26] (see Chapter 5. Hemato-poietic Stem Cells). In contrast, stem cells in the small intestine are stationary, and are physically separated from the mature cell types they generate. Gut epi-thelial stem cells (or precursors) occur at the bases of crypts—deep invaginations between the mature, differentiated epithelial cells that line the lumen of the intestine. These epithelial crypt cells divide fairly often, but remain part of the stationary group of cells they generate [93].

Unlike embryonic stem cells, which are defined by their origin (the inner cell mass of the blastocyst), adult stem cells share no such definitive means of characterization. In fact, no one knows the origin of adult stem cells in any mature tissue. Some have proposed that stem cells are somehow set aside during fetal development and restrained from differentiating. Definitions of adult stem cells vary in the scientific literature range from a simple descrip-tion of the cells to a rigorous set of experimental criteria that must be met before characterizing a

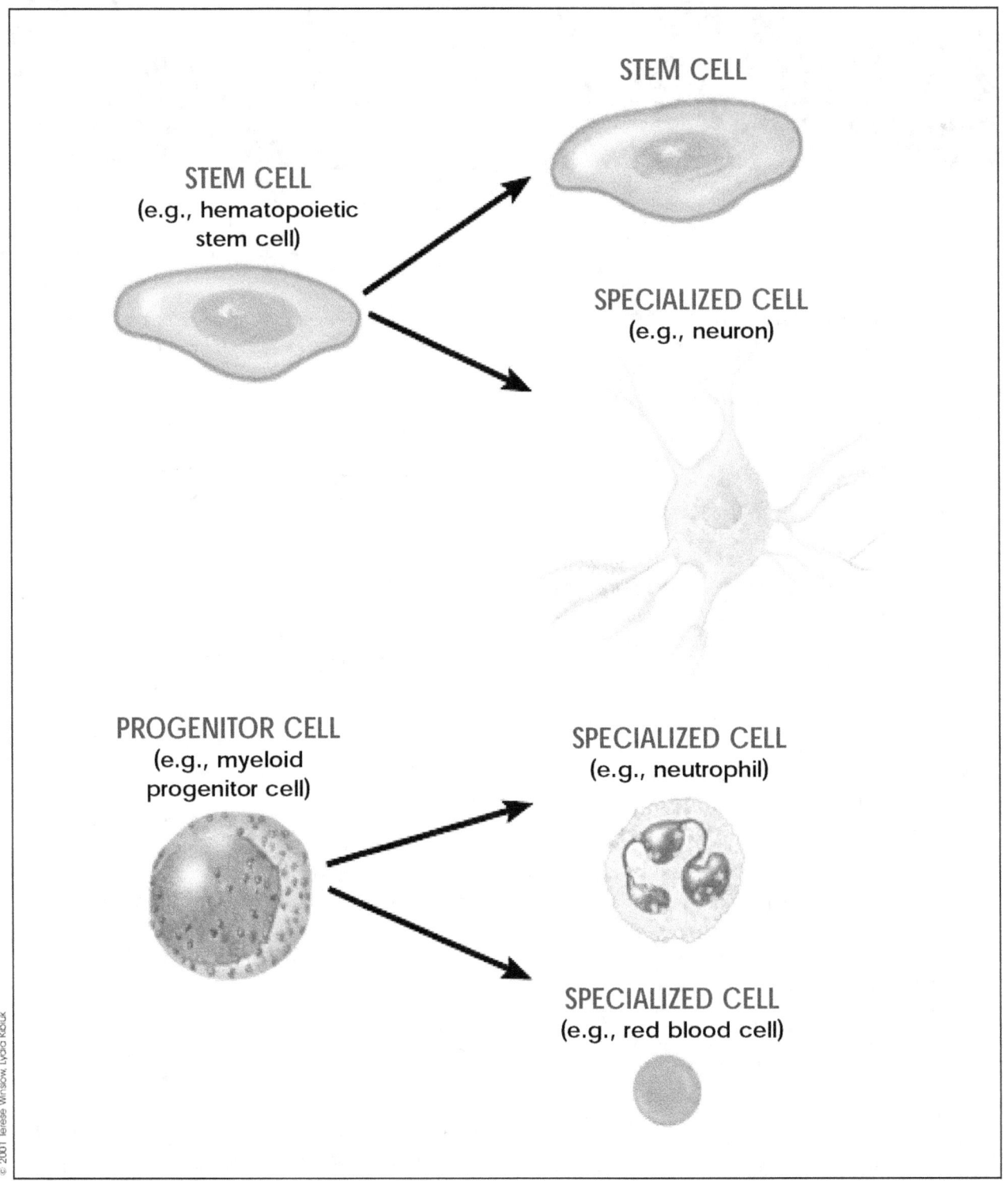

STEM CELL

STEM CELL
(e.g., hematopoietic
stem cell)

SPECIALIZED CELL
(e.g., neuron)

PROGENITOR CELL
(e.g., myeloid
progenitor cell)

SPECIALIZED CELL
(e.g., neutrophil)

SPECIALIZED CELL
(e.g., red blood cell)

© 2001 Terese Winslow, Lydia Kibiuk

Figure 4.1. Distinguishing Features of Progenitor/Precursor Cells and Stem Cells. A stem cell is an unspecialized cell that is capable of replicating or self renewing itself and developing into specialized cells of a variety of cell types. The product of a stem cell undergoing division is at least one additional stem cell that has the same capabilities of the originating cell. Shown here is an example of a hematopoietic stem cell producing a second generation stem cell and a neuron. A progenitor cell (also known as a precursor cell) is unspecialized or has partial characteristics of a specialized cell that is capable of undergoing cell division and yielding two specialized cells. Shown here is an example of a myeloid progenitor/precursor undergoing cell division to yield two specialized cells (a neutrophil and a red blood cell).

particular cell as an adult stem cell. Most of the information about adult stem cells comes from studies of mice. The list of adult tissues reported to contain stem cells is growing and includes bone marrow, peripheral blood, brain, spinal cord, dental pulp, blood vessels, skeletal muscle, epithelia of the skin and digestive system, cornea, retina, liver, and pancreas.

In order to be classified as an adult stem cell, the cell should be capable of self-renewal for the lifetime of the organism. This criterion, although fundamental to the nature of a stem cell, is difficult to prove *in vivo*. It is nearly impossible, in an organism as complex as a human, to design an experiment that will allow the fate of candidate adult stem cells to be identified *in vivo* and tracked over an individual's entire lifetime.

Ideally, adult stem cells should also be clonogenic. In other words, a single adult stem cell should be able to generate a line of genetically identical cells, which then gives rise to all the appropriate, differentiated cell types of the tissue in which it resides. Again, this property is difficult to demonstrate *in vivo*; in practice, scientists show either that a stem cell is clonogenic *in vitro*, or that a purified population of candidate stem cells can repopulate the tissue.

An adult stem cell should also be able to give rise to fully differentiated cells that have mature phenotypes, are fully integrated into the tissue, and are capable of specialized functions that are appropriate for the tissue. The term phenotype refers to all the observable characteristics of a cell (or organism); its shape (morphology); interactions with other cells and the non-cellular environment (also called the extracellular matrix); proteins that appear on the cell surface (surface markers); and the cell's behavior (e.g., secretion, contraction, synaptic transmission).

The majority of researchers who lay claim to having identified adult stem cells rely on two of these characteristics—appropriate cell morphology, and the demonstration that the resulting, differentiated cell types display surface markers that identify them as belonging to the tissue. Some studies demonstrate that the differentiated cells that are derived from adult stem cells are truly functional, and a few studies show that cells are integrated into the differentiated tissue *in vivo* and that they interact appropriately with neighboring cells. At present, there is, however, a paucity of research, with a few notable exceptions, in which researchers were able to conduct studies of

genetically identical (clonal) stem cells. In order to fully characterize the regenerating and self-renewal capabilities of the adult stem cell, and therefore to truly harness its potential, it will be important to demonstrate that a single adult stem cell can, indeed, generate a line of genetically identical cells, which then gives rise to all the appropriate, differentiated cell types of the tissue in which it resides.

EVIDENCE FOR THE PRESENCE OF ADULT STEM CELLS

Adult stem cells have been identified in many animal and human tissues. In general, three methods are used to determine whether candidate adult stem cells give rise to specialized cells. Adult stem cells can be labeled *in vivo* and then they can be tracked. Candidate adult stem cells can also be isolated and labeled and then transplanted back into the organism to determine what becomes of them. Finally, candidate adult stem cells can be isolated, grown *in vitro* and manipulated, by adding growth factors or introducing genes that help determine what differentiated cells types they will yield. For example, currently, scientists believe that stem cells in the fetal and adult brain divide and give rise to more stem cells or to several types of precursor cells, which give rise to nerve cells (neurons), of which there are many types.

It is often difficult—if not impossible—to distinguish adult, tissue-specific stem cells from progenitor cells, which are found in fetal or adult tissues and are partly differentiated cells that divide and give rise to differentiated cells. These are cells found in many organs that are generally thought to be present to replace cells and maintain the integrity of the tissue. Progenitor cells give rise to certain types of cells—such as the blood cells known as T lymphocytes, B lymphocytes, and natural killer cells—but are not thought to be capable of developing into all the cell types of a tissue and as such are not truly stem cells. The current wave of excitement over the existence of stem cells in many adult tissues is perhaps fueling claims that progenitor or precursor cells in those tissues are instead stem cells. Thus, there are reports of endothelial progenitor cells, skeletal muscle stem cells, epithelial precursors in the skin and digestive system, as well as some reports of progenitors or stem cells in the pancreas and liver. A detailed summary of some of the evidence for the existence of stem cells in various tissues and organs is presented later in the chapter.

ADULT STEM CELL PLASTICITY

It was not until recently that anyone seriously considered the possibility that stem cells in adult tissues could generate the specialized cell types of another type of tissue from which they normally reside—either a tissue derived from the same embryonic germ layer or from a different germ layer (see Table 1.1. Embryonic Germ Layers From Which Differentiated Tissues Develop). For example, studies have shown that blood stem cells (derived from mesoderm) may be able to generate both skeletal muscle (also derived from mesoderm) and neurons (derived from ectoderm). That realization has been triggered by a flurry of papers reporting that stem cells derived from one adult tissue can change their appearance and assume characteristics that resemble those of differentiated cells from other tissues.

The term plasticity, as used in this report, means that a stem cell from one adult tissue can generate the differentiated cell types of another tissue. At this time, there is no formally accepted name for this phenomenon in the scientific literature. It is variously referred to as "plasticity" [15, 52], "unorthodox differentiation" [10] or "transdifferentiation" [7, 54].

Approaches for Demonstrating Adult Stem Cell Plasticity

To be able to claim that adult stem cells demonstrate plasticity, it is first important to show that a cell population exists in the starting tissue that has the identifying features of stem cells. Then, it is necessary to show that the adult stem cells give rise to cell types that normally occur in a different tissue. Neither of these criteria is easily met. Simply proving the existence of an adult stem cell population in a differentiated tissue is a laborious process. It requires that the candidate stem cells are shown to be self-renewing, and that they can give rise to the differentiated cell types that are characteristic of that tissue.

To show that the adult stem cells can generate other cell types requires them to be tracked in their new environment, whether it is in vitro or in vivo. In general, this has been accomplished by obtaining the stem cells from a mouse that has been genetically engineered to express a molecular tag in all its cells. It is then necessary to show that the labeled adult stem

cells have adopted key structural and biochemical characteristics of the new tissue they are claimed to have generated. Ultimately—and most importantly—it is necessary to demonstrate that the cells can integrate into their new tissue environment, survive in the tissue, and function like the mature cells of the tissue.

In the experiments reported to date, adult stem cells may assume the characteristics of cells that have developed from the same primary germ layer or a different germ layer (see Figure 4.2. Preliminary Evidence of Plasticity Among Nonhuman Adult Stem Cells). For example, many plasticity experiments involve stem cells derived from bone marrow, which is a mesodermal derivative. The bone marrow stem cells may then differentiate into another mesodermally derived tissue such as skeletal muscle [28, 43], cardiac muscle [51, 71] or liver [4, 54, 97].

Alternatively, adult stem cells may differentiate into a tissue that—during normal embryonic development—would arise from a different germ layer. For example, bone marrow-derived cells may differentiate into neural tissue, which is derived from embryonic ectoderm [15, 65]. And—reciprocally—neural stem cell lines cultured from adult brain tissue may differentiate to form hematopoietic cells [13], or even give rise to many different cell types in a chimeric embryo [17]. In both cases cited above, the cells would be deemed to show plasticity, but in the case of bone marrow stem cells generating brain cells, the finding is less predictable.

In order to study plasticity within and across germ layer lines, the researcher must be sure that he/she is using only one kind of adult stem cell. The vast majority of experiments on plasticity have been conducted with adult stem cells derived either from the bone marrow or the brain. The bone marrow-derived cells are sometimes sorted—using a panel of surface markers—into populations of hematopoietic stem cells or bone marrow stromal cells [46, 54, 71]. The HSCs may be highly purified or partially purified, depending on the conditions used. Another way to separate population of bone marrow cells is by fractionation to yield cells that adhere to a growth substrate (stromal cells) or do not adhere (hematopoietic cells) [28].

To study plasticity of stem cells derived from the brain, the researcher must overcome several problems. Stem cells from the central nervous system (CNS),

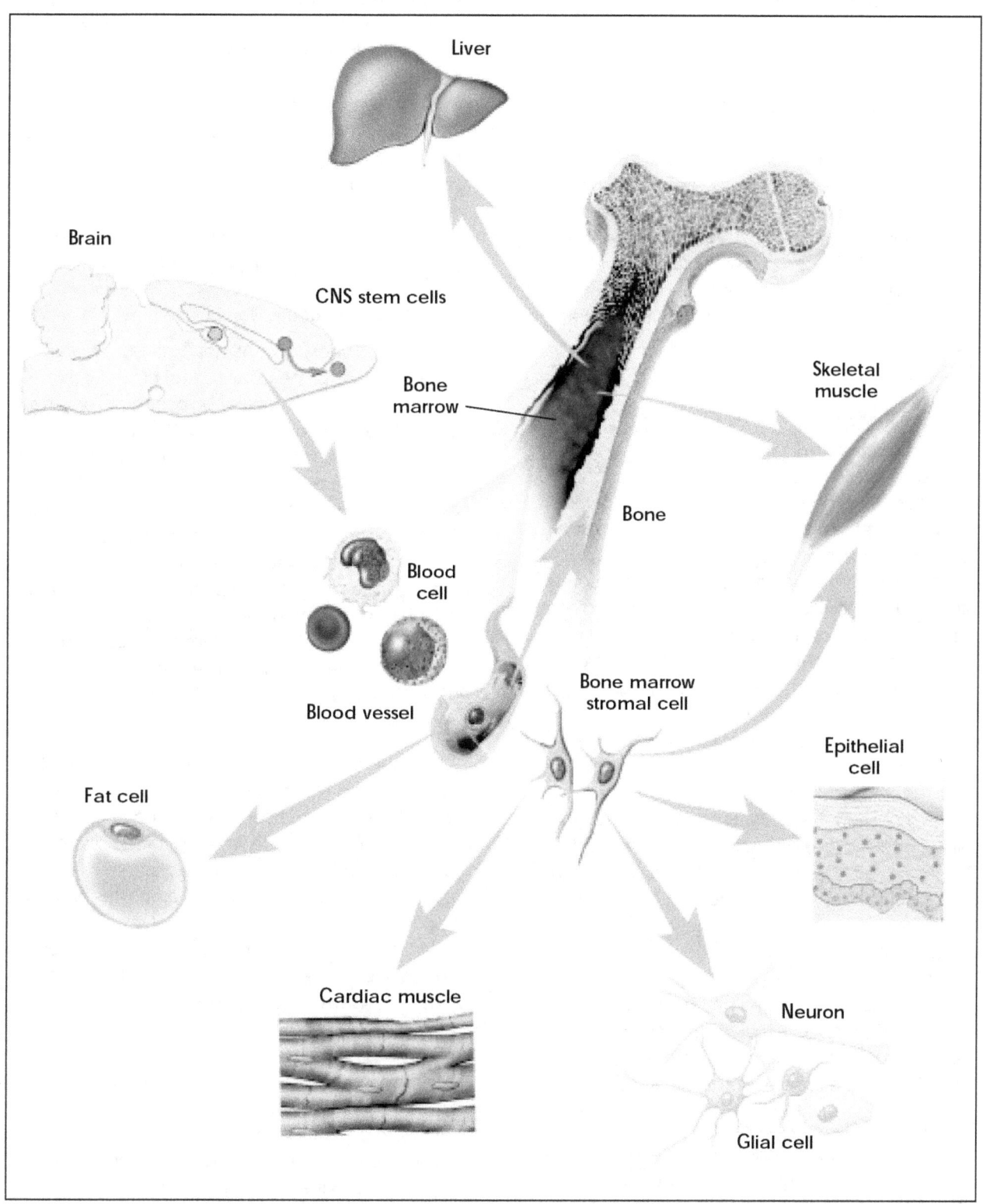

Figure 4.2. Preliminary Evidence of Plasticity Among Nonhuman Adult Stem Cells.

© 2001 Terese Winslow, Lydia Kibiuk, Caitlin Duckwall

unlike bone marrow cells, do not occur in a single, accessible location. Instead, they are scattered in three places, at least in rodent brain—the tissue around the lateral ventricles in the forebrain, a migratory pathway for the cells that leads from the ventricles to the olfactory bulbs, and the hippocampus. Many of the experiments with CNS stem cells involve the formation of neurospheres, round aggregates of cells that are sometimes clonally derived. But it is not possible to observe cells in the center of a neurosphere, so to study plasticity *in vitro*, the cells are usually dissociated and plated in monolayers. To study plasticity *in vivo*, the cells may be dissociated before injection into the circulatory system of the recipient animal [13], or injected as neurospheres [17].

What is the Evidence for Plasticity?

The differentiated cell types that result from plasticity are usually reported to have the morphological characteristics of the differentiated cells and to display their characteristic surface markers. In reports that transplanted adult stem cells show plasticity *in vivo*, the stem cells typically are shown to have integrated into a mature host tissue and assumed at least some of its characteristics [15, 28, 51, 65, 71]. Many plasticity experiments involve injury to a particular tissue, which is intended to model a particular human disease or injury [13, 54, 71]. However, there is limited evidence to date that such adult stem cells can generate mature, fully functional cells or that the cells have restored lost function *in vivo* [54]. Most of the studies that show the plasticity of adult stem cells involve cells that are derived from the bone marrow [15, 28, 54, 65, 77] or brain [13, 17]. To date, adult stem cells are best characterized in these two tissues, which may account for the greater number of plasticity studies based on bone marrow and brain. Collectively, studies on plasticity suggest that stem cell populations in adult mammals are not fixed entities, and that after exposure to a new environment, they may be able to populate other tissues and possibly differentiate into other cell types.

It is not yet possible to say whether plasticity occurs normally *in vivo*. Some scientists think it may [14, 64], but as yet there is no evidence to prove it. Also, it is not yet clear to what extent plasticity can occur in experimental settings, and how—or whether—the phenomenon can be harnessed to generate tissues that may be useful for therapeutic transplantation. If the phenomenon of plasticity is to be used as a basis for generating tissue for transplantation, the techniques for doing it will need to be reproducible and reliable (see Chapter 10. Assessing Human Stem Cell Safety). In some cases, debate continues about observations that adult stem cells yield cells of tissue types different than those from which they were obtained [7, 68].

EXPERIMENTAL EVIDENCE OF ADULT STEM CELLS AND PLASTICITY

Adult Stem Cells of the Nervous System

More than 30 years ago, Altman and Das showed that two regions of the postnatal rat brain, the hippocampus and the olfactory bulb, contain dividing cells that become neurons [5, 6]. Despite these reports, the prevailing view at the time was that nerve cells in the adult brain do not divide. In fact, the notion that stem cells in the adult brain can generate its three major cell types—astrocytes and oligodendrocytes, as well as neurons—was not accepted until far more recently. Within the past five years, a series of studies has shown that stem cells occur in the adult mammalian brain and that these cells can generate its three major cell lineages [35, 48, 63, 66, 90, 96, 104] (see Chapter 8. Rebuilding the Nervous System with Stem Cells).

Today, scientists believe that stem cells in the fetal and adult brain divide and give rise to more stem cells or to several types of precursor cells. Neuronal precursors (also called neuroblasts) divide and give rise to nerve cells (neurons), of which there are many types. Glial precursors give rise to astrocytes or oligodendrocytes. Astrocytes are a kind of glial cell, which lend both mechanical and metabolic support for neurons; they make up 70 to 80 percent of the cells of the adult brain. Oligodendrocytes make myelin, the fatty material that ensheathes nerve cell axons and speeds nerve transmission. Under normal, *in vivo* conditions, neuronal precursors do not give rise to glial cells, and glial precursors do not give rise to neurons. In contrast, a fetal or adult CNS (central nervous system—the brain and spinal cord) stem cell may give rise to neurons, astrocytes, or oligodendrocytes, depending on the signals it receives and its three-dimensional environment within the brain tissue.

There is now widespread consensus that the adult mammalian brain does contain stem cells. However, there is no consensus about how many populations of CNS stem cells exist, how they may be related, and how they function in vivo. Because there are no markers currently available to identify the cells in vivo, the only method for testing whether a given population of CNS cells contains stem cells is to isolate the cells and manipulate them in vitro, a process that may change their intrinsic properties [67].

Despite these barriers, three groups of CNS stem cells have been reported to date. All occur in the adult rodent brain and preliminary evidence indicates they also occur in the adult human brain. One group occupies the brain tissue next to the ventricles, regions known as the ventricular zone and the subventricular zone (see discussion below). The ventricles are spaces in the brain filled with cerebrospinal fluid. During fetal development, the tissue adjacent to the ventricles is a prominent region of actively dividing cells. By adulthood, however, this tissue is much smaller, although it still appears to contain stem cells [70].

A second group of adult CNS stem cells, described in mice but not in humans, occurs in a streak of tissue that connects the lateral ventricle and the olfactory bulb, which receives odor signals from the nose. In rodents, olfactory bulb neurons are constantly being replenished via this pathway [59, 61]. A third possible location for stem cells in adult mouse and human brain occurs in the hippocampus, a part of the brain thought to play a role in the formation of certain kinds of memory [27, 34].

Central Nervous System Stem Cells in the Subventricular Zone. CNS stem cells found in the forebrain that surrounds the lateral ventricles are heterogeneous and can be distinguished morphologically. Ependymal cells, which are ciliated, line the ventricles. Adjacent to the ependymal cell layer, in a region sometimes designated as the subependymal or subventricular zone, is a mixed cell population that consists of neuroblasts (immature neurons) that migrate to the olfactory bulb, precursor cells, and astrocytes. Some of the cells divide rapidly, while others divide slowly. The astrocyte-like cells can be identified because they contain glial fibrillary acidic protein (GFAP), whereas the ependymal cells stain positive for nestin, which is regarded as a marker of neural stem cells. Which of these cells best qualifies as a CNS stem cell is a matter of debate [76].

A recent report indicates that the astrocytes that occur in the subventricular zone of the rodent brain act as neural stem cells. The cells with astrocyte markers appear to generate neurons in vivo, as identified by their expression of specific neuronal markers. The in vitro assay to demonstrate that these astrocytes are, in fact, stem cells involves their ability to form neurospheres—groupings of undifferentiated cells that can be dissociated and coaxed to differentiate into neurons or glial cells [25]. Traditionally, these astrocytes have been regarded as differentiated cells, not as stem cells and so their designation as stem cells is not universally accepted.

A series of similar in vitro studies based on the formation of neurospheres was used to identify the subependymal zone as a source of adult rodent CNS stem cells. In these experiments, single, candidate stem cells derived from the subependymal zone are induced to give rise to neurospheres in the presence of mitogens—either epidermal growth factor (EGF) or fibroblast growth factor-2 (FGF-2). The neurospheres are dissociated and passaged. As long as a mitogen is present in the culture medium, the cells continue forming neurospheres without differentiating. Some populations of CNS cells are more responsive to EGF, others to FGF [100]. To induce differentiation into neurons or glia, cells are dissociated from the neurospheres and grown on an adherent surface in serum-free medium that contains specific growth factors. Collectively, the studies demonstrate that a population of cells derived from the adult rodent brain can self-renew and differentiate to yield the three major cell types of the CNS cells [41, 69, 74, 102].

Central Nervous System Stem Cells in the Ventricular Zone. Another group of potential CNS stem cells in the adult rodent brain may consist of the ependymal cells themselves [47]. Ependymal cells, which are ciliated, line the lateral ventricles. They have been described as non-dividing cells [24] that function as part of the blood-brain barrier [22]. The suggestion that ependymal cells from the ventricular zone of the adult rodent CNS may be stem cells is therefore unexpected. However, in a recent study, in which two molecular tags—the fluorescent marker DiI, and an adenovirus vector carrying lacZ tags—were used to label the ependymal cells that line the entire CNS ventricular system of adult rats, it was shown that these cells could, indeed, act as stem cells. A few days after labeling, fluorescent or *lacZ*+ cells were observed in the rostral migratory stream (which leads from the lateral ventricle to the olfactory bulb), and then in the olfactory bulb itself. The labeled cells in the olfactory bulb also stained for the neuronal markers βIII tubulin and Map2, which indicated that ependymal cells from the ventricular zone of the adult rat brain had migrated along the rostral migratory stream to generate olfactory bulb neurons *in vivo* [47].

To show that Dil+ cells were neural stem cells and could generate astrocytes and oligodendrocytes as well as neurons, a neurosphere assay was performed *in vitro*. Dil-labeled cells were dissociated from the ventricular system and cultured in the presence of mitogen to generate neurospheres. Most of the neurospheres were Dil+; they could self-renew and generate neurons, astrocytes, and oligodendrocytes when induced to differentiate. Single, Dil+ ependymal cells isolated from the ventricular zone could also generate self-renewing neurospheres and differentiate into neurons and glia.

To show that ependymal cells can also divide *in vivo*, bromodeoxyuridine (BrdU) was administered in the drinking water to rats for a 2- to 6-week period. Bromodeoxyuridine (BrdU) is a DNA precursor that is only incorporated into dividing cells. Through a series of experiments, it was shown that ependymal cells divide slowly *in vivo* and give rise to a population of progenitor cells in the subventricular zone [47]. A different pattern of scattered BrdU-labeled cells was observed in the spinal cord, which suggested that ependymal cells along the central canal of the cord occasionally divide and give rise to nearby ependymal cells, but do not migrate away from the canal.

Collectively, the data suggest that CNS ependymal cells in adult rodents can function as stem cells. The cells can self-renew, and most proliferate via asymmetrical division. Many of the CNS ependymal cells are not actively dividing (quiescent), but they can be stimulated to do so *in vitro* (with mitogens) or *in vivo* (in response to injury). After injury, the ependymal cells in the spinal cord only give rise to astrocytes, not to neurons. How and whether ependymal cells from the ventricular zone are related to other candidate populations of CNS stem cells, such as those identified in the hippocampus [34], is not known.

Are ventricular and subventricular zone CNS stem cells the same population? These studies and other leave open the question of whether cells that directly line the ventricles—those in the ventricular zone—or cells that are at least a layer removed from this zone—in the subventricular zone are the same population of CNS stem cells. A new study, based on the finding that they express different genes, confirms earlier reports that the ventricular and subventricular zone cell populations are distinct. The new research utilizes a technique called representational difference analysis, together with cDNA microarray analysis, to monitor the patterns of gene expression in the complex tissue of the developing and postnatal mouse brain. The study revealed the expression of a panel of genes known to be important in CNS development, such as *L3-PSP* (which encodes a phosphoserine phosphatase important in cell signaling), *cyclin D2* (a cell cycle gene), and *ERCC-1* (which is important in DNA excision repair). All of these genes in the recent study were expressed in cultured neurospheres, as well as the ventricular zone, the subventricular zone, and a brain area outside those germinal zones. This analysis also revealed the expression of novel genes such as *A16F10*, which is similar to a gene in an embryonic cancer cell line. A16F10 was expressed in neurospheres and at high levels in the subventricular zone, but not significantly in the ventricular zone. Interestingly, several of the genes identified in cultured neurospheres were also expressed in hematopoietic cells, suggesting that neural stem cells and blood-forming cells may share aspects of their genetic programs or signaling systems [38]. This finding may help explain recent reports that CNS stem cells derived from mouse brain can give rise to hematopoietic cells after injection into irradiated mice [13].

Central Nervous System Stem Cells in the Hippocampus. The hippocampus is one of the oldest parts of the cerebral cortex, in evolutionary terms, and is thought to play an important role in certain forms of memory. The region of the hippocampus in which stem cells apparently exist in mouse and human brains is the subgranular zone of the dentate gyrus. In mice, when BrdU is used to label dividing cells in this region, about 50% of the labeled cells differentiate into cells that appear to be dentate gyrus granule neurons, and 15% become glial cells. The rest of the BrdU-labeled cells do not have a recognizable phenotype [90]. Interestingly, many, if not all the BrdU-labeled cells in the adult rodent hippocampus occur next to blood vessels [33].

In the human dentate gyrus, some BrdU-labeled cells express NeuN, neuron-specific enolase, or calbindin, all of which are neuronal markers. The labeled neuron-like cells resemble dentate gyrus granule cells, in terms of their morphology (as they did in mice). Other BrdU-labeled cells express glial fibrillary acidic protein (GFAP) an astrocyte marker. The study involved autopsy material, obtained with family consent, from five cancer patients who had been injected with BrdU dissolved in saline prior to their death for diagnostic purposes. The patients ranged in age from 57 to 72 years. The greatest number of BrdU-labeled cells were identified in the oldest patient, suggesting that new neuron formation in the hippocampus can continue late in life [27].

Fetal Central Nervous System Stem Cells. Not surprisingly, fetal stem cells are numerous in fetal tissues, where they are assumed to play an important role in the expansion and differentiation of all tissues of the developing organism. Depending on the developmental stage of an animal, fetal stem cells and precursor cells—which arise from stem cells—may make up the bulk of a tissue. This is certainly true in the brain [48], although it has not been demonstrated experimentally in many tissues.

It may seem obvious that the fetal brain contains stem cells that can generate all the types of neurons in the brain as well as astrocytes and oligodendrocytes, but it was not until fairly recently that the concept was proven experimentally. There has been a long-standing question as to whether or not the same cell type gives rise to both neurons and glia. In studies of the developing rodent brain, it has now been shown that all the major cell types in the fetal brain arise from a common population of progenitor cells [20, 34, 48, 80, 108].

Neural stem cells in the mammalian fetal brain are concentrated in seven major areas: olfactory bulb, ependymal (ventricular) zone of the lateral ventricles (which lie in the forebrain), subventricular zone (next to the ependymal zone), hippocampus, spinal cord, cerebellum (part of the hindbrain), and the cerebral cortex. Their number and pattern of development

vary in different species. These cells appear to represent different stem cell populations, rather than a single population of stem cells that is dispersed in multiple sites. The normal development of the brain depends not only on the proliferation and differentiation of these fetal stem cells, but also on a genetically programmed process of selective cell death called apoptosis [76].

Little is known about stem cells in the human fetal brain. In one study, however, investigators derived clonal cell lines from CNS stem cells isolated from the diencephalon and cortex of human fetuses, 10.5 weeks post-conception [103]. The study is unusual, not only because it involves human CNS stem cells obtained from fetal tissue, but also because the cells were used to generate clonal cell lines of CNS stem cells that generated neurons, astrocytes, and oligodendrocytes, as determined on the basis of expressed markers. In a few experiments described as "preliminary," the human CNS stem cells were injected into the brains of immunosuppressed rats where they apparently differentiated into neuron-like cells or glial cells.

In a 1999 study, a serum-free growth medium that included EGF and FGF2 was devised to grow the human fetal CNS stem cells. Although most of the cells died, occasionally, single CNS stem cells survived, divided, and ultimately formed neurospheres after one to two weeks in culture. The neurospheres could be dissociated and individual cells replated. The cells resumed proliferation and formed new neurospheres, thus establishing an in vitro system that (like the system established for mouse CNS neurospheres) could be maintained up to 2 years. Depending on the culture conditions, the cells in the neurospheres could be maintained in an undifferentiated dividing state (in the presence of mitogen), or dissociated and induced to differentiate (after the removal of mitogen and the addition of specific growth factors to the culture medium). The differentiated cells consisted mostly of astrocytes (75%), some neurons (13%) and rare oligodendrocytes (1.2%). The neurons generated under these conditions expressed markers indicating they were GABAergic, [the major type of inhibitory neuron in the mammalian CNS responsive to the amino acid neurotransmitter, gamma-aminobutyric acid (GABA)]. However, catecholamine-like cells that express tyrosine hydroxylase (TH, a critical enzyme in the dopamine-synthesis pathway) could be generated, if the culture conditions were altered to include different medium conditioned by a rat glioma line (BB49). Thus, the report indicates that human CNS stem cells obtained from early fetuses can be maintained *in vitro* for a long time without differentiating, induced to differentiate into the three major lineages of the CNS (and possibly two kinds of neurons, GABAergic and TH-positive), and engraft (in rats) *in vivo* [103].

Central Nervous System Neural Crest Stem Cells.
Neural crest cells differ markedly from fetal or adult neural stem cells. During fetal development, neural crest cells migrate from the sides of the neural tube as it closes. The cells differentiate into a range of tissues, not all of which are part of the nervous system [56, 57, 91]. Neural crest cells form the sympathetic and parasympathetic components of the peripheral nervous system (PNS), including the network of nerves that innervate the heart and the gut, all the sensory ganglia (groups of neurons that occur in pairs along the dorsal surface of the spinal cord), and Schwann cells, which (like oligodendrocytes in the CNS) make myelin in the PNS. The non-neural tissues that arise from the neural crest are diverse. They populate certain hormone-secreting glands—including the adrenal medulla and Type I cells in the carotid body—pigment cells of the skin (melanocytes), cartilage and bone in the face and skull, and connective tissue in many parts of the body [76].

Thus, neural crest cells migrate far more extensively than other fetal neural stem cells during development, form mesenchymal tissues, most of which develop from embryonic mesoderm as well as the components of the CNS and PNS which arises from embryonic ectoderm. This close link, in neural crest development, between ectodermally derived tissues and mesodermally derived tissues accounts in part for the interest in neural crest cells as a kind of stem cell. In fact, neural crest cells meet several criteria of stem cells. They can self-renew (at least in the fetus) and can differentiate into multiple cells types, which include cells derived from two of the three embryonic germ layers [76].

Recent studies indicate that neural crest cells persist late into gestation and can be isolated from E14.5 rat sciatic nerve, a peripheral nerve in the hindlimb. The cells incorporate BrdU, indicating that they are dividing *in vivo*. When transplanted into chick embryos, the rat neural crest cells develop into neurons and glia, an indication of their stem cell-like properties [67]. However, the ability of rat E14.5 neural crest cells taken from sciatic nerve to generate nerve and glial cells in chick is more limited than neural crest cells derived from younger, E10.5 rat embryos. At the earlier stage of development, the neural tube has formed, but neural crest cells have not yet migrated to their final destinations. Neural crest cells from early developmental stages are more sensitive to bone morphogenetic protein 2 (BMP2) signaling, which may help explain their greater differentiation potential [106].

Stem Cells in the Bone Marrow and Blood
The notion that the bone marrow contains stem cells is not new. One population of bone marrow cells, the hematopoietic stem cells (HSCs), is responsible for forming all of the types of blood cells in the body. HSCs were recognized as a stem cells more than 40 years ago [9, 99]. Bone marrow stromal cells—a mixed cell population that generates bone, cartilage, fat, fibrous connective tissue, and the reticular network that supports blood cell formation—were described shortly after the discovery of HSCs [30, 32, 73]. The mesenchymal stem cells of the bone marrow also give rise to these tissues, and may constitute the same population of cells as the bone marrow stromal cells [78]. Recently, a population of progenitor cells that differentiates into endothelial cells, a type of cell that lines the blood vessels, was isolated from circulating blood [8] and identified as originating in bone marrow [89]. Whether these endothelial progenitor cells, which resemble the angioblasts that give rise to blood vessels during embryonic development, represent a bona fide population of adult bone marrow stem cells remains uncertain. Thus, the bone marrow appears to contain three stem cell populations—hematopoietic stem cells, stromal cells, and (possibly) endothelial progenitor cells (see Figure 4.3. Hematopoietic and Stromal Stem Cell Differentiation).

Two more apparent stem cell types have been reported in circulating blood, but have not been shown to originate from the bone marrow. One population, called pericytes, may be closely related to bone marrow stromal cells, although their origin remains elusive [12]. The second population of blood-born stem cells, which occur in four species of

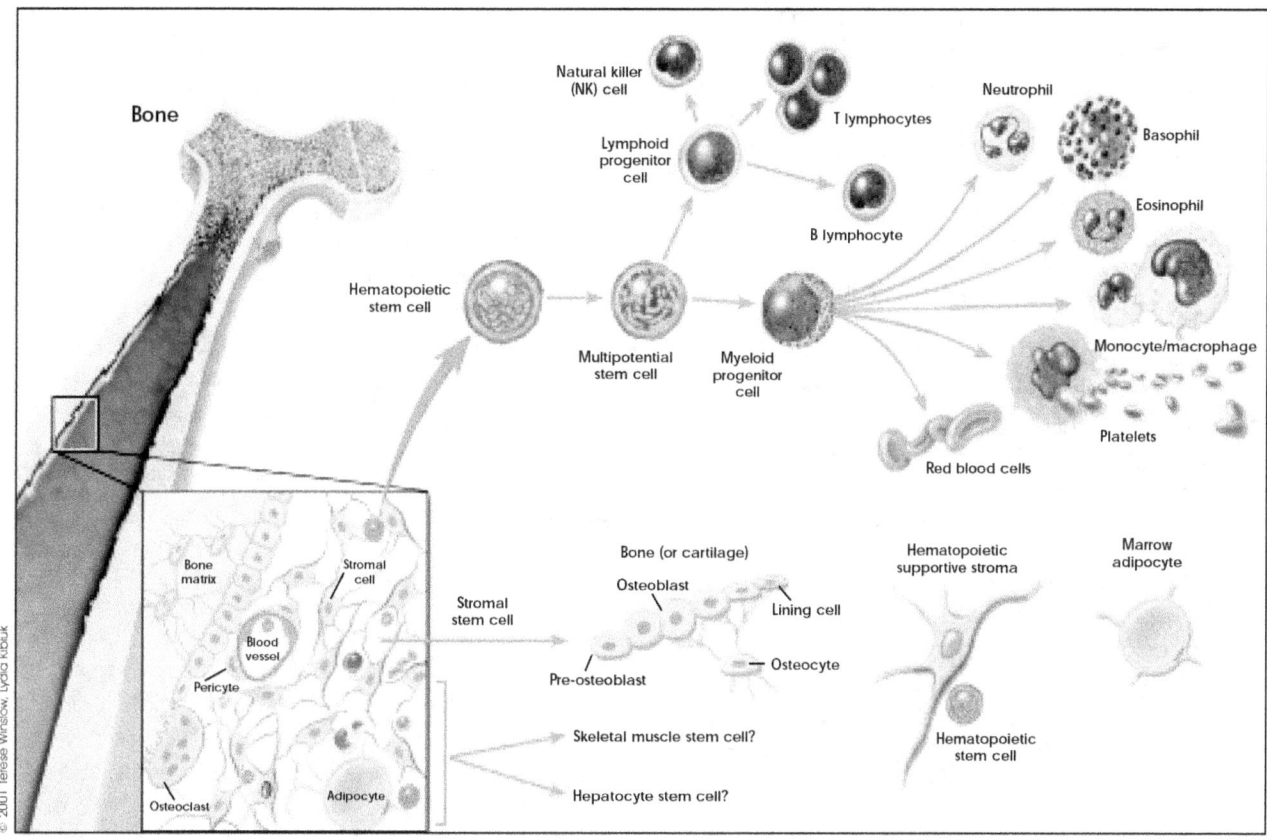

Figure 4.3. Hematopoietic and Stromal Stem Cell Differentiation.

animals tested—guinea pigs, mice, rabbits, and humans—resemble stromal cells in that they can generate bone and fat [53].

Hematopoietic Stem Cells. Of all the cell types in the body, those that survive for the shortest period of time are blood cells and certain kinds of epithelial cells. For example, red blood cells (erythrocytes), which lack a nucleus, live for approximately 120 days in the bloodstream. The life of an animal literally depends on the ability of these and other blood cells to be replenished continuously. This replenishment process occurs largely in the bone marrow, where HSCs reside, divide, and differentiate into all the blood cell types. Both HSCs and differentiated blood cells cycle from the bone marrow to the blood and back again, under the influence of a barrage of secreted factors that regulate cell proliferation, differentiation, and migration (see Chapter 5. Hematopoietic Stem Cells).

HSCs can reconstitute the hematopoietic system of mice that have been subjected to lethal doses of radiation to destroy their own hematopoietic systems. This test, the rescue of lethally irradiated mice, has become a standard by which other candidate stem cells are measured because it shows, without question, that HSCs can regenerate an entire tissue system—in this case, the blood [9, 99]. HSCs were first proven to be blood-forming stem cells in a series of experiments in mice; similar blood-forming stem cells occur in humans. HSCs are defined by their ability to self-renew and to give rise to all the kinds of blood cells in the body. This means that a single HSC is capable of regenerating the entire hematopoietic system, although this has been demonstrated only a few times in mice [72].

Over the years, many combinations of surface markers have been used to identify, isolate, and purify HSCs derived from bone marrow and blood. Undifferentiated HSCs and hematopoietic progenitor cells express c-kit, CD34, and H-2K. These cells usually lack the lineage marker Lin, or express it at very low levels (Lin$^{-/low}$). And for transplant purposes, cells that are CD34$^+$ Thy1$^+$ Lin$^-$ are most likely to contain stem cells and result in engraftment.

Two kinds of HSCs have been defined. Long-term HSCs proliferate for the lifetime of an animal. In young adult mice, an estimated 8 to 10 % of long-term HSCs enter the cell cycle and divide each day. Short-term HSCs proliferate for a limited time, possibly a few months. Long-term HSCs have high levels of telomerase activity. Telomerase is an enzyme that helps maintain the length of the ends of chromosomes, called telomeres, by adding on nucleotides. Active telomerase is a characteristic of undifferentiated, dividing cells and cancer cells. Differentiated, human somatic cells do not show telomerase activity. In adult humans, HSCs occur in the bone marrow, blood, liver, and spleen, but are extremely rare in any of these tissues. In mice, only 1 in 10,000 to 15,000 bone marrow cells is a long-term HSC [105].

Short-term HSCs differentiate into lymphoid and myeloid precursors, the two classes of precursors for the two major lineages of blood cells. Lymphoid precursors differentiate into T cells, B cells, and natural killer cells. The mechanisms and pathways that lead to their differentiation are still being investigated [1, 2]. Myeloid precursors differentiate into monocytes and macrophages, neutrophils, eosinophils, basophils, megakaryocytes, and erythrocytes [3]. *In vivo*, bone marrow HSCs differentiate into mature, specialized blood cells that cycle constantly from the bone marrow to the blood, and back to the bone marrow [26]. A recent study showed that short-term HSCs are a heterogeneous population that differ significantly in terms of their ability to self-renew and repopulate the hematopoietic system [42].

Attempts to induce HSC to proliferate *in vitro*—on many substrates, including those intended to mimic conditions in the stroma—have frustrated scientists for many years. Although HSCs proliferate readily *in vivo*, they usually differentiate or die *in vitro* [26]. Thus, much of the research on HSCs has been focused on understanding the factors, cell-cell interactions, and cell-matrix interactions that control their proliferation and differentiation *in vivo*, with the hope that similar conditions could be replicated *in vitro*. Many of the soluble factors that regulate HSC differentiation *in vivo* are cytokines, which are made by different cell types and are then concentrated in the bone marrow by the extracellular matrix of stromal cells—the sites of blood formation [45, 107]. Two of the most-studied cytokines are granulocyte-macrophage colony-stimulating factor (GM-CSF) and interleukin-3 (IL-3) [40, 81].

Also important to HSC proliferation and differentiation are interactions of the cells with adhesion molecules in the extracellular matrix of the bone marrow stroma [83, 101, 110].

Bone Marrow Stromal Cells. Bone marrow (BM) stromal cells have long been recognized for playing an important role in the differentiation of mature blood cells from HSCs (see Figure 4.3. Hematopoietic and Stromal Stem Cell Differentiation). But stromal cells also have other important functions [30, 31]. In addition to providing the physical environment in which HSCs differentiate, BM stromal cells generate cartilage, bone, and fat. Whether stromal cells are best classified as stem cells or progenitor cells for these tissues is still in question. There is also a question as to whether BM stromal cells and so-called mesenchymal stem cells are the same population [78].

BM stromal cells have many features that distinguish them from HSCs. The two cell types are easy to separate *in vitro*. When bone marrow is dissociated, and the mixture of cells it contains is plated at low density, the stromal cells adhere to the surface of the culture dish, and the HSCs do not. Given specific *in vitro* conditions, BM stromal cells form colonies from a single cell called the colony forming unit-F (CFU-F). These colonies may then differentiate as adipocytes or myelosupportive stroma, a clonal assay that indicates the stem cell-like nature of stromal cells. Unlike HSCs, which do not divide *in vitro* (or proliferate only to a limited extent), BM stromal cells can proliferate for up to 35 population doublings *in vitro* [16]. They grow rapidly under the influence of such mitogens as platelet-derived growth factor (PDGF), epidermal growth factor (EGF), basic fibroblast growth factor (bFGF), and insulin-like growth factor-1 (IGF-1) [12].

To date, it has not been possible to isolate a population of pure stromal cells from bone marrow. Panels of markers used to identify the cells include receptors for certain cytokines (interleukin-1, 3, 4, 6, and 7) receptors for proteins in the extracellular matrix, (ICAM-1 and 2, VCAM-1, the alpha-1, 2, and 3 integrins, and the beta-1, 2, 3 and 4 integrins), etc. [64]. Despite the use of these markers and another stromal cell marker called Stro-1, the origin and specific identity of stromal cells have remained elusive. Like HSCs, BM stromal cells arise from embryonic mesoderm during development, although no specific precursor or stem cell for stromal cells has been isolated and identified.

One theory about their origin is that a common kind of progenitor cell—perhaps a primordial endothelial cell that lines embryonic blood vessels—gives rise to both HSCs and to mesodermal precursors. The latter may then differentiate into myogenic precursors (the satellite cells that are thought to function as stem cells in skeletal muscle), and the BM stromal cells [10].

In vivo, the differentiation of stromal cells into fat and bone is not straightforward. Bone marrow adipocytes and myelosupportive stromal cells—both of which are derived from BM stromal cells—may be regarded as interchangeable phenotypes [10, 11]. Adipocytes do not develop until postnatal life, as the bones enlarge and the marrow space increases to accommodate enhanced hematopoiesis. When the skeleton stops growing, and the mass of HSCs decreases in a normal, age-dependent fashion, BM stromal cells differentiate into adipocytes, which fill the extra space. New bone formation is obviously greater during skeletal growth, although bone "turns over" throughout life. Bone forming cells are osteoblasts, but their relationship to BM stromal cells is not clear. New trabecular bone, which is the inner region of bone next to the marrow, could logically develop from the action of BM stromal cells. But the outside surface of bone also turns over, as does bone next to the Haversian system (small canals that form concentric rings within bone). And neither of these surfaces is in contact with BM stromal cells [10, 11].

Adult Stem Cells in Other Tissues

It is often difficult—if not impossible—to distinguish adult, tissue-specific stem cells from progenitor cells. With that caveat in mind, the following summary identifies reports of stem cells in various adult tissues.

Endothelial Progenitor Cells. Endothelial cells line the inner surfaces of blood vessels throughout the body, and it has been difficult to identify specific endothelial stem cells in either the embryonic or the adult mammal. During embryonic development, just after gastrulation, a kind of cell called the hemangioblast, which is derived from mesoderm, is presumed to be the precursor of both the hematopoietic and endothelial cell lineages. The embryonic vasculature formed at this stage is transient and consists of blood islands in the yolk sac. But hemangioblasts, per se, have not been isolated from the embryo and their existence remains in question. The process of forming new blood vessels in the embryo is called vasculogenesis. In the adult, the process of forming blood vessels from pre-existing blood vessels is called angiogenesis [50].

Evidence that hemangioblasts do exist comes from studies of mouse embryonic stem cells that are directed to differentiate in vitro. These studies have shown that a precursor cell derived from mouse ES cells that express Flk-1 [the receptor for vascular endothelial growth factor (VEGF) in mice] can give rise to both blood cells and blood vessel cells [88, 109]. Both VEGF and fibroblast growth factor-2 (FGF-2) play critical roles in endothelial cell differentiation in vivo [79].

Several recent reports indicate that the bone marrow contains cells that can give rise to new blood vessels in tissues that are ischemic (damaged due to the deprivation of blood and oxygen) [8, 29, 49, 94]. But it is unclear from these studies what cell type(s) in the bone marrow induced angiogenesis. In a study which sought to address that question, researchers found that adult human bone marrow contains cells that resemble embryonic hemangioblasts, and may therefore be called endothelial stem cells.

In more recent experiments, human bone marrow-derived cells were injected into the tail veins of rats with induced cardiac ischemia. The human cells migrated to the rat heart where they generated new blood vessels in the infarcted muscle (a process akin to vasculogenesis), and also induced angiogenesis. The candidate endothelial stem cells are CD34+ (a marker for HSCs), and they express the transcription factor GATA-2 [51]. A similar study using transgenic mice that express the gene for enhanced green fluorescent protein (which allows the cells to be tracked), showed that bone-marrow-derived cells could repopulate an area of infarcted heart muscle in mice, and generate not only blood vessels, but also cardiomyocytes that integrated into the host tissue [71] (see Chapter 9. Can Stem Cells Repair a Damaged Heart?).

And, in a series of experiments in adult mammals, progenitor endothelial cells were isolated from peripheral blood (of mice and humans) by using antibodies against CD34 and Flk-1, the receptor for VEGF. The cells were mononuclear blood cells (meaning they have a nucleus) and are referred to as MB^{CD34+} cells and MB^{Flk1+} cells. When plated in tissue-culture dishes, the cells attached to the substrate, became spindle-shaped, and formed tube-like structures that resemble blood vessels. When transplanted into mice of the same species (autologous transplants) with induced ischemia in one limb, the MB^{CD34+} cells promoted the formation of new blood vessels [8]. Although the adult MB^{CD34+} and MB^{Flk1+} cells function in some ways like stem cells, they are usually regarded as progenitor cells.

Skeletal Muscle Stem Cells. Skeletal muscle, like the cardiac muscle of the heart and the smooth muscle in the walls of blood vessels, the digestive system, and the respiratory system, is derived from embryonic mesoderm. To date, at least three populations of skeletal muscle stem cells have been identified: satellite cells, cells in the wall of the dorsal aorta, and so-called "side population" cells.

Satellite cells in skeletal muscle were identified 40 years ago in frogs by electron microscopy [62], and thereafter in mammals [84]. Satellite cells occur on the surface of the basal lamina of a mature muscle cell, or myofiber. In adult mammals, satellite cells mediate muscle growth [85]. Although satellite cells are normally non-dividing, they can be triggered to proliferate as a result of injury, or weight-bearing exercise. Under either of these circumstances, muscle satellite cells give rise to myogenic precursor cells, which then differentiate into the myofibrils that typify skeletal muscle. A group of transcription factors called myogenic regulatory factors (MRFs) play important roles in these differentiation events. The so-called primary MRFs, MyoD and Myf5, help regulate myoblast formation during embryogenesis. The secondary MRFs, myogenin and MRF4, regulate the terminal differentiation of myofibrils [86].

With regard to satellite cells, scientists have been addressing two questions. Are skeletal muscle satellite cells true adult stem cells or are they instead precursor cells? Are satellite cells the only cell type that can regenerate skeletal muscle. For example, a recent report indicates that muscle stem cells may also occur in the dorsal aorta of mouse embryos, and constitute a cell type that gives rise both to muscle satellite cells and endothelial cells. Whether the dorsal aorta cells meet the criteria of a self-renewing muscle stem cell is a matter of debate [21].

Another report indicates that a different kind of stem cell, called an SP cell, can also regenerate skeletal muscle may be present in muscle and bone marrow. SP stands for a side population of cells that can be separated by fluorescence-activated cell sorting analysis. Intravenously injecting these muscle-derived stem cells restored the expression of dystrophin in mdx mice. Dystrophin is the protein that is defective in people with Duchenne's muscular dystrophy; mdx mice provide a model for the human disease. Dystrophin expression in the SP cell-treated mice was lower than would be needed for clinical benefit. Injection of bone marrow- or muscle-derived SP cells into the dystrophic muscle of the mice yielded equivocal results that the transplanted cells had integrated into the host tissue. The authors conclude that a similar population of SP stem cells can be derived from either adult mouse bone marrow or skeletal muscle, and suggest "there may be some direct relationship between bone marrow-derived stem cells and other tissue- or organ-specific cells" [43]. Thus, stem cell or progenitor cell types from various mesodermally-derived tissues may be able to generate skeletal muscle.

Epithelial Cell Precursors in the Skin and Digestive System. Epithelial cells, which constitute 60 percent of the differentiated cells in the body are responsible for covering the internal and external surfaces of the body, including the lining of vessels and other cavities. The epithelial cells in skin and the digestive tract are replaced constantly. Other epithelial cell populations—in the ducts of the liver or pancreas, for example—turn over more slowly. The cell population that renews the epithelium of the small intestine occurs in the intestinal crypts, deep invaginations in the lining of the gut. The crypt cells are often regarded as stem cells; one of them can give rise to an organized cluster of cells called a structural-proliferative unit [93].

The skin of mammals contains at least three populations of epithelial cells: epidermal cells, hair follicle cells, and glandular epithelial cells, such as those that make up the sweat glands. The replacement patterns for epithelial cells in these three compartments differ, and in all the compartments, a stem cell population has been postulated. For example, stem cells in the bulge region of the hair follicle appear to give rise to multiple cell types. Their progeny can migrate down to the base of the follicle where they become matrix cells, which may then give rise to different cell types in the hair follicle, of which there are seven [39]. The bulge stem cells of the follicle may also give rise to the epidermis of the skin [95].

Another population of stem cells in skin occurs in the basal layer of the epidermis. These stem cells proliferate in the basal region, and then differentiate as they move toward the outer surface of the skin. The keratinocytes in the outermost layer lack nuclei and act as a protective barrier. A dividing skin stem cell can divide asymmetrically to produce two kinds of daughter cells. One is another self-renewing stem cell. The second kind of daughter cell is an intermediate precursor cell which is then committed to replicate a few times before differentiating into keratinocytes. Self-renewing stem cells can be distinguished from this intermediate precursor cell by their higher level of $\beta 1$ integrin expression, which signals keratinocytes to proliferate via a mitogen-activated protein (MAP) kinase [112]. Other signaling pathways include that triggered by β-catenin, which helps maintain the stem-cell state [111], and the pathway regulated by the oncoprotein c-Myc, which triggers stem cells to give rise to transit amplifying cells [36].

Stem Cells in the Pancreas and Liver. The status of stem cells in the adult pancreas and liver is unclear. During embryonic development, both tissues arise from endoderm. A recent study indicates that a single precursor cell derived from embryonic endoderm may generate both the ventral pancreas and the liver [23]. In adult mammals, however, both the pancreas and the liver contain multiple kinds of differentiated cells that may be repopulated or regenerated by multiple types of stem cells. In the pancreas, endocrine (hormone-producing) cells occur in the islets of Langerhans. They include the beta cells (which produce insulin), the alpha cells (which secrete glucagon), and cells that release the peptide hormones somatostatin and pancreatic polypeptide. Stem cells in the adult pancreas are postulated to occur in the pancreatic ducts or in the islets themselves. Several recent reports indicate that stem cells that express nestin—which is usually regarded as a marker of neural stem cells—can generate all of the cell types in the islets [60, 113] (see Chapter 7. Stem Cells and Diabetes).

The identity of stem cells that can repopulate the liver of adult mammals is also in question. Recent studies in rodents indicate that HSCs (derived from mesoderm) may be able to home to liver after it is damaged, and demonstrate plasticity in becoming

into hepatocytes (usually derived from endoderm) [54, 77, 97]. But the question remains as to whether cells from the bone marrow normally generate hepatocytes in vivo. It is not known whether this kind of plasticity occurs without severe damage to the liver or whether HSCs from the bone marrow generate oval cells of the liver [18]. Although hepatic oval cells exist in the liver, it is not clear whether they actually generate new hepatocytes [87, 98]. Oval cells may arise from the portal tracts in liver and may give rise to either hepatocytes [19, 55] and to the epithelium of the bile ducts [37, 92]. Indeed, hepatocytes themselves, may be responsible for the well-know regenerative capacity of liver.

SUMMARY

What Do We Know About Adult Stem Cells?

- Adult stem cells can proliferate without differentiating for a long period (a characteristic referred to as long-term self-renewal), and they can give rise to mature cell types that have characteristic shapes and specialized functions.

- Some adult stem cells have the capability to differentiate into tissues other than the ones from which they originated; this is referred to as plasticity.

- Adult stem cells are rare. Often they are difficult to identify and their origins are not known. Current methods for characterizing adult stem cells are dependent on determining cell surface markers and observations about their differentiation patterns in test tubes and culture dishes.

- To date, published scientific literature indicates that adult stem cells have been derived from brain, bone marrow, peripheral blood, dental pulp, spinal cord, blood vessels, skeletal muscle, epithelia of the skin and digestive system, cornea, retina, liver, and pancreas; thus, adult stem cells have been found in tissues that develop from all three embryonic germ layers.

- Hematopoietic stem cells from bone marrow are the most studied and used for clinical applications in restoring various blood and immune components to the bone marrow via transplantation. There are at least two other populations of adult stem cells that have been identified from bone marrow and blood.

- Several populations of adult stem cells have been identified in the brain, particularly the hippocampus. Their function is unknown. Proliferation and differentiation of brain stem cells are influenced by various growth factors.

- There are now several reports of adult stem cells in other tissues (muscle, blood, and fat) that demonstrate plasticity. Very few published research reports on plasticity of adult stem cells have, however, included clonality studies. That is, there is limited evidence that a single adult stem cell or genetically identical line of adult stem cells demonstrates plasticity.

- Rarely have experiments that claim plasticity demonstrated that the adult stem cells have generated mature, fully functional cells or that the cells have restored lost function *in vivo*.

What Do We Need to Know About Adult Stem Cells?

- What are the sources of adult stem cells in the body? Are they "leftover" embryonic stem cells, or do they arise in some other way? And if the latter is true—which seems to be the case—exactly how do adult stem cells arise, and why do they remain in an undifferentiated state, when all the cells around them have differentiated?

- Is it possible to manipulate adult stem cells to increase their ability to proliferate *in vitro*, so that adult stem cells can be used as a sufficient source of tissue for transplants?

- How many kinds of adult stem cells exist, and in which tissues do they exist? Evidence is accumulating that, although they occur in small numbers, adult stem cells are present in many differentiated tissues.

- What is the best evidence that adult stem cells show plasticity and generate cell types of other tissues?

- Is it possible to manipulate adult stem cells to increase their ability to proliferate *in vitro* so that adult stem cells can be used as a sufficient source of tissue for transplants?

- Is there a universal stem cell? An emerging concept is that, in adult mammals, there may be a population of "universal" stem cells. Although largely theoretical, the concept has some experimental basis. A candidate, universal adult stem cell may be one that circulates in the blood stream, can escape from the blood, and populate various adult tissues. In more than one experimental system, researchers have noted that dividing cells in adult tissues often appear near a blood vessel, such as candidate stem cells in the hippocampus, a region of the brain [75].

- Do adult stem cells exhibit plasticity as a normal event *in vivo*? If so, is this true of all adult stem cells? What are the signals that regulate the proliferation and differentiation of stem cells that demonstrate plasticity?

REFERENCES

1. Akashi, K., Traver, D., Kondo, M., and Weissman, I.L. (1999). Lymphoid development from hematopoietic stem cells. Int. J. Hematol. 69, 217-226.

2. Akashi, K., Kondo, M., Cheshier, S., Shizuru, J., Gandy, K., Domen, J., Mebius, R., Traver, D., and Weissman, I.L. (1999). Lymphoid development from stem cells and the common lymphocyte progenitors. Cold Spring Harb. Symp. Quant. Biol. 64, 1-12.

3. Akashi, K., Traver, D., Miyamoto, T., and Weissman, I.L. (2000). A clonogenic common myeloid progenitor that gives rise to all myeloid lineages. Nature. 404, 193-197.

4. Alison, M.R., Poulsom, R., Jeffery, R., Dhillon, A.P., Quaglia, A., Jacob, J., Novelli, M., Prentice, G., Williamson, J., and Wright, N.A. (2000). Hepatocytes from non-hepatic adult stem cells. Nature. 406, 257.

5. Altman, J. and Das, G.D. (1965). Autoradiographic and histological evidence of postnatal hippocampal neurogenesis in rats. J. Comp. Neurol. 124, 319-335.

6. Altman, J. (1969). Autoradiographic and histological studies of postnatal neurogenesis. IV. Cell proliferation and migration in the anterior forebrain, with special reference to persisting neurogenesis in the olfactory bulb. J. Comp. Neurol. 137, 433-457.

7. Anderson, D.J., Gage, F.H., and Weissman, I.L. (2001). Can stem cells cross lineage boundaries? Nat. Med. 7, 393-395.

8. Asahara, T., Murohara, T., Sullivan, A., Silver, M., van der Zee R., Li, T., Witzenbichler, B., Schatteman, G., and Isner, J.M. (1997). Isolation of putative progenitor endothelial cells for angiogenesis. Science. 275, 964-967.

9. Becker, A.J., McCullough, E.A., and Till, J.E. (1963). Cytological demonstration of the clonal nature of spleen colonies derived from transplanted mouse marrow cells. Nature. 197, 452-454.

10. Bianco, P. and Cossu, G. (1999). Uno, nessuno e centomila: searching for the identity of mesodermal progenitors. Exp. Cell Res. 251, 257-263.

11. Bianco, P., Riminucci, M., Kuznetsov, S., and Robey, P.G. (1999). Multipotential cells in the bone marrow stroma: regulation in the context of organ physiology. Crit. Rev. Eukaryotic. Gene Expr. 9, 159-173.

12. Bianco, P., Riminucci, M., Gronthos, S., and Robey, P.G. (2001). Bone marrow stromal stem cells: nature, biology, and potential applications. Stem Cells. 19, 180-192.

13. Bjornson, C.R., Rietze, R.L., Reynolds, B.A., Magli, M.C., and Vescovi, A.L. (1999). Turning brain into blood: a hematopoietic fate adopted by adult neural stem cells in vivo. Science. 283, 534-537.

14. Blau, H., personal communication.

15. Brazelton, T.R., Rossi, F.M., Keshet, G.I., and Blau, H.M. (2000). From marrow to brain: expression of neuronal phenotypes in adult mice. Science. 290, 1775-1779.

16. Bruder, S.P., Jaiswal, N., and Haynesworth, S.E. (1997). Growth kinetics, self-renewal, and the osteogenic potential of purified human mesenchymal stem cells during extensive subcultivation and following cryopreservation. J. Cell. Biochem. 64, 278-294.

17. Clarke, D.L., Johansson, C.B., Wilbertz, J., Veress, B., Nilsson, E., Karlström, H., Lendahl, U., and Frisen, J. (2000). Generalized potential of adult neural stem cells. Science. 288, 1660-1663.

18. Crosby, H.A. and Strain, A.J. (2001). Adult liver stem cells: bone marrow, blood, or liver derived? Gut. 48, 153-154.

19. Dabeva, M.D. and Shafritz, D.A. (1993). Activation, proliferation, and differentiation of progenitor cells into hepatocytes in the D-galactosamine model of liver regeneration. Am. J. Pathol. 143, 1606-1620.

20. Davis, A.A. and Temple, S. (1994). A self-renewing multipotential stem cell in embryonic rat cerebral cortex. Nature. 372, 263-266.

21. De Angelis, L., Berghella, L., Coletta, M., Lattanzi, L., Zanchi, M., Cusella-De Angelis, M.G., Ponzetto, C., and Cossu, G. (1999). Skeletal myogenic progenitors originating from embryonic dorsal aorta coexpress endothelial and myogenic markers and contribute to postnatal muscle growth and regeneration. J. Cell Biol. 147, 869-877.

22. Del Bigio, M.R. (1995). The ependyma: a protective barrier between brain and cerebrospinal fluid. Glia. 14, 1-13.

23. Deutsch, G., Jung, J., Zheng, M., Lora, J., and Zaret, K.S. (2001). A bipotential precursor population for pancreas and liver within the embryonic endoderm. Development. 128, 871-881.

24. Doetsch, F., Garcia-Verdugo, J.M., and Alvarez-Buylla, A. (1997). Cellular composition and three-dimensional organization of the subventricular germinal zone in the adult mammalian brain. J. Neurosci. 17, 5046-5061.

25. Doetsch, F., Caille, I., Lim, D.A., Garcia-Verdugo, J.M., and Alvarez-Buylla, A. (1999). Subventricular zone astrocytes are neural stem cells in the adult mammalian brain. Cell. 97, 703-716.

26. Domen, J. and Weissman, I.L. (1999). Self-renewal, differentiation or death: regulation and manipulation of hematopoietic stem cell fate. Mol. Med. Today. 5, 201-208.

27. Eriksson, P.S., Perfilieva, E., Bjork-Eriksson, T., Alborn, A.M., Nordborg, C., Peterson, D.A., and Gage, F.H. (1998). Neurogenesis in the adult human hippocampus. Nat. Med. 4, 1313-1317.

28. Ferrari, G., Cusella-De Angelis, G., Coletta, M., Paolucci, E., Stornaiuolo, A., Cossu, G., and Mavilio, F. (1998). Muscle regeneration by bone marrow-derived myogenic progenitors. Science. 279, 1528-1530.

29. Folkman, J. (1998). Therapeutic angiogenesis in ischemic limbs. Circulation. 97, 1108-1110.

30. Friedenstein, A.J., Piatetzky-Shapiro, I.I., and Petrakova, K.V. (1966). Osteogenesis in transplants of bone marrow cells. J. Embryol. Exp. Morphol. 16, 381-390.

31. Friedenstein, A.J., Petrakova, K.V., Kurolesova, A.I., and Frolova, G.P. (1968). Heterotopic of bone marrow. Analysis of precursor cells for osteogenic and hematopoietic tissues. Transplantation. 6, 230-247.

32. Friedenstein, A.J., Chailakhjan, R.K., and Lalykina, K.S. (1970). The development of fibroblast colonies in monolayer cultures of guinea-pig bone marrow and spleen cells. Cell Tissue Kinet. 3, 393-403.

33. Gage, F., personal communication.

34. Gage, F.H., Ray, J., and Fisher, L.J. (1995). Isolation, characterization, and use of stem cells from the CNS. Annu. Rev. Neurosci. 18, 159-192.

35. Gage, F.H., Coates, P.W., Palmer, T.D., Kuhn, H.G., Fisher, L.J., Suhonen, J.O., Peterson, D.A., Suhr, S.T., and Ray, J. (1995). Survival and differentiation of adult neuronal progenitor cells transplanted to the adult brain. Proc. Natl. Acad. Sci. U. S. A. 92, 11879-11883.

36. Gandarillas, A. and Watt, F.M. (1997). c-Myc promotes differentiation of human epidermal stem cells. Genes Dev. 11, 2869-2882.

37. Germain, L., Noel, M., Gourdeau, H., and Marceau, N. (1988). Promotion of growth and differentiation of rat ductular oval cells in primary culture. Cancer Res. 48, 368-378.

38. Geschwind, D.H., Ou, J., Easterday, M.C., Dougherty, J.D., Jackson, R.L., Chen, Z., Antoine, H., Terskikh, A., Weissman, I.L., Nelson, S.F., and Kornblum, H.I. (2001). A genetic analysis of neural progenitor differentiation. Neuron. 29, 325-339.

39. Ghazizadeh, S. and Taichman, L.B. (2001). Multiple classes of stem cells in cutaneous epithelium: a lineage analysis of adult mouse skin. EMBO J. 20, 1215-1222.

40. Gordon, M.Y., Riley, G.P., Watt, S.M., and Greaves, M.F. (1987). Compartmentalization of a haematopoietic growth factor (GM-CSF) by glycosaminoglycans in the bone marrow microenvironment. Nature. 326, 403-405.

41. Gritti, A., Parati, E.A., Cova, L., Frolichsthal, P., Galli, R., Wanke, E., Faravelli, L., Morassutti, D.J., Roisen, F., Nickel, D.D., and Vescovi, A.L. (1996). Multipotential stem cells from the adult mouse brain proliferate and self-renew in response to basic fibroblast growth factor. J. Neurosci. *16*, 1091-1100.

42. Guenechea, G., Gan, O.I., Dorrell, C., and Dick, J.E. (2001). Distinct classes of human stem cells that differ in proliferative and self-renewal potential. Nat. Immunol. *2*, 75-82.

43. Gussoni, E., Soneoka, Y., Strickland, C.D., Buzney, E.A., Khan, M.K., Flint, A.F., Kunkel, L.M., and Mulligan, R.C. (1999). Dystrophin expression in the mdx mouse restored by stem cell transplantation. Nature. *401*, 390-394.

44. Holtzer. H. (1978). Cell lineages, stem cells and the 'quantal' cell cycle concept. In: Stem cells and tissue homeostasis. Eds: B.I. Lord, C.S. Potten, and R.J. Cole. (Cambridge, New York: Cambridge University Press). 1-28.

45. Hunt, P., Robertson, D., Weiss, D., Rennick, D., Lee, F., and Witte, O.N. (1987). A single bone marrow-derived stromal cell type supports the *in vitro* growth of early lymphoid and myeloid cells. Cell. *48*, 997-1007.

46. Jackson, K., Majka SM, Wang H, Pocius J, Hartley CJ, Majesky MW, Entman ML, Michael LH, Hirschi KK, and Goodell MA (2001). Regeneration of ischemic cardiac muscle and vascular endothelium by adult stem cells. J. Clin. Invest. *107*, 1-8.

47. Johansson, C.B., Momma, S., Clarke, D.L., Risling, M., Lendahl, U., and Frisen, J. (1999). Identification of a neural stem cell in the adult mammalian central nervous system. Cell. *96*, 25-34.

48. Johe, K.K., Hazel, T.G., Muller, T., Dugich-Djordjevic, M.M., and McKay, R.D. (1996). Single factors direct the differentiation of stem cells from the fetal and adult central nervous system. Genes Dev. *10*, 3129-3140.

49. Kalka, C., Masuda, H., Takahashi, T., Kalka-Moll, W.M., Silver, M., Kearney, M., Li, T., Isner, J.M., and Asahara, T. (2000). Transplantation of ex vivo expanded endothelial progenitor cells for therapeutic neovascularization. Proc. Natl. Acad. Sci. U. S. A. *97*, 3422-3427.

50. Keller, G. (2001). The hemangioblast. Marshak, D.R., Gardner, D.K., and Gottlieb, D. eds. (Cold Spring Harbor, New York: Cold Spring Harbor Laboratory Press). 329-348.

51. Kocher, A.A., Schuster, M.D., Szabolcs, M.J., Takuma, S., Burkhoff, D., Wang, J., Homma, S., Edwards, N.M., and Itescu, S. (2001). Neovascularization of ischemic myocardium by human bone-marrow-derived angioblasts prevents cardiomyocyte apoptosis, reduces remodeling and improves cardiac function. Nat. Med. *7*, 430-436.

52. Krause, D.S., Theise, N.D., Collector, M.I., Henegariu, O., Hwang, S., Gardner, R., Neutzel, S., and Sharkis, S.J. (2001). Multi-organ, multi-lineage engraftment by a single bone marrow-derived stem cell. Cell. *105*, 369-377.

53. Kuznetsov, S.A., Mankani, M.H., Gronthos, S., Satomura, K., Bianco, P., and Robey P.G. (2001). Circulating skeletal stem cells. J. Cell Biol. *153*, 1133-1140.

54. Lagasse, E., Connors, H., Al Dhalimy, M., Reitsma, M., Dohse, M., Osborne, L., Wang, X., Finegold, M., Weissman, I.L., and Grompe, M. (2000). Purified hematopoietic stem cells can differentiate into hepatocytes *in vivo*. Nat. Med. *6*, 1229-1234.

55. Lazaro, C.A., Rhim, J.A., Yamada, Y., and Fausto, N. (1998). Generation of hepatocytes from oval cell precursors in culture. Cancer Res. *58*, 5514-5522.

56. Le Douarin, N.M. (1980). The ontogeny of the neural crest in avian embryo chimaeras. Nature. *286*, 663-669.

57. Le Douarin, N.M. and Kalcheim, C. (1999). The migration of neural crest cells. In: The neural crest. (Cambridge, New York: Cambridge University Press). 23-59.

58. Leblond, C.P. (1964). Classification of cell populations on the basis of their proliferative behavior. National Cancer Institute. *14*, 119-150.

59. Lois, C. and Alvarez-Buylla, A. (1994). Long-distance neuronal migration in the adult mammalian brain. Science. *264*, 1145-1148.

60. Lumelsky, N., Blondel, O., Laeng, P., Velasco, I., Ravin, R., and McKay, R. (2001). Differentiation of Embryonic Stem Cells to Insulin-Secreting Structures Similiar to Pancreatic Islets. Science. *292*, 1309-1599.

61. Luskin, M.B. (1993). Restricted proliferation and migration of postnatally generated neurons derived from the forebrain subventricular zone. Neuron. *11*, 173-189.

62. Mauro, A. (1961). Satellite cell of skeletal muscle fibers. J. Biophys. Biochem. Cytol. 9, 493-495.

63. McKay, R. (1997). Stem cells in the central nervous system. Science. *276*, 66-71.

64. McKay, R., personal communication.

65. Mezey, E., Chandross, K.J., Harta, G., Maki, R.A., and McKercher, S.R. (2000). Turning blood into brain: cells bearing neuronal antigens generated *in vivo* from bone marrow. Science. *290*, 1779-1782.

66. Momma, S., Johansson, C.B., and Frisen, J. (2000). Get to know your stem cells. Curr. Opin. Neurobiol. *10*, 45-49.

67. Morrison, S.J., White, P.M., Zock, C., and Anderson, D.J. (1999). Prospective identification, isolation by flow cytometry, and *in vivo* self-renewal of multipotent mammalian neural crest stem cells. Cell. *96*, 737-749.

68. Morrison, S.J. (2001). Neuronal differentiation: Proneural genes inhibit gliogenesis. Curr. Biol. *11*, R349-R351.

69. Morshead, C.M., Reynolds, B.A., Craig, C.G., McBurney, M.W., Staines, W.A., Morassutti, D., Weiss, S., and van der, K.D. (1994). Neural stem cells in the adult mammalian forebrain: a relatively quiescent subpopulation of subependymal cells. Neuron. *13*, 1071-1082.

70. Morshead, C.M. and van der Kooy, K.D. (2001). A new 'spin' on neural stem cells? Curr. Opin. Neurobiol. *11*, 59-65.

71. Orlic, D., Kajstura, J., Chimenti, S., Jakoniuk, I., Anderson, S.M., Li, B., Pickel, J., McKay, R., Nadal-Ginard, B., Bodine, D.M., Leri, A., and Anversa, P. (2001). Bone marrow cells regenerate infarcted myocardium. Nature. *410*, 701-705.

72. Osawa, M., Hanada, K., Hamada, H., and Nakauchi, H. (1996). Long-term lymphohematopoietic reconstitution by a single CD34- low/negative hematopoietic stem cell. Science. *273*, 242-245.

73. Owen, M. (1988). Marrow derived stromal stem cells. J. Cell Science Supp. *10*, 63-76.

74. Palmer, T.D., Takahashi, J., and Gage, F.H. (1997). The adult rat hippocampus contains primordial neural stem cells. Mol. Cell. Neurosci. *8*, 389-404.

75. Palmer, T.D., Willhoite, A.R., and Gage, F.H. (2000). Vascular niche for adult hippocampal neurogenesis. J. Comp. Neurol. *425*, 479-494.

76. Panicker, M. and Rao, M. (2001). Stem cells and neurogenesis. Marshak, D.R., Gardner, D.K., and Gottlieb, D. eds. (Cold Spring Harbor, New York: Cold Spring Harbor Laboratory Press). 399-438.

77. Petersen, B.E., Bowen, W.C., Patrene, K.D., Mars, W.M., Sullivan, A.K., Murase, N., Boggs, S.S., Greenberger, J.S., and Goff, J.P. (1999). Bone marrow as a potential source of hepatic oval cells. Science. *284*, 1168-1170.

78. Pittenger, M.F. and Marshak, D.R. (2001). Mesenchymal stem cells of human adult bone marrow. Marshak, D.R., Gardner, D.K., and Gottlieb, D. eds. (Cold Spring Harbor, New York: Cold Spring Harbor Laboratory Press). 349-374.

79. Poole, T.J., Finkelstein, E.B., and Cox, C.M. (2001). The role of FGF and VEGF in angioblast induction and migration during vascular development. Dev. Dyn. *220*, 1-17.

80. Reynolds, B.A. and Weiss, S. (1992). Generation of neurons and astrocytes from isolated cells of the adult mammalian central nervous system. Science. *255*, 1707-1710.

81. Roberts, R., Gallagher, J., Spooncer, E., Allen, T.D., Bloomfield, F., and Dexter, T.M. (1988). Heparan sulphate bound growth factors: a mechanism for stromal cell mediated haemopoiesis. Nature. *332*, 376-378.

82. Robey, P.G. (2000). Stem cells near the century mark. J. Clin. Invest. *105*, 1489-1491.

83. Roy, V. and Verfaillie, C.M. (1999). Expression and function of cell adhesion molecules on fetal liver, cord blood and bone marrow hematopoietic progenitors: implications for anatomical localization and developmental stage specific regulation of hematopoiesis. Exp. Hematol. *27*, 302-312.

84. Schultz, E. (1976). Fine structure of satellite cells in growing skeletal muscle. Am. J. Anat. *147*, 49-70.

85. Schultz, E. (1996). Satellite cell proliferative compartments in growing skeletal muscles. Dev. Biol. *175*, 84-94.

86. Seale, P. and Rudnicki, M.A. (2000). A new look at the origin, function, and "stem-cell" status of muscle satellite cells. Dev. Biol. *218*, 115-124.

87. Sell, S. (1990). Is there a liver stem cell? Cancer Res. *50*, 3811-3815.

88. Shalaby, F., Rossant, J., Yamaguchi, T.P., Gertsenstein, M., Wu, X.F., Breitman, M.L., and Schuh, A.C. (1995). Failure of blood-island formation and vasculogenesis in Flk-1-deficient mice. Nature. *376*, 62-66.

89. Shi, Q., Rafii, S., Wu, M.H., Wijelath, E.S., Yu, C., Ishida, A., Fujita, Y., Kothari, S., Mohle, R., Sauvage, L.R., Moore, M.A., Storb, R.F., and Hammond, W.P. (1998). Evidence for circulating bone marrow-derived endothelial cells. Blood. *92*, 362-367.

90. Shihabuddin, L.S., Palmer, T.D., and Gage, F.H. (1999). The search for neural progenitor cells: prospects for the therapy of neurodegenerative disease. Mol. Med. Today. *5*, 474-480.

91. Sieber-Blum, M. (2000). Factors controlling lineage specification in the neural crest. Int. Rev. Cytol. *197*, 1-33.

92. Sirica, A.E., Mathis, G.A., Sano, N., and Elmore, L.W. (1990). Isolation, culture, and transplantation of intrahepatic biliary epithelial cells and oval cells. Pathobiology. *58*, 44-64.

93. Slack, J.M. (2000). Stem Cells in Epithelial Tissues. Science. *287*, 1431-1433.

94. Takahashi, T., Kalka, C., Masuda, H., Chen, D., Silver, M., Kearney, M., Magner, M., Isner, J.M., and Asahara, T. (1999). Ischemia- and cytokine-induced mobilization of bone marrow-derived endothelial progenitor cells for neovascularization. Nat. Med. *5*, 434-438.

95. Taylor, G., Lehrer, M.S., Jensen, P.J., Sun, T.T., and Lavker, R.M. (2000). Involvement of follicular stem cells in forming not only the follicle but also the epidermis. Cell. *102*, 451-461.

96. Temple, S. and Alvarez-Buylla, A. (1999). Stem cells in the adult mammalian central nervous system. Curr. Opin. Neurobiol. *9*, 135-141.

97. Theise, N.D., Nimmakayalu, M., Gardner, R., Illei, P.B., Morgan, G., Teperman, L., Henegariu, O., and Krause, D.S. (2000). Liver from bone marrow in humans. Hepatology. *32*, 11-16.

98. Thorgeirsson, S.S. (1993). Hepatic stem cells. Am. J. Pathol. *142*, 1331-1333.

99. Till, J.E. and McCullough, E.A. (1961). A direct measurement of the radiation sensitivity of normal mouse bone marrow cells. Radiat. Res. *14*, 213-222.

100. Tropepe, V., Sibilia, M., Ciruna, B.G., Rossant, J., Wagner, E.F., and van der Kooy D. (1999). Distinct neural stem cells proliferate in response to EGF and FGF in the developing mouse telencephalon. Dev. Biol. *208*, 166-188.

101. Verfaillie, C.M. (1998). Adhesion receptors as regulators of the hematopoietic process. Blood. *92*, 2609-2612.

102. Vescovi, A.L., Reynolds, B.A., Fraser, D.D., and Weiss, S. (1993). bFGF regulates the proliferative fate of unipotent (neuronal) and bipotent (neuronal/astroglial) EGF-generated CNS progenitor cells. Neuron. *11*, 951-966.

103. Vescovi, A.L., Gritti, A., Galli, R., and Parati, E.A. (1999). Isolation and intracerebral grafting of nontransformed multipotential embryonic human CNS stem cells. J. Neurotrauma. *16*, 689-693.

104. Weiss, S. and van der Kooy D. (1998). CNS stem cells: where's the biology (a.k.a. beef)? J. Neurobiol. *36*, 307-314.

105. Weissman, I.L. (2000). Stem cells: units of development, units of regeneration, and units in evolution. Cell. *100*, 157-168.

106. White, P.M., Morrison, S.J., Orimoto, K., Kubu, C.J., Verdi, J.M., and Anderson, D.J. (2001). Neural crest stem cells undergo cell-intrinsic developmental changes in sensitivity to instructive differentiation signals. Neuron. *29*, 57-71.

107. Whitlock, C.A., Tidmarsh, G.F., Muller-Sieburg, C., and Weissman, I.L. (1987). Bone marrow stromal cell lines with lymphopoietic activity express high levels of a pre-B neoplasia-associated molecule. Cell. *48*, 1009-1021.

108. Williams, B.P., Read, J., and Price, J. (1991). The generation of neurons and oligodendrocytes from a common precursor cell. Neuron. *7*, 685-693.

109. Yamashita, J., Itoh, H., Hirashima, M., Ogawa, M., Nishikawa, S., Yurugi, T., Naito, M., Nakao, K., and Nishikawa, S. (2000). Flk1-positive cells derived from embryonic stem cells serve as vascular progenitors. Nature. *408*, 92-96.

110. Zandstra, P.W., Lauffenburger, D.A., and Eaves, C.J. (2000). A ligand-receptor signaling threshold model of stem cell differentiation control: a biologically conserved mechanism applicable to hematopoiesis. Blood. *96*, 1215-1222.

111. Zhu, A.J. and Watt, F.M. (1999). beta-catenin signalling modulates proliferative potential of human epidermal keratinocytes independently of intercellular adhesion. Development. *126*, 2285-2298.

112. Zhu, A.J., Haase, I., and Watt, F.M. (1999). Signaling via beta1 integrins and mitogen-activated protein kinase determines human epidermal stem cell fate *in vitro*. Proc. Natl. Acad. Sci. U. S. A. *96*, 6728-6733.

113. Zulewski, H., Abraham, E.J., Gerlach, M.J., Daniel, P.B., Moritz, W., Muller, B., Vallejo, M., Thomas, M.K., and Habener, J.F. (2001). Multipotential nestin-positive stem cells isolated from adult pancreatic islets differentiate ex vivo into pancreatic endocrine, exocrine, and hepatic phenotypes. Diabetes. *50*, 521-533.

5. HEMATOPOIETIC STEM CELLS

With more than 50 years of experience studying blood-forming stem cells called hematopoietic stem cells, scientists have developed sufficient understanding to actually use them as a therapy. Currently, no other type of stem cell, adult, fetal or embryonic, has attained such status. Hematopoietic stem cell transplants are now routinely used to treat patients with cancers and other disorders of the blood and immune systems. Recently, researchers have observed in animal studies that hematopoietic stem cells appear to be able to form other kinds of cells, such as muscle, blood vessels, and bone. If this can be applied to human cells, it may eventually be possible to use hematopoietic stem cells to replace a wider array of cells and tissues than once thought.

Despite the vast experience with hematopoietic stem cells, scientists face major roadblocks in expanding their use beyond the replacement of blood and immune cells. First, hematopoietic stem cells are unable to proliferate (replicate themselves) and differentiate (become specialized to other cell types) in vitro (in the test tube or culture dish). Second, scientists do not yet have an accurate method to distinguish stem cells from other cells recovered from the blood or bone marrow. Until scientists overcome these technical barriers, they believe it is unlikely that hematopoietic stem cells will be applied as cell replacement therapy in diseases such as diabetes, Parkinson's Disease, spinal cord injury, and many others.

INTRODUCTION

Blood cells are responsible for constant maintenance and immune protection of every cell type of the body. This relentless and brutal work requires that blood cells, along with skin cells, have the greatest powers of self-renewal of any adult tissue.

The stem cells that form blood and immune cells are known as hematopoietic stem cells (HSCs). They are ultimately responsible for the constant renewal of blood—the production of billions of new blood cells each day. Physicians and basic researchers have known and capitalized on this fact for more than 50 years in treating many diseases. The first evidence and definition of blood-forming stem cells came from studies of people exposed to lethal doses of radiation in 1945.

Basic research soon followed. After duplicating radiation sickness in mice, scientists found they could rescue the mice from death with bone marrow transplants from healthy donor animals. In the early 1960s, Till and McCulloch began analyzing the bone marrow to find out which components were responsible for regenerating blood [56]. They defined what remain the two hallmarks of an HSC: it can renew itself and it can produce cells that give rise to all the different types of blood cells (see Chapter 4. The Adult Stem Cell).

WHAT IS A HEMATOPOIETIC STEM CELL?

A hematopoietic stem cell is a cell isolated from the blood or bone marrow that can renew itself, can differentiate to a variety of specialized cells, can mobilize out of the bone marrow into circulating blood, and can undergo programmed cell death, called apoptosis—a process by which cells that are detrimental or unneeded self-destruct.

A major thrust of basic HSC research since the 1960s has been identifying and characterizing these stem cells. Because HSCs look and behave in culture like ordinary white blood cells, this has been a difficult challenge and this makes them difficult to identify by morphology (size and shape). Even today, scientists must rely on cell surface proteins, which serve, only roughly, as markers of white blood cells.

Identifying and characterizing properties of HSCs began with studies in mice, which laid the groundwork for human studies. The challenge is formidable as about 1 in every 10,000 to 15,000 bone marrow cells is thought to be a stem cell. In the blood stream the proportion falls to 1 in 100,000 blood cells. To this end, scientists began to develop tests for proving the self-renewal and the plasticity of HSCs.

The "gold standard" for proving that a cell derived from mouse bone marrow is indeed an HSC is still based on the same proof described above and used in mice many years ago. That is, the cells are injected into a mouse that has received a dose of irradiation sufficient to kill its own blood-producing cells. If the mouse recovers and all types of blood cells reappear (bearing a genetic marker from the donor animal), the transplanted cells are deemed to have included stem cells.

These studies have revealed that there appear to be two kinds of HSCs. If bone marrow cells from the transplanted mouse can, in turn, be transplanted to another lethally irradiated mouse and restore its

hematopoietic system over some months, they are considered to be *long-term stem cells* that are capable of self-renewal. Other cells from bone marrow can immediately regenerate all the different types of blood cells, but under normal circumstances cannot renew themselves over the long term, and these are referred to as *short-term progenitor or precursor cells.* Progenitor or precursor cells are relatively immature cells that are precursors to a fully differentiated cell of the same tissue type. They are capable of proliferating, but they have a limited capacity to differentiate into more than one cell type as HSCs do. For example, a blood progenitor cell may only be able to make a red blood cell (see Figure 5.1. Hematopoietic and Stromal Stem Cell Differentiation).

Harrison et al. write that short-term blood-progenitor cells in a mouse may restore hematopoiesis for three to four months [36]. The longevity of short-term stem cells for humans is not firmly established. A true stem cell, capable of self-renewal, must be able to renew itself for the entire lifespan of an organism. It is these

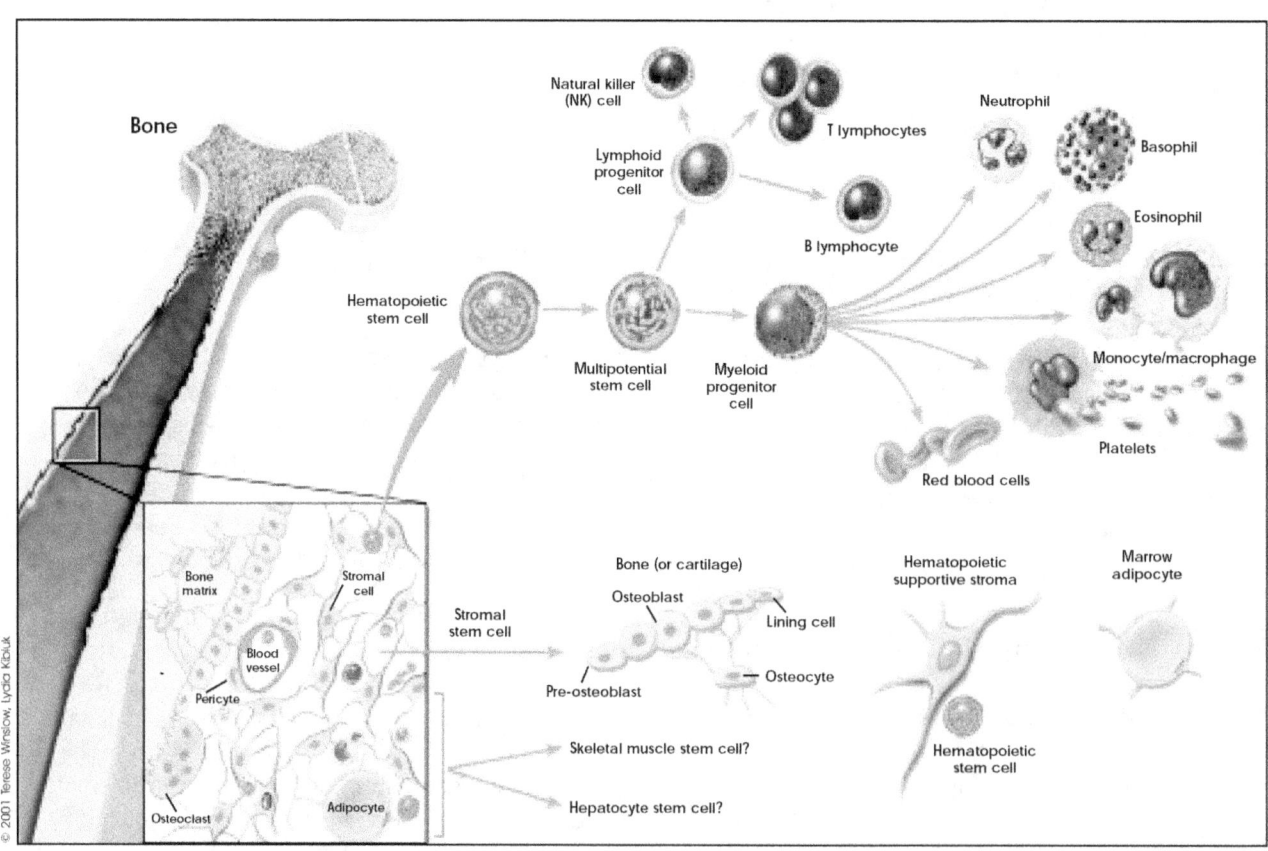

Figure 5.1. Hematopoietic and Stromal Stem Cell Differentiation.

long-term replicating HSCs that are most important for developing HSC-based cell therapies. Unfortunately, to date, researchers cannot distinguish the long-term from the short-term cells when they are removed from the bloodstream or bone marrow.

The central problem of the assays used to identify long-term stem cells and short-term progenitor cells is that they are difficult, expensive, and time-consuming and cannot be done in humans. A few assays are now available that test cells in culture for their ability to form primitive and long-lasting colonies of cells, but these tests are not accepted as proof that a cell is a long-term stem cell. Some genetically altered mice can receive transplanted human HSCs to test the cells' self-renewal and hematopoietic capabilities during the life of a mouse, but the relevance of this test for the cells in humans—who may live for decades—is open to question.

The difficulty of HSC assays has contributed to two mutually confounding research problems: definitively identifying the HSC and getting it to proliferate, or increase its numbers, in a culture dish. More rapid research progress on characterizing and using HSCs would be possible if they could be readily grown in the laboratory. Conversely, progress in identifying growth conditions suitable for HSCs and getting the cells to multiply would move more quickly if scientists could reliably and readily identify true HSCs.

CAN CELL MARKERS BE USED TO IDENTIFY HEMATOPOIETIC STEM CELLS?

HSCs have an identity problem. First, the ones with long-term replicating ability are rare. Second, there are multiple types of stem cells. And, third, the stem cells look like many other blood or bone marrow cells. So how do researchers find the desired cell populations? The most common approach is through markers that appear on the surface of cells. (For a more detailed discussion, see Appendix E.i. Markers: How Do Researchers Use Them to Identify Stem Cells?) These are useful, but not perfect tools for the research laboratory.

In 1988, in an effort to develop a reliable means of identifying these cells, Irving Weissman and his collaborators focused attention on a set of protein markers on the surface of mouse blood cells that were associated with increased likelihood that the

cell was a long-term HSC [50]. Four years later, the laboratory proposed a comparable set of markers for the human stem cell [3]. Weissman proposes the markers shown in Table 5.1 as the closest markers for mouse and human HSCs [62].

Table 5.1. Proposed cell-surface markers of undifferentiated hematopoietic stem cells.

Listed here are cell surface markers found on mouse and human hematopoietic stem cells as they exist in their undifferentiated state *in vivo* and *in vitro*. As these cells begin to develop as distinct cell lineages the cell surface markers are no longer identified.

Mouse	Human
CD34$^{low/-}$	CD 34$^+$
SCA-1$^+$	CD59^{+*}
Thy1$^{+/low}$	Thy1$^+$
CD38$^+$	CD38$^{low/-}$
C-kit$^+$	C-kit$^{-/low}$
lin^{-*}	lin^{-**}

* Only one of a family of CD59 markers has thus far been evaluated.

** Lin- cells lack 13 to 14 different mature blood-lineage markers.

Such cell markers can be tagged with monoclonal antibodies bearing a fluorescent label and culled out of bone marrow with fluorescence-activated cell sorting (FACS).

The groups of cells thus sorted by surface markers are heterogeneous and include some cells that are true, long-term self-renewing stem cells, some shorter-term progenitors, and some non-stem cells. Weissman's group showed that as few as five genetically tagged cells, injected along with larger doses of stem cells into lethally irradiated mice, could establish themselves and produce marked donor cells in all blood cell lineages for the lifetime of the mouse. A single tagged cell could produce all lineages for as many as seven weeks, and 30 purified cells were sufficient to rescue mice and fully repopulate the bone marrow without extra doses of backup cells to rescue the mice [49]. Despite these efforts, researchers remain divided on the most consistently expressed set of HSC markers [27, 32]. Connie Eaves of the University of British Columbia says none of the markers are tied to unique stem cell functions or truly define the stem cell [14]. "Almost every marker I am aware of has been shown to be fickle," she says.

More recently, Diane Krause and her colleagues at Yale University, New York University, and Johns Hopkins University, used a new technique to home in on a single cell capable of reconstituting all blood cell lineages of an irradiated mouse [27]. After marking bone marrow cells from donor male mice with a nontoxic dye, they injected the cells into female recipient mice that had been given a lethal dose of radiation. Over the next two days, some of the injected cells migrated, or homed, to the bone marrow of the recipients and did not divide; when transplanted into a second set of irradiated female mice, they eventually proved to be a concentrated pool of self-renewing stem cells. The cells also reconstituted blood production. The scientists estimate that their technique concentrated the long-term stem cells 500 to 1,000-fold compared with bone marrow.

WHAT ARE THE SOURCES OF HEMATOPOIETIC STEM CELLS?

Bone Marrow

The classic source of hematopoietic stem cells (HSCs) is bone marrow. For more than 40 years, doctors performed bone marrow transplants by anesthetizing the stem cell donor, puncturing a bone—typically a hipbone—and drawing out the bone marrow cells with a syringe. About 1 in every 100,000 cells in the marrow is a long-term, blood-forming stem cell; other cells present include stromal cells, stromal stem cells, blood progenitor cells, and mature and maturing white and red blood cells.

Peripheral Blood

As a source of HSCs for medical treatments, bone marrow retrieval directly from bone is quickly fading into history. For clinical transplantation of human HSCs, doctors now prefer to harvest donor cells from peripheral, circulating blood. It has been known for decades that a small number of stem and progenitor cells circulate in the bloodstream, but in the past 10 years, researchers have found that they can coax the cells to migrate from marrow to blood in greater numbers by injecting the donor with a cytokine, such as granulocyte-colony stimulating factor (GCSF). The donor is injected with GCSF a few days before the cell harvest. To collect the cells, doctors insert an intravenous tube into the donor's vein and pass his blood through a filtering system that pulls out CD34+ white blood cells and returns the red blood cells to the donor. Of the cells collected, just 5 to 20 percent

will be true HSCs. Thus, when medical researchers commonly refer to peripherally harvested "stem cells," this is something of a misnomer. As is true for bone marrow, the CD34+ cells are a mixture of stem cells, progenitors, and white blood cells of various degrees of maturity.

In the past three years, the majority of autologous (where the donor and recipient are the same person) and allogeneic (where the donor and recipient are different individuals) "bone marrow" transplants have actually been white blood cells drawn from peripheral circulation, not bone marrow. Richard Childs, an intramural investigator at the NIH, says peripheral harvest of cells is easier on the donor—with minimal pain, no anesthesia, and no hospital stay—but also yields better cells for transplants [6]. Childs points to evidence that patients receiving peripherally harvested cells have higher survival rates than bone marrow recipients do. The peripherally harvested cells contain twice as many HSCs as stem cells taken from bone marrow and engraft more quickly. This means patients may recover white blood cells, platelets, and their immune and clotting protection several days faster than they would with a bone marrow graft. Scientists at Stanford report that highly purified, mobilized peripheral cells that have CD34+ and Thy-1+ surface markers engraft swiftly and without complication in breast cancer patients receiving an autologous transplant of the cells after intensive chemotherapy [41].

Umbilical Cord Blood

In the late 1980s and early 1990s, physicians began to recognize that blood from the human umbilical cord and placenta was a rich source of HSCs. This tissue supports the developing fetus during pregnancy, is delivered along with the baby, and, is usually discarded. Since the first successful umbilical cord blood transplants in children with Fanconi anemia, the collection and therapeutic use of these cells has grown quickly. The New York Blood Center's Placental Blood Program, supported by NIH, is the largest U.S. public umbilical cord blood bank and now has 13,000 donations available for transplantation into small patients who need HSCs. Since it began collecting umbilical cord blood in 1992, the center has provided thousands of cord blood units to patients. Umbilical cord blood recipients—typically children—have now lived in excess of eight years, relying on the HSCs from an umbilical cord blood transplant [31, 57].

There is a substantial amount of research being conducted on umbilical cord blood to search for ways to expand the number of HSCs and compare and contrast the biological properties of cord blood with adult bone marrow stem cells. There have been suggestions that umbilical cord blood contains stem cells that have the capability of developing cells of multiple germ layers (multipotent) or even all germ layers, e.g., endoderm, ectoderm, and mesoderm (pluripotent). To date, there is no published scientific evidence to support this claim. While umbilical cord blood represents a valuable resource for HSCs, research data have not conclusively shown qualitative differences in the differentiated cells produced between this source of HSCs and peripheral blood and bone marrow.

Fetal Hematopoietic System

An important source of HSCs in research, but not in clinical use, is the developing blood-producing tissues of fetal animals. Hematopoietic cells appear early in the development of all vertebrates. Most extensively studied in the mouse, HSC production sweeps through the developing embryo and fetus in waves. Beginning at about day 7 in the life of the mouse embryo, the earliest hematopoietic activity is indicated by the appearance of blood islands in the yolk sac (see Appendix A. Early Development). The point is disputed, but some scientists contend that yolk sac blood production is transient and will generate some blood cells for the embryo, but probably not the bulk of the HSCs for the adult animal [12, 26, 44]. According to this proposed scenario, most stem cells that will be found in the adult bone marrow and circulation are derived from cells that appear slightly later and in a different location. This other wave of hematopoietic stem cell production occurs in the AGM—the region where the aorta, gonads, and fetal kidney (mesonephros) begin to develop. The cells that give rise to the HSCs in the AGM may also give rise to endothelial cells that line blood vessels. [13]. These HSCs arise at around days 10 to 11 in the mouse embryo (weeks 4 to 6 in human gestation), divide, and within a couple of days, migrate to the liver [11]. The HSCs in the liver continue to divide and migrate, spreading to the spleen, thymus, and—near the time of birth—to the bone marrow.

Whereas an increasing body of fetal HSC research is emerging from mice and other animals, there is much less information about human fetal and embryonic HSCs. Scientists in Europe, including Coulombel, Peault, and colleagues, first described hematopoietic precursors in human embryos only a few years ago [20, 53]. Most recently, Gallacher and others reported finding HSCs circulating in the blood of 12- to 18-week aborted human fetuses [16, 28, 54] that was rich in HSCs. These circulating cells had different markers than did cells from fetal liver, fetal bone marrow, or umbilical cord blood.

Embryonic Stem Cells and Embryonic Germ Cells

In 1985, it was shown that it is possible to obtain precursors to many different blood cells from mouse embryonic stem cells [9]. Perkins was able to obtain all the major lineages of progenitor cells from mouse embryoid bodies, even without adding hematopoietic growth factors [45].

Mouse embryonic stem cells in culture, given the right growth factors, can generate most, if not all, the different blood cell types [19], but no one has yet achieved the "gold standard" of proof that they can produce long-term HSCs from these sources—namely by obtaining cells that can be transplanted into lethally irradiated mice to reconstitute long-term hematopoiesis [32].

The picture for human embryonic stem and germ cells is even less clear. Scientists from James Thomson's laboratory reported in 1999 that they were able to direct human embryonic stem cells—which can now be cultured in the lab—to produce blood progenitor cells [23]. Israeli scientists reported that they had induced human ES cells to produce hematopoietic cells, as evidenced by their production of a blood protein, gamma-globin [21]. Cell lines derived from human embryonic germ cells (cultured cells derived originally from cells in the embryo that would ultimately give rise to eggs or sperm) that are cultured under certain conditions will produce CD34+ cells [47]. The blood-producing cells derived from human ES and embryonic germ (EG) cells have not been rigorously tested for long-term self-renewal or the ability to give rise to all the different blood cells.

As sketchy as data may be on the hematopoietic powers of human ES and EG cells, blood experts are intrigued by their clinical potential and their potential to answer basic questions on renewal and differentiation of HSCs [19]. Connie Eaves, who has made comparisons of HSCs from fetal liver, cord blood,

The Stem Cell Database
http://stemcell.princeton.edu

Ihor Lemischka and colleagues at Princeton University and the Computational Biology and Informatics Laboratory at the University of Pennsylvania are collaborating to record all the findings about hematopoietic stem cell (HSC) genes and markers in the Stem Cell Database.

The collaborators started the database five years ago. Its goal is listing and annotating all the genes that are differentially expressed in mouse liver HSCs and their cellular progeny. The database is growing to include human HSCs from different blood sources, and a

related database, constructed in collaboration with Kateri A. Moore, also at Princeton University, will document all genes active in stromal cells, which provide the microenvironment in which stem cells are maintained. The combined power of the two databases, along with new tools and methods for studying molecular biology, will help researchers put together a complete portrait of the hematopoietic stem cell and how it works. The databases will continue to grow and take advantage of other efforts, such as those to complete the gene sequences of mammals. Data will be publicly available to researchers around the world.

and adult bone marrow, expects cells derived from embryonic tissues to have some interesting traits. She says actively dividing blood-producing cells from ES cell culture—if they are like other dividing cells—will not themselves engraft or rescue hematopoiesis in an animal whose bone marrow has been destroyed. However, they may play a critical role in developing an abundant supply of HSCs grown in the lab. Indications are that the dividing cells will also more readily lend themselves to gene manipulations than do adult HSCs. Eaves anticipates that HSCs derived from early embryo sources will be developmentally more "plastic" than later HSCs, and more capable of self-renewal [14].

HOW DO HSCs FROM VARYING SOURCES DIFFER?

Scientists in the laboratory and clinic are beginning to measure the differences among HSCs from different sources. In general, they find that HSCs taken from tissues at earlier developmental stages have a greater ability to self-replicate, show different homing and surface characteristics, and are less likely to be rejected by the immune system—making them potentially more useful for therapeutic transplantation.

Stem cell populations of the bone marrow
When do HSCs move from the early locations in the developing fetus to their adult "home" in the bone marrow? European scientists have found that the relative number of CD34+ cells in the collections of cord blood declined with gestational age, but expression of cell-adhesion molecules on these cells increased.

The authors believe these changes reflect preparations for the cells to relocate—from homing in fetal liver to homing in bone marrow [52].

The point is controversial, but a paper by Chen et al. provides evidence that at least in some strains of mice, HSCs from old mice are less able to repopulate bone marrow after transplantation than are cells from young adult mice [5]. Cells from fetal mice were 50 to 100 percent better at repopulating marrow than were cells from young adult mice were. The specific potential for repopulating marrow appears to be strain-specific, but the scientists found this potential declined with age for both strains. Other scientists find no decreases or sometimes increases in numbers of HSCs with age [51]. Because of the difficulty in identifying a long-term stem cell, it remains difficult to quantify changes in numbers of HSCs as a person ages.

Effectiveness of Transplants of Adult versus Umbilical Cord Blood Stem Cells
A practical and important difference between HSCs collected from adult human donors and from umbilical cord blood is simply quantitative. Doctors are rarely able to extract more than a few million HSCs from a placenta and umbilical cord—too few to use in a transplant for an adult, who would ideally get 7 to 10 million CD34+ cells per kilogram body weight, but often adequate for a transplant for a child [33, 48].

Leonard Zon says that HSCs from cord blood are less likely to cause a transplantation complication called graft-versus-host disease, in which white blood cells from a donor attack tissues of the recipient [65]. In a recent review of umbilical cord blood transplantation, Laughlin cites evidence that cord blood causes less graft-versus-host disease [31]. Laughlin writes that it is yet to be determined whether umbilical cord blood HSCs are, in fact, longer lived in a transplant recipient.

In lab and mouse-model tests comparing CD34+ cells from human cord with CD34+ cells derived from adult bone marrow, researchers found cord blood had greater proliferation capacity [24]. White blood cells from cord blood engrafted better in a mouse model, which was genetically altered to tolerate the human cells, than did their adult counterparts.

Effectiveness in Transplants of Peripheral Versus Bone Marrow Stem Cells

In addition to being far easier to collect, peripherally harvested white blood cells have other advantages over bone marrow. Cutler and Antin's review says that peripherally harvested cells engraft more quickly, but are more likely to cause graft-versus-host disease [8]. Prospecting for the most receptive HSCs for gene therapy, Orlic and colleagues found that mouse HSCs mobilized with cytokines were more likely to take up genes from a viral vector than were non-mobilized bone marrow HSCs [43].

WHAT DO HEMATOPOIETIC STEM CELLS DO AND WHAT FACTORS ARE INVOLVED IN THESE ACTIVITIES?

As stated earlier, an HSC in the bone marrow has four actions in its repertoire: 1) it can renew itself, 2) it can differentiate, 3) it can mobilize out of the bone marrow into circulation (or the reverse), or 4) it can undergo programmed cell death, or apoptosis. Understanding the how, when, where, which, and why of this simple repertoire will allow researchers to manipulate and use HSCs for tissue and organ repair.

Self-renewal of Hematopoietic Stem Cells

Scientists have had a tough time trying to grow— or even maintain—true stem cells in culture. This is an important goal because cultures of HSCs that could maintain their characteristic properties of self-renewal and lack of differentiation could provide an unlimited source of cells for therapeutic transplantation and study. When bone marrow or blood cells are observed in culture, one often observes large increases in the number of cells. This usually reflects an increase in

differentiation of cells to progenitor cells that can give rise to different lineages of blood cells but cannot renew themselves. True stem cells divide and replace themselves slowly in adult bone marrow.

New tools for gene-expression analysis will now allow scientists to study developmental changes in telomerase activity and telomeres. Telomeres are regions of DNA found at the end of chromosomes that are extended by the enzyme telomerase. Telomerase activity is necessary for cells to proliferate and activity decreases with age leading to shortened telomeres. Scientists hypothesize that declines in stem cell renewal will be associated with declines in telomere length and telomerase activity. Telomerase activity in hematopoietic cells is associated with self-renewal potential [40].

Because self-renewal divisions are rare, hard to induce in culture, and difficult to prove, scientists do not have a definitive answer to the burning question: what puts—or perhaps keeps—HSCs in a self-renewal division mode? HSCs injected into an anemic patient or mouse—or one whose HSCs have otherwise been suppressed or killed—will home to the bone marrow and undergo active division to both replenish all the different types of blood cells and yield additional self-renewing HSCs. But exactly how this happens remains a mystery that scientists are struggling to solve by manipulating cultures of HSCs in the laboratory.

Two recent examples of progress in the culturing studies of mouse HSCs are by Ema and coworkers and Audet and colleagues [2, 15]. Ema et al. found that two cytokines—stem cell factor and thrombopoietin—efficiently induced an unequal first cell division in which one daughter cell gave rise to repopulating cells with self-renewal potential. Audet et al. found that activation of the signaling molecule gp130 is critical to survival and proliferation of mouse HSCs in culture.

Work with specific cytokines and signaling molecules builds on several earlier studies demonstrating modest increases in the numbers of stem cells that could be induced briefly in culture. For example, Van Zant and colleagues used continuous-perfusion culture and bioreactors in an attempt to boost human HSC numbers in single cord blood samples incubated for one to two weeks [58]. They obtained a 20-fold increase in "long-term culture initiating cells."

More clues on how to increase numbers of stem cells may come from looking at other animals and various developmental stages. During early developmental stages—in the fetal liver, for example—HSCs may undergo more active cell division to increase their numbers, but later in life, they divide far less often [30, 42]. Culturing HSCs from 10- and 11-day-old mouse embryos, Elaine Dzierzak at Erasmus University in the Netherlands finds she can get a 15-fold increase in HSCs within the first 2 or 3 days after she removes the AGM from the embryos [38]. Dzierzak recognizes that this is dramatically different from anything seen with adult stem cells and suggests it is a difference with practical importance. She suspects that the increase is not so much a response to what is going on in the culture but rather, it represents the developmental momentum of this specific embryonic tissue. That is, it is the inevitable consequence of divisions that were cued by that specific embryonic microenvironment. After five days, the number of HSCs plateaus and can be maintained for up to a month. Dzierzak says that the key to understanding how adult-derived HSCs can be expanded and manipulated for clinical purposes may very well be found by defining the cellular composition and complex molecular signals in the AGM region during development [13].

In another approach, Lemischka and coworkers have been able to maintain mouse HSCs for four to seven weeks when they are grown on a clonal line of cells (AFT024) derived from the stroma, the other major cellular constituent of bone marrow [39]. No one knows which specific factors secreted by the stromal cells maintain the stem cells. He says ongoing gene cloning is rapidly zeroing in on novel molecules from the stromal cells that may "talk" to the stem cells and persuade them to remain stem cells—that is, continue to divide and not differentiate.

If stromal factors provide the key to stem cell self-renewal, research on maintaining stromal cells may be an important prerequisite. In 1999, researchers at Osiris Therapeutics and Johns Hopkins University reported culturing and expanding the numbers of mesenchymal stem cells, which produce the stromal environment [46]. Whereas cultured HSCs rush to differentiate and fail to retain primitive, self-renewing cells, the mesenchymal stem cells could be increased in numbers and still retained their powers to generate the full repertoire of descendant lineages.

Differentiation of HSCs into Components of the Blood and Immune System

Producing differentiated white and red blood cells is the real work of HSCs and progenitor cells. M.C. MacKey calculates that in the course of producing a mature, circulating blood cell, the original hematopoietic stem cell will undergo between 17 and 19.5 divisions, "giving a net amplification of between ~170,000 and ~720,000" [35].

Through a series of careful studies of cultured cells—often cells with mutations found in leukemia patients or cells that have been genetically altered—investigators have discovered many key growth factors and cytokines that induce progenitor cells to make different types of blood cells. These factors interact with one another in complex ways to create a system of exquisite genetic control and coordination of blood cell production.

Migration of Hematopoietic Stem Cells Into and Out of Marrow and Tissues

Scientists know that much of the time, HSCs live in intimate connection with the stroma of bone marrow in adults (see Chapter 4. The Adult Stem Cell). But HSCs may also be found in the spleen, in peripheral blood circulation, and other tissues. Connection to the interstices of bone marrow is important to both the engraftment of transplanted cells and to the maintenance of stem cells as a self-renewing population. Connection to stroma is also important to the orderly proliferation, differentiation, and maturation of blood cells [63].

Weissman says HSCs appear to make brief forays out of the marrow into tissues, then duck back into marrow [62]. At this time, scientists do not understand why or how HSCs leave bone marrow or return to it [59]. Scientists find that HSCs that have been mobilized into peripheral circulation are mostly non-dividing cells [64]. They report that adhesion molecules on the stroma, play a role in mobilization, in attachment to the stroma, and in transmitting signals that regulate HSC self-renewal and progenitor differentiation [61].

Apoptosis and Regulation of Hematopoietic Stem Cell Populations

The number of blood cells in the bone marrow and blood is regulated by genetic and molecular mechanisms. How do hematopoietic stem cells know when to stop proliferating? Apoptosis is the process of programmed cell death that leads cells to self-destruct when they are unneeded or detrimental. If there are too few HSCs in the body, more cells divide and boost the numbers. If excess stem cells were injected into an animal, they simply wouldn't divide or would undergo apoptosis and be eliminated [62]. Excess numbers of stem cells in an HSC transplant actually seem to improve the likelihood and speed of engraftment, though there seems to be no rigorous identification of a mechanism for this empirical observation.

The particular signals that trigger apoptosis in HSCs are as yet unknown. One possible signal for apoptosis might be the absence of life-sustaining signals from bone marrow stroma. Michael Wang and others found that when they used antibodies to disrupt the adhesion of HSCs to the stroma via VLA-4/VCAM-1, the cells were predisposed to apoptosis [61].

Understanding the forces at play in HSC apoptosis is important to maintaining or increasing their numbers in culture. For example, without growth factors, supplied in the medium or through serum or other feeder layers of cells, HSCs undergo apoptosis. Domen and Weissman found that stem cells need to get two growth factor signals to continue life and avoid apoptosis: one via a protein called BCL-2, the other from steel factor, which, by itself, induces HSCs to produce progenitor cells but not to self-renew [10].

WHAT ARE THE CLINICAL USES OF HEMATOPOIETIC STEM CELLS?

Leukemia and Lymphoma

Among the first clinical uses of HSCs were the treatment of cancers of the blood—leukemia and lymphoma, which result from the uncontrolled proliferation of white blood cells. In these applications, the patient's own cancerous hematopoietic cells were destroyed via radiation or chemotherapy, then replaced with a bone marrow transplant, or, as is done now, with a transplant of HSCs collected from the peripheral circulation of a matched donor. A matched donor is typically a sister or brother of the patient who has inherited similar human leukocyte antigens (HLAs) on the surface of their cells. Cancers of the blood include acute lymphoblastic leukemia, acute myeloblastic leukemia, chronic myelogenous leukemia (CML), Hodgkin's disease, multiple myeloma, and non-Hodgkin's lymphoma.

Thomas and Clift describe the history of treatment for chronic myeloid leukemia as it moved from largely ineffective chemotherapy to modestly successful use of a cytokine, interferon, to bone marrow transplants—first in identical twins, then in HLA-matched siblings [55]. Although there was significant risk of patient death soon after the transplant either from infection or from graft-versus-host disease, for the first time, many patients survived this immediate challenge and had survival times measured in years or even decades, rather than months. The authors write, "In the space of 20 years, marrow transplantation has contributed to the transformation of [chronic myelogenous leukemia] CML from a fatal disease to one that is frequently curable. At the same time, experience acquired in this setting has improved our understanding of many transplant-related problems. It is now clear that morbidity and mortality are not inevitable consequences of allogeneic transplantation, [and] that an allogeneic effect can add to the anti-leukemic power of conditioning regimens..."

In a recent development, CML researchers have taken their knowledge of hematopoietic regulation one step farther. On May 10, 2001, the Food and Drug Administration approved Gleevec™ (imatinib mesylate), a new, rationally designed oral drug for treatment of CML. The new drug specifically targets a mutant protein, produced in CML cancer cells, that sabotages the cell signals controlling orderly division of progenitor cells. By silencing this protein, the new drug turns off cancerous overproduction of white blood cells, so doctors do not have to resort to bone marrow transplantation. At this time, it is unknown whether the new drug will provide sustained remission or will prolong life for CML patients.

Inherited Blood Disorders

Another use of allogeneic bone marrow transplants is in the treatment of hereditary blood disorders, such as different types of inherited anemia (failure to produce blood cells), and inborn errors of metabolism (genetic disorders characterized by defects in key enzymes need to produce essential body components or degrade chemical byproducts). The blood disorders include aplastic anemia, beta-thalassemia, Blackfan-Diamond syndrome, globoid cell leukodystrophy, sickle-cell anemia, severe combined immunodeficiency, X-linked lymphoproliferative syndrome, and Wiskott-Aldrich syndrome. Inborn errors of metabolism that are treated with bone marrow

The National Marrow Donor Program
http://www.marrow.org

Launched in 1987, the National Marrow Donor Program (NMDP) was created to connect patients who need blood-forming stem cells or bone marrow with potential nonrelated donors. About 70 percent of patients who need a life-saving HSC transplant cannot find a match in their own family.

The NMDP is made up of an international network of centers and banks that collect cord blood, bone marrow, and peripherally harvested stem cells and that recruit potential donors. As of February 28, 2001, the NMDP listed 4,291,434 potential donors. Since its start, the Minneapolis-based group has facilitated almost 12,000 transplants—75 percent of them for leukemia. Major recruiting efforts have led to substantial increases in the number of donations from minorities, but the chance that African Americans, Native Americans, Asian/Pacific Islanders, or Hispanics will find a match is still lower than it is for Caucasians.

transplants include: Hunter's syndrome, Hurler's syndrome, Lesch Nyhan syndrome, and osteopetrosis. Because bone marrow transplantation has carried a significant risk of death, this is usually a treatment of last resort for otherwise fatal diseases.

Hematopoietic Stem Cell Rescue in Cancer Chemotherapy
Chemotherapy aimed at rapidly dividing cancer cells inevitably hits another target—rapidly dividing hematopoietic cells. Doctors may give cancer patients an autologous stem cell transplant to replace the cells destroyed by chemotherapy. They do this by mobilizing HSCs and collecting them from peripheral blood. The cells are stored while the patient undergoes intensive chemotherapy or radiotherapy to destroy the cancer cells. Once the drugs have washed out of a patient's body, the patient receives a transfusion of his or her stored HSCs. Because patients get their own cells back, there is no chance of immune mismatch or graft-versus-host disease. One problem with the use of autologous HSC transplants in cancer therapy has been that cancer cells are sometimes inadvertently collected and reinfused back into the patient along with the stem cells. One team of investigators finds that they can prevent reintroducing cancer cells by purifying the cells and preserving only the cells that are CD34+, Thy-1+ [41].

Graft-Versus-Tumor Treatment of Cancer
One of the most exciting new uses of HSC transplantation puts the cells to work attacking otherwise untreatable tumors. A group of researchers in NIH's intramural research program recently described this approach to treating metastatic kidney cancer [7]. Just under half of the 38 patients treated so far have had their tumors reduced. The research protocol is now expanding to treatment of other solid tumors that resist standard therapy, including cancer of the lung, prostate, ovary, colon, esophagus, liver, and pancreas.

This experimental treatment relies on an allogeneic stem cell transplant from an HLA-matched sibling whose HSCs are collected peripherally. The patient's own immune system is suppressed, but not totally destroyed. The donor's cells are transfused into the patient, and for the next three months, doctors closely monitor the patient's immune cells, using DNA fingerprinting to follow the engraftment of the donor's cells and regrowth of the patient's own blood cells. They must also judiciously suppress the patient's immune system as needed to deter his/her T cells from attacking the graft and to reduce graft-versus-host disease.

A study by Joshi et al. shows that umbilical cord blood and peripherally harvested human HSCs show antitumor activity in the test tube against leukemia cells and breast cancer cells [22]. Grafted into a mouse model that tolerates human cells, HSCs attack human leukemia and breast cancer cells. Although untreated cord blood lacks natural killer (NK) lymphocytes capable of killing tumor cells, researchers have found that at least in the test tube and in mice, they can greatly enhance the activity and numbers of these cells with cytokines IL-15 [22, 34].

Other Applications of Hematopoietic Stem Cells
Substantial basic and limited clinical research exploring the experimental uses of HSCs for other diseases is underway. Among the primary applications are autoimmune diseases, such as diabetes, rheumatoid

arthritis, and system lupus erythematosis. Here, the body's immune system turns to destroying body tissues. Experimental approaches similar to those applied above for cancer therapies are being conducted to see if the immune system can be reconstituted or reprogrammed. More detailed discussion on this application is provided in Chapter 6. Autoimmune Diseases and the Promise of Stem Cell-Based Therapies. The use of HSCs as a means to deliver genes to repair damaged cells is another application being explored. The use of HSCs for gene therapies is discussed in detail in Chapter 11. Use of Genetically Modified Stem Cells in Experimental Gene Therapies.

PLASTICITY OF HEMATOPOIETIC STEM CELLS

A few recent reports indicate that scientists have been able to induce bone marrow or HSCs to differentiate into other types of tissue, such as brain, muscle, and liver cells. These concepts and the experimental evidence supporting this concept are discussed in Chapter 4. The Adult Stem Cell.

Research in a mouse model indicates that cells from grafts of bone marrow or selected HSCs may home to damaged skeletal and cardiac muscle or liver and regenerate those tissues [4, 29]. One recent advance has been in the study of muscular dystrophy, a genetic disease that occurs in young people and leads to progressive weakness of the skeletal muscles. Bittner and colleagues used *mdx* mice, a genetically modified mouse with muscle cell defects similar to those in human muscular dystrophy. Bone marrow from non-*mdx* male mice was transplanted into female *mdx* mice with chronic muscle damage; after 70 days, researchers found that nuclei from the males had taken up residence in skeletal and cardiac muscle cells.

Lagasse and colleagues' demonstration of liver repair by purified HSCs is a similarly encouraging sign that HSCs may have the potential to integrate into and grow in some non-blood tissues. These scientists lethally irradiated female mice that had an unusual genetic liver disease that could be halted with a drug. The mice were given transplants of genetically marked, purified HSCs from male mice that did not have the liver disease. The transplants were given a chance to engraft for a couple of months while the

mice were on the liver-protective drug. The drug was then removed, launching deterioration of the liver—and a test to see whether cells from the transplant would be recruited and rescue the liver. The scientists found that transplants of as few as 50 cells led to abundant growth of marked, donor-derived liver cells in the female mice.

Recently, Krause has shown in mice that a *single* selected donor hematopoietic stem cell could do more than just repopulate the marrow and hematopoietic system of the recipient [27]. These investigators also found epithelial cells derived from the donors in the lungs, gut, and skin of the recipient mice. This suggests that HSCs may have grown in the other tissues in response to infection or damage from the irradiation the mice received.

In humans, observations of male liver cells in female patients who have received bone marrow grafts from males, and in male patients who have received liver transplants from female donors, also suggest the possibility that some cells in bone marrow have the capacity to integrate into the liver and form hepatocytes [1].

WHAT ARE THE BARRIERS TO THE DEVELOPMENT OF NEW AND IMPROVED TREATMENTS USING HEMATOPOIETIC STEM CELLS?

Boosting the Numbers of Hematopoietic Stem Cells

Clinical investigators share the same fundamental problem as basic investigators—limited ability to grow and expand the numbers of human HSCs. Clinicians repeatedly see that larger numbers of cells in stem cell grafts have a better chance of survival in a patient than do smaller numbers of cells. The limited number of cells available from a placenta and umbilical cord blood transplant currently means that cord blood banks are useful to pediatric but not adult patients. Investigators believe that the main cause of failure of HSCs to engraft is host-versus-graft disease, and larger grafts permit at least some donor cells to escape initial waves of attack from a patient's residual or suppressed immune system [6]. Ability to expand numbers of human HSCs *in vivo* or *in vitro* would clearly be an enormous boost to all current and future medical uses of HSC transplantation.

Once stem cells and their progeny can be multiplied in culture, gene therapists and blood experts could combine their talents to grow limitless quantities of "universal donor" stem cells, as well as progenitors and specific types of red and white blood cells. If the cells were engineered to be free of markers that provoke rejection, these could be transfused to any recipient to treat any of the diseases that are now addressed with marrow, peripheral, cord, or other transfused blood. If gene therapy and studies of the plasticity of HSCs succeed, the cells could also be grown to repair other tissues and treat non-blood-related disorders [32].

Several research groups in the United States, Canada, and abroad have been striving to find the key factor or factors for boosting HSC production. Typical approaches include comparing genes expressed in primitive HSCs versus progenitor cells; comparing genes in actively dividing fetal HSCs versus adult HSCs; genetic screening of hematopoietically mutated zebrafish; studying dysregulated genes in cancerous hematopoietic cells; analyzing stromal or feeder-layer factors that appear to boost HSC division; and analyzing factors promoting homing and attachment to the stroma. Promising candidate factors have been tried singly and in combination, and researchers claim they can now increase the number of long-term stem cells 20-fold, albeit briefly, in culture.

The specific assays researchers use to prove that their expanded cells are stem cells vary, which makes it difficult to compare the claims of different research groups. To date, there is only a modest ability to expand true, long-term, self-renewing human HSCs. Numbers of progenitor cells are, however, more readily increased. Kobari et al., for example, can increase progenitor cells for granulocytes and macrophages 278-fold in culture [25].

Some investigators are now evaluating whether these comparatively modest increases in HSCs are clinically useful. At this time, the increases in cell numbers are not sustainable over periods beyond a few months, and the yield is far too low for mass production. In addition, the cells produced are often not rigorously characterized. A host of other questions remain— from how well the multiplied cells can be altered for gene therapy to their potential longevity, immunogenicity, ability to home correctly, and susceptibility to

cancerous transformation. Glimm et al. [17] highlight some of these problems, for example, with their confirmation that human stem cells lose their ability to repopulate the bone marrow as they enter and progress through the cell cycleælike mouse stem cells that have been stimulated to divide lose their transplantability [18]. Observations on the inverse relationship between progenitor cell division rate and longevity in strains of mice raise an additional concern that culture tricks or selection of cells that expand rapidly may doom the cells to a short life.

Pragmatically, some scientists say it may not be necessary to be able to induce the true, long-term HSC to divide in the lab. If they can manipulate progenitors and coax them into division on command, gene uptake, and differentiation into key blood cells and other tissues, that may be sufficient to accomplish clinical goals. It might be sufficient to boost HSCs or subpopulations of hematopoietic cells within the body by chemically prodding the bone marrow to supply the as-yet-elusive factors to rejuvenate cell division.

Outfoxing the Immune System in Host, Graft, and Pathogen Attacks

Currently, the risks of bone marrow transplants—graft rejection, host-versus-graft disease, and infection during the period before HSCs have engrafted and resumed full blood cell production—restrict their use to patients with serious or fatal illnesses. Allogeneic grafts must come from donors with a close HLA match to the patient (see Chapter 6. Autoimmune Diseases and the Promise of Stem Cell-Based Therapies). If doctors could precisely manipulate immune reactions and protect patients from pathogens before their transplants begin to function, HSC transplants could be extended to less ill patients and patients for whom the HLA match was not as close as it must now be. Physicians might use transplants with greater impunity in gene therapy, autoimmune disease, HIV/AIDS treatment, and the preconditioning of patients to accept a major organ transplant.

Scientists are zeroing in on subpopulations of T cells that may cause or suppress potentially lethal host-versus-graft rejection and graft-versus-host disease in allogeneic-transplant recipients. T cells in a graft are a two-edged sword. They fight infections and help the graft become established, but they also can cause graft-versus-host disease. Identifying sub-populations of T cells responsible for deleterious and beneficial effects—in the graft, but also in residual cells surviving or returning in the host—could allow clinicians to make grafts safer and to ratchet up graft-versus-tumor effects [48]. Understanding the presentation of antigens to the immune system and the immune system's healthy and unhealthy responses to these antigens and maturation and programmed cell death of T cells is crucial.

The approach taken by investigators at Stanford—purifying peripheral blood—may also help eliminate the cells causing graft-versus-host disease. Transplants in mouse models support the idea that purified HSCs, cleansed of mature lymphocytes, engraft readily and avoid graft-versus-host disease [60].

Knowledge of the key cellular actors in autoimmune disease, immune grafting, and graft rejection could also permit scientists to design gentler "minitrans-plants." Rather than obliterating and replacing the patient's entire hematopoietic system, they could replace just the faulty components with a selection of cells custom tailored to the patient's needs. Clinicians are currently experimenting with deletion of T cells from transplants in some diseases, for example, thereby reducing graft-versus-host disease.

Researchers are also experimenting with the possibility of knocking down the patient's immune system—but not knocking it out. A blow that is sublethal to the patient's hematopoietic cells given before an allo-geneic transplant can be enough to give the graft a chance to take up residence in the bone marrow. The cells replace some or all of the patient's original stem cells, often making their blood a mix of donor and original cells. For some patients, this mix of cells will be enough to accomplish treatment objectives but without subjecting them to the vicious side effects and infection hazards of the most powerful treatments used for total destruction of their hemato-poietic systems [37].

Understanding the Differentiating Environment and Developmental Plasticity

At some point in embryonic development, all cells are plastic, or developmentally flexible enough to grow into a variety of different tissues. Exactly what is it about the cell or the embryonic environment that instructs cells to grow into one organ and not another?

Could there be embryological underpinnings to the apparent plasticity of adult cells? Researchers have suggested that a lot of the tissues that are showing plasticity are adjacent to one another after gastru-lation in the sheet of mesodermal tissue that will go on to form blood—muscle, blood vessels, kidney, mesenchyme, and notochord. Plasticity may reflect derivation from the mesoderm, rather than being a fixed trait of hematopoietic cells. One lab is now studying the adjacency of embryonic cells and how the developing embryo makes the decision to make one tissue instead of another—and whether the decision is reversible [65].

In vivo studies of the plasticity of bone marrow or purified stem cells injected into mice are in their infancy. Even if follow-up studies confirm and more precisely characterize and quantify plasticity potential of HSCs in mice, there is no guarantee that it will occur or can be induced in humans.

SUMMARY

Grounded in half a century of research, the study of hematopoietic stem cells is one of the most exciting and rapidly advancing disciplines in biomedicine today. Breakthrough discoveries in both the laboratory and clinic have sharply expanded the use and supply of life-saving stem cells. Yet even more promising applications are on the horizon and scientists' current inability to grow HSCs outside the body could delay or thwart progress with these new therapies. New treatments include graft-versus-tumor therapy for currently incurable cancers, autologous transplants for autoimmune diseases, and gene therapy and tissue repair for a host of other problems. The techniques, cells, and knowledge that researchers have now are inadequate to realize the full promise of HSC-based therapy.

Key issues for tapping the potential of hematopoietic stem cells will be finding ways to safely and efficiently expand the numbers of transplantable human HSCs in vitro or in vivo. It will also be important to gain a better understanding of the fundamentals of how immune cells work—in fighting infections, in causing transplant rejection, and in graft-versus-host disease as well as master the basics of HSC differentiation. Concomitant advances in gene therapy techniques and the understanding of cellular plasticity could make HSCs one of the most powerful tools for healing.

REFERENCES

1. Alison, M.R., Poulsom, R., Jeffery, R., Dhillon, A.P., Quaglia, A., Jacob, J., Novelli, M., Prentice, G., Williamson, J., and Wright, N.A. (2000). Hepatocytes from non-hepatic adult stem cells. Nature. *406*, 257.

2. Audet, J., Miller, C.L., Rose-John, S., Piret, J.M., and Eaves, C.J. (2001). Distinct role of gp130 activation in promoting self-renewal divisions by mitogenically stimulated murine hematopoietic stem cells. Proc. Natl. Acad. Sci. U. S. A. *98*, 1757-1762.

3. Baum, C.M., Weissman, I.L., Tsukamoto, A.S., Buckle, A.M., and Peault, B. (1992). Isolation of a candidate human hematopoietic stem-cell population. Proc. Natl. Acad. Sci. U. S. A. *89*, 2804-2808.

4. Bittner, R.E., Schofer, C., Weipoltshammer, K., Ivanova, S., Streubel, B., Hauser, E., Freilinger, M., Hoger, H., Elbe-Burger, A., and Wachtler, F. (1999). Recruitment of bone-marrow-derived cells by skeletal and cardiac muscle in adult dystrophic mdx mice. Anat. Embryol. (Berl) *199*, 391-396.

5. Chen, J., Astle, C.M., and Harrison, D.E. (1999). Development and aging of primitive hematopoietic stem cells in BALB/cBy mice. Exp. Hematol. *27*, 928-935.

6. Childs, R., personal communication.

7. Childs, R., Chernoff, A., Contentin, N., Bahceci, E., Schrump, D., Leitman, S., Read, E.J., Tisdale, J., Dunbar, C., Linehan, W.M., Young, N.S., and Barrett, A.J. (2000). Regression of metastatic renal-cell carcinoma after nonmyeloablative allogeneic peripheral-blood stem-cell transplantation. N. Engl. J. Med. *343*, 750-758.

8. Cutler, C. and Antin, J.H. (2001). Peripheral blood stem cells for allogeneic transplantation: a review. Stem Cells. *19*, 108-117.

9. Doetschman, T., Eistetter, H., Katz, M., Schmit, W., and Kemler, R. (1985). The *in vitro* development of blastocyst-derived embryonic stem cell lines: formation of visceral yolk sac, blood islands and myocardium. J. Embryol. Exp. Morph. *87*, 27-45.

10. Domen, J. and Weissman, I.L. (2000). Hematopoietic stem cells need two signals to prevent apoptosis; BCL-2 can provide one of these, Kitl/c-Kit signaling the other. J. Exp. Med. *192*, 1707-1718.

11. Dzierzak, E., Medvinsky, A., and de Bruijn, M. (1998). Qualitative and quantitative aspects of haematopoietic cell development in the mammalian embryo. Immunol. Today. *19*, 228-236.

12. Dzierzak, E. (1999). Embryonic beginnings of definitive hematopoietic stem cells. Ann. N. Y. Acad. Sci. *872*, 256-262.

13. Dzierzak, E., personal communication.

14. Eaves, C. J., personal communication.

15. Ema, H., Takano, H., Sudo, K., and Nakauchi, H. (2000). *In vitro* self-renewal division of hematopoietic stem cells. J. Exp. Med. *192*, 1281-1288.

16. Gallacher, L., Murdoch, B., Wu, D., Karanu, F., Fellows, F., and Bhatia, M. (2000). Identification of novel circulating human embryonic blood stem cells. Blood. *96*, 1740-1747.

17. Glimm, H., Oh, I.H., and Eaves, C.J. (2000). Human hematopoietic stem cells stimulated to proliferate *in vitro* lose engraftment potential during their S/G(2)/M transit and do not reenter G(0). Blood. *96*, 4185-4193.

18. Gothot, A., van der Loo, J.C., Clapp, D.W., and Srour, E.F. (1998). Cell cycle-related changes in repopulating capacity of human mobilized peripheral blood CD34+ cells in non-obese diabetic/severe combined immune-deficient mice. Blood. *92*, 2641-2649.

19. Hole, N. (1999). Embryonic stem cell-derived haematopoiesis. Cells Tissues Organs. *165*, 181-189.

20. Huyhn, A., Dommergues, M., Izac, B., Croisille, L., Katz, A., Vainchenker, W., and Coulombel, L. (1995). Characterization of hematopoietic progenitors from human yolk sacs and embryos. Blood. *86*, 4474-4485.

21. Itskovitz-Eldor, J., Schuldiner, M., Karsenti, D., Eden, A., Yanuka, O., Amit, M., Soreq, H., and Benvenisty, N. (2000). Differentiation of human embryonic stem cells into embryoid bodies comprising the three embryonic germ layers. Mol. Med. *6*, 88-95.

22. Joshi, S.S., Tarantolo, S.R., Kuszynski, C.A., and Kessinger, A. (2000). Antitumor therapeutic potential of activated human umbilical cord blood cells against leukemia and breast cancer. Clin. Cancer Res. *6*, 4351-4358.

23. Kaufman, D.S., Lewis, R.L., Auerbach, R., and Thomson, J.A. (1999). Directed differentiation of human embryonic stem cells into hematopoietic colony forming cells. Blood. *94 (Supplement part 1)*, 34a.

24. Kim, D.K., Fujiki, Y., Fukushima, T., Ema, H., Shibuya, A., and Nakauchi, H. (1999). Comparison of hematopoietic activities of human bone marrow and umbilical cord blood CD34 positive and negative cells. Stem Cells. *17*, 286-294.

25. Kobari, L., Pflumio, F., Giarratana, M., Li, X., Titeux, M., Izac, B., Leteurtre, F., Coulombel, L., and Douay, L. (2000). *In vitro* and *in vivo* evidence for the long-term multilineage (myeloid, B, NK, and T) reconstitution capacity of ex vivo expanded human CD34+ cord blood cells. Exp. Hematol. *28*, 1470-1480.

26. Koichi, T., Akashi, K., and Weissman, I.L. (2001). Stem cells and hematolymphoic development. Zon, L.I. ed. Oxford Press.

27. Krause, D.S., Theise, N.D., Collector, M.I., Henegariu, O., Hwang, S., Gardner, R., Neutzel, S., and Sharkis, S.J. (2001). Multi-organ, multi-lineage engraftment by a single bone marrow-derived stem cell. Cell. *105*, 369-377.

28. Labastie, M.C., Cortes, F., Romeo, P.H., Dulac, C., and Peault, B. (1998). Molecular identity of hematopoietic precursor cells emerging in the human embryo. Blood. *92*, 3624-3635.

29. Lagasse, E., Connors, H., Al Dhalimy, M., Reitsma, M., Dohse, M., Osborne, L., Wang, X., Finegold, M., Weissman, I.L., and Grompe, M. (2000). Purified hematopoietic stem cells can differentiate into hepatocytes in vivo. Nat. Med. 6, 1229-1234.

30. Lansdorp, P.M., Dragowska, W., and Mayani, H. (1993). Ontogeny-related changes in proliferative potential of human hematopoietic cells. J. Exp. Med. 178, 787-791.

31. Laughlin, M.J. (2001). Umbilical cord blood for allogeneic transplantation in children and adults. Bone Marrow Transplant. 27, 1-6.

32. Lemischka, I. R., personal communication.

33. Lickliter, J.D., McGlave, P.B., DeFor, T.E., Miller, J.S., Ramsay, N.K., Verfaillie, C.M., Burns, L.J., Wagner, J.E., Eastlund, T., Dusenbery, K., and Weisdorf, D.J. (2000). Matched-pair analysis of peripheral blood stem cells compared to marrow for allogeneic transplantation. Bone Marrow Transplant. 26, 723-728.

34. Lin, S.J., Yang, M.H., Chao, H.C., Kuo, M.L., and Huang, J.L. (2000). Effect of interleukin-15 and Flt3-ligand on natural killer cell expansion and activation: umbilical cord vs. adult peripheral blood mononuclear cells. Pediatr. Allergy Immunol. 11, 168-174.

35. MacKey, M.C. (2001). Cell kinetic status of haematopoietic stem cells. Cell. Prolif. 34, 71-83.

36. Marshak, D.R., Gottlieb, D., Kiger, A.A., Fuller, M.T., Kunath, T., Hogan, B., Gardner, R.L., Smith, A., Klar, A.J.S., Henrique, D., D'Urso, G., Datta, S., Holliday, R., Astle, C.M., Chen, J., Harrison, D.E., Xie, T., Spradling, A., Andrews, P.W., Przyborski, S.A., Thomson, J.A., Kunath, T., Strumpf, D., Rossant, J., Tanaka, S., Orkin, S.H., Melchers, F., Rolink, A., Keller, G., Pittenger, M.F., Marshak, D.R., Flake, A.W., Panicker, M.M., Rao, M., Watt, F.M., Grompe, M., Finegold, M.J., Kritzik, M.R., Sarvetnick, N., and Winton, D.J. (2001). Stem cell biology, Marshak, D.R., Gardner, R.L., and Gottlieb, D. eds. (Cold Spring Harbor, New York: Cold Spring Harbor Laboratory Press).

37. McSweeney, P.A. and Storb, R. (1999). Mixed chimerism: preclinical studies and clinical applications. Biol. Blood Marrow Transplant. 5, 192-203.

38. Medvinsky, A. and Dzierzak, E. (1996). Definitive hematopoiesis is autonomously initiated by the AGM region. Cell. 86, 897-906.

39. Moore, K.A., Ema, H., and Lemischka, I.R. (1997). In vitro maintenance of highly purified, transplantable hematopoietic stem cells. Blood. 89, 4337-4347.

40. Morrison, S.J., Prowse, K.R., Ho, P., and Weissman, I.L. (1996). Telomerase activity in hematopoietic cells is associated with self- renewal potential. Immunity. 5, 207-216.

41. Negrin, R.S., Atkinson, K., Leemhuis, T., Hanania, E., Juttner, C., Tierney, K., Hu, W.W., Johnston, L.J., Shizurn, J.A., Stockerl-Goldstein, K.E., Blume, K.G., Weissman, I.L., Bower, S., Baynes, R., Dansey, R., Karanes, C., Peters, W., and Klein, J. (2000). Transplantation of highly purified CD34+ Thy-1+ hematopoietic stem cells in patients with metastatic breast cancer. Biol. Blood Marrow Transplant. 6, 262-271.

42. Oh, I.H., Lau, A., and Eaves, C.J. (2000). During ontogeny primitive (CD34+ CD38-) hematopoietic cells show altered expression of a subset of genes associated with early cytokine and differentiation responses of their adult counterparts. Blood. 96, 4160-4168.

43. Orlic, D., Girard, L.J., Anderson, S.M., Pyle, L.C., Yoder, M.C., Broxmeyer, H.E., and Bodine, D.M. (1998). Identification of human and mouse hematopoietic stem cell populations expressing high levels of mRNA encoding retrovirus receptors. Blood. 91, 3247-3254.

44. Orlic, D., Bock, T.A., and Kanz, L. (1999). Hematopoietic stem cells biology and transplantation. Annals of The New York Academy of Sciences (New York, NY).

45. Perkins, A.C. (1998). Enrichment of blood from embryonic stem cells in vitro. Reprod. Fertil. Dev. 10, 563-572.

46. Pittenger, M.F., Mackay, A.M., Beck, S.C., Jaiswal, R.K., Douglas, R., Mosca, J.D., Moorman, M.A., Simonetti, D.W., Craig, S., and Marshak, D.R. (1999). Multilineage potential of adult human mesenchymal stem cells. Science. 284, 143-147.

47. Shamblott, M.J., Axelman, J., Littlefield, J.W., Blumenthal, P.D., Huggins, G.R., Cui, Y., Cheng, L., and Gearhart, J.D. (2001). Human embryonic germ cell derivatives express a broad range of developmentally distinct markers and proliferate extensively in vitro. Proc. Natl. Acad. Sci. U. S. A. 98, 113-118.

48. Sharp, J.G., Kessinger, A., Lynch, J.C., Pavletic, Z.S., and Joshi, S.S. (2000). Blood stem cell transplantation: factors influencing cellular immunological reconstitution. J. Hematother. Stem Cell Res. 9, 971-981.

49. Smith, L.G., Weissman, I.L., and Heimfeld, S. (1991). Clonal analysis of hematopoietic stem-cell differentiation in vivo. Proc. Natl. Acad. Sci. U. S. A. 88, 2788-2792.

50. Spangrude, G.J., Heimfeld, S., and Weissman, I.L. (1988). Purification and characterization of mouse hematopoietic stem cells. Science. 241, 58-62.

51. Sudo, K., Ema, H., Morita, Y., and Nakauchi, H. (2000). Age-associated characteristics of murine hematopoietic stem cells. J. Exp. Med. 192, 1273-1280.

52. Surbek, D.V., Steinmann, C., Burk, M., Hahn, S., Tichelli, A., and Holzgreve, W. (2000). Developmental changes in adhesion molecule expressions in umbilical cord blood CD34+ hematopoietic progenitor and stem cells. Am. J. Obstet. Gynecol. 183, 1152-1157.

53. Tavian, M., Coulombel, L., Luton, D., Clemente, H.S., Dieterlen-Lievre, F., and Peault, B. (1996). Aorta-associated CD34+ hematopoietic cells in the early human embryo. Blood. 87, 67-72.

54. Tavian, M., Hallais, M.F., and Peault, B. (1999). Emergence of intraembryonic hematopoietic precursors in the pre-liver human embryo. Development. 126, 793-803.

55. Thomas, E.D. and Clift, R.A. (1999). Allogenic transplantation for chronic myeloid leukemia. Thomas, E.D., Blume, K.G., and Forman, S.J. eds. Blackwell Sci., 807-815.

56. Till, J.E. and McCullough, E.A. (1961). A direct measurement of the radiation sensitivity of normal mouse bone marrow cells. Radiat. Res. 14, 213-222.

57. U.S. Department of Health and Human Services. (2000). Report to Congress on the Status of Umbilical Cord Blood Transplantation.

58. Van Zant, G., Rummel, S.A., Koller, M.R., Larson, D.B., Drubachevsky, I., Palsson, M., and Emerson, S.G. (1994). Expansion in bioreactors of human progenitor populations from cord blood and mobilized peripheral blood. Blood Cells. 20, 482-490.

59. Verfaillie, C. M., personal communication.

60. Verlinden, S.F., Mulder, A.H., de Leeuw, J.P., and van Bekkum, D.W. (1998). T lymphocytes determine the development of xeno GVHD and of human hemopoiesis in NOD/SCID mice following human umbilical cord blood transplantation. Stem Cells. 16, Suppl. 1, 205-217.

61. Wang, M.W., Consoli, U., Lane, C.M., Durett, A., Lauppe, M.J., Champlin, R., Andreeff, M., and Deisseroth, A.B. (1998). Rescue from apoptosis in early (CD34-selected) versus late (non-CD34- selected) human hematopoietic cells by very late antigen 4- and vascular cell adhesion molecule (VCAM) 1-dependent adhesion to bone marrow stromal cells. Cell Growth Differ. 9, 105-112.

62. Weissman, I. L., personal communication.

63. Whetton, A.D. and Graham, G.J. (1999). Homing and mobilization in the stem cell niche. Trends Cell. Biol. 9, 233-238.

64. Wright, D.E., Cheshier, S.H., Wagers, A.J., Randall, T.D., Christensen, J.L., and Weissman, I.L. (2001). Cyclophosphamide/granulocyte colony-stimulating factor causes selective mobilization of bone marrow hematopoietic stem cells into the blood after M-phase of the cell cycle.

65. Zon, L. I., personal communication.

6. AUTOIMMUNE DISEASES AND THE PROMISE OF STEM CELL-BASED THERAPIES

One of the more perplexing questions in biomedical research is—why does the body's protective shield against infections, the immune system, attack its own vital cells, organs, and tissues? The answer to this question is central to understanding an array of autoimmune diseases, such as rheumatoid arthritis, type 1 diabetes, systemic lupus erythematosus, and Sjogren's syndrome. When some of the body's cellular proteins are recognized as "foreign" by immune cells called T lymphocytes, a destructive cascade of inflammation is set in place. Current therapies to combat these cases of cellular mistaken identity dampen the body's immune response and leave patients vulnerable to life-threatening infections. Research on stem cells is now providing new approaches to strategically remove the misguided immune cells and restore normal immune cells to the body. Presented here are some of the basic research investigations that are being guided by adult and embryonic stem cell discoveries.

INTRODUCTION

The body's main line of defense against invasion by infectious organisms is the immune system. To succeed, an immune system must distinguish the many cellular components of its own body (self) from the cells or components of invading organisms (nonself). "Nonself" should be attacked while "self" should not. Therefore, two general types of errors can be made by the immune system. If the immune system fails to quickly detect and destroy an invading organism, an infection will result. However, if the immune system fails to recognize self cells or components and mistakenly attacks them, the result is known as an autoimmune disease. Common autoimmune diseases include rheumatoid arthritis, systemic lupus erythematosis (lupus), type 1 diabetes, multiple sclerosis, Sjogren's syndrome and inflammatory bowel disease. Although each of these diseases has

different symptoms, they share the unfortunate reality that, for some reason, the body's immune system has turned against itself (see Box 6.1. Immune System Components: Common Terms and Definitions).

HOW DOES THE IMMUNE SYSTEM NORMALLY KEEP US HEALTHY?

The "soldiers" of the immune system are white blood cells, including T and B lymphocytes, which originate in the bone marrow from hematopoietic stem cells. Every day the body comes into contact with many organisms such as bacteria, viruses, and parasites. Unopposed, these organisms have the potential to cause serious infections, such as pneumonia or AIDS. When a healthy individual is infected, the body responds by activating a variety of immune cells. Initially, invading bacteria or viruses are engulfed by an antigen presenting cell (APC), and their component proteins (antigens) are cut into pieces and displayed on the cell's surface. Pieces of the foreign protein (antigen) bind to the major histocompatibility complex (MHC) proteins, also known as human leukocyte antigen (HLA) molecules, on the surface of the APCs (see Figure 6.1 Immune Response to Self or Foreign Antigens). This complex, formed by a foreign protein and an MHC protein, then binds to a T cell receptor on the surface of another type of immune cell, the CD4 helper T cell. They are so named because they "help" immune responses proceed and have a protein called CD4 on their surface. This complex enables these T cells to focus the immune response to a specific invading organism. The antigen-specific CD4 helper T cells divide and multiply while secreting substances called cytokines, which cause inflammation and help activate other immune cells. The particular cytokines secreted by the CD4 helper T cells act on cells known as the CD8 "cytotoxic" T cells (because they can kill the cells that are infected by the invading organism and have the CD8

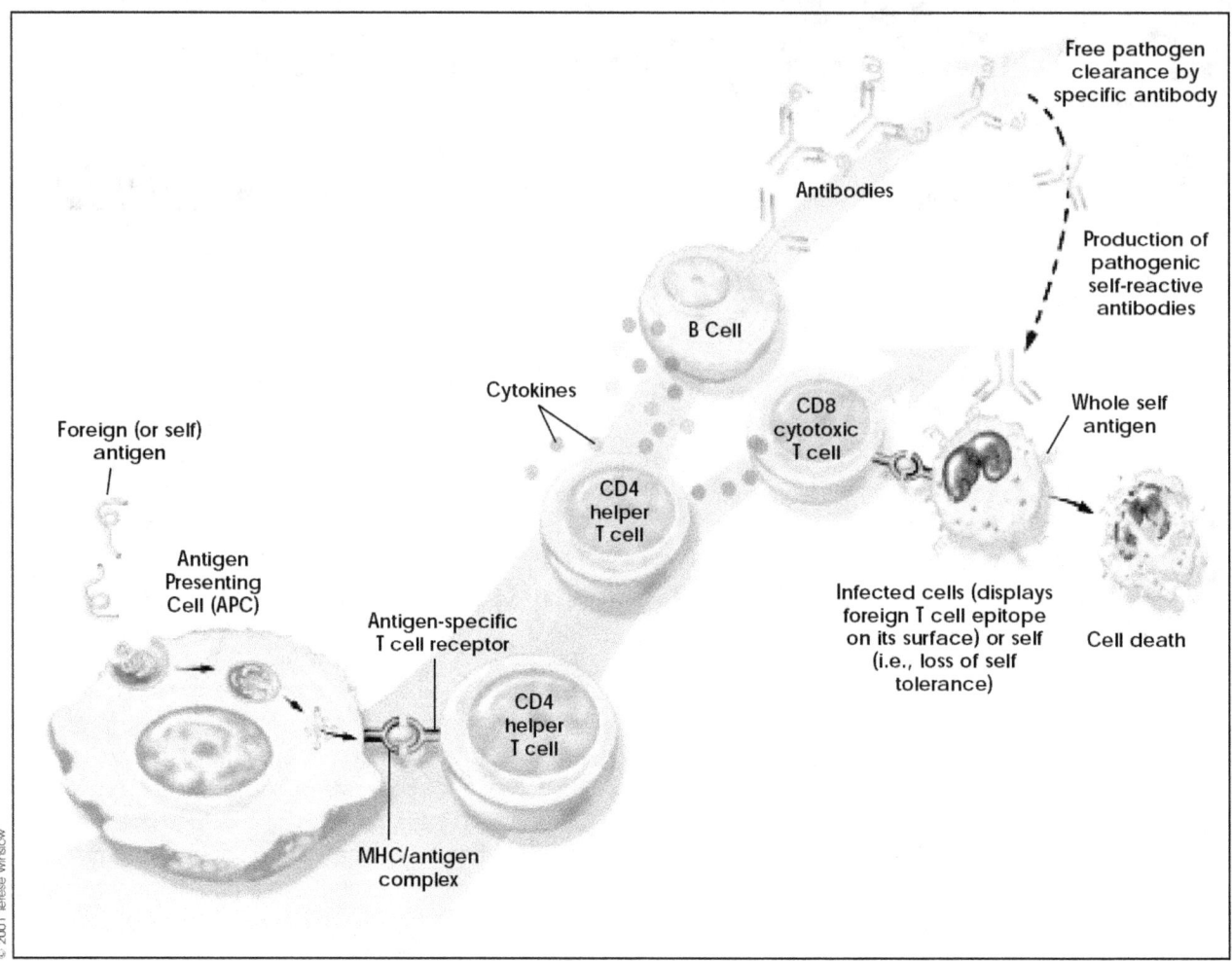

Figure 6.1. Immune Response to Self or Foreign Antigens.

protein on their surface). The helper T cells can also activate antigen-specific B cells to produce antibodies, which can neutralize and help eliminate bacteria and viruses from the body. Some of the antigen-specific T and B cells that are activated to rid the body of infectious organisms become long-lived "memory" cells. Memory cells have the capacity to act quickly when confronted with the same infectious organism at later times. It is the memory cells that cause us to become "immune" from later reinfections with the same organism.

HOW DO THE IMMUNE CELLS OF THE BODY KNOW WHAT TO ATTACK AND WHAT NOT TO?

All immune and blood cells develop from multipotent hematopoietic stem cells that originate in the bone

marrow. Upon their departure from the bone marrow, immature T cells undergo a final maturation process in the thymus, a small organ located in the upper chest, before being dispersed to the body with the rest of the immune cells (e.g., B cells). Within the thymus, T cells undergo an important process that "educates" them to distinguish between self (the proteins of their own body) and nonself (the invading organism's) antigens. Here, the T cells are selected for their ability to bind to the particular MHC proteins expressed by the individual. The particular array of MHCs varies slightly between individuals, and this variation is the basis of the immune response when a transplanted organ is rejected. MHCs and other less easily characterized molecules called minor histocompatibility antigens are genetically determined and this is the reason why donor organs from relatives of the recipient are preferred over unrelated donors.

Box 6.1

Immune System Components: Common Terms and Definitions

Antibody — A Y-shaped protein secreted by B cells in response to an antigen. An antibody binds specifically to the antigen that induced its production. Antibodies directed against antigens on the surface of infectious organisms help eliminate those organisms from the body.

Antigen — A substance (often a protein) that induces the formation of an antibody. Antigens are commonly found on the surface of infectious organisms, transfused blood cells, and organ transplants.

Antigen presenting cells (APC) — One of a variety of cells within the body that can process antigens and display them on their surface in a form recognizable by T cells.

Autoantibody — An antibody that reacts with antigens found on the cells and tissues of an individual's own body. Autoantibodies can cause autoimmune diseases.

Autoimmune disease — A condition that results from the formation of antibodies that attack the cells or tissues of an individual's own body.

B cells — Also known as B lymphocytes. Each B cell is capable of making one specific antibody. When stimulated by antigen and helper T cells, B cells mature into plasma cells that secrete large amounts of their specific antibody

Bone marrow — The soft, living tissue that fills most bone cavities and contains hematopoietic stem cells, from which all red and white blood cells evolve. The bone marrow also contains mesenchymal stem cells that a number of cell types come from, including chondrocytes, which produce cartilage.

Cytokines — A generic term for a large variety of regulatory proteins produced and secreted by cells and used to communicate with other cells. One class of cytokines is the interleukins, which act as intercellular mediators during the generation of an immune response.

Immune system cells — White blood cells or leukocytes that originate from the bone marrow. They include antigen presenting cells, such as dendritic cells, T and B lymphocytes, and neutrophils, among many others.

Lymphatic system — A network of lymph vessels and nodes that drain and filter antigens from tissue fluids before returning lymphocytes to the blood.

Memory cells — A subset of antigen-specific T or B cells that "recall" prior exposure to an antigen and respond quickly without the need to be activated again by CD4 helper T cells.

Major histocompatibility complex (MHC) — A group of genes that code for cell-surface histocompatibility antigens. These antigens are the primary reason why organ and tissue transplants from incompatible donors fail.

T cells — Also known as T lymphocytes. There are two primary subsets of T cells. CD4 helper T cells (identified by the presence of the CD4 protein on their surfaces) are instrumental in initiating an immune response by supplying special cytokines. CD8 cytotoxic (killer) T cells (identified by the presence of the CD8 protein on their surfaces), after being activated by the CD4 helper cells, are capable of killing infected cells in the body. CD4 helper T cells are destroyed by the HIV virus in AIDS patients, resulting in an ineffective immune system.

Thymus — A lymphoid organ located in the upper chest cavity. Maturing T cells leave the bone marrow and go directly to the thymus, where they are educated to discriminate between self and nonself proteins. (See tolerance.)

Tolerance — A state of specific immunologic unresponsiveness. Individuals should normally be tolerant of the cells and tissues that make up our own bodies. Should tolerance fail, an autoimmune disease may result.

In the bone marrow, a highly diverse and random array of T cells is produced. Collectively, these T cells are capable of recognizing an almost unlimited number of antigens. Because the process of generating a T cell's antigen specificity is a random one, many immature T cells have the potential to react with the body's own (self) proteins. To avoid this potential disaster, the thymus provides an environment where T cells that recognize self-antigens (autoreactive or self-reactive T cells) are deleted or inactivated in a process called tolerance induction.

Tolerance usually ensures that T cells do not attack the "autoantigens" (self-proteins) of the body. Given the importance of this task, it is not surprising that there are multiple checkpoints for destroying or inactivating T cells that might react to auto-antigens.

Autoimmune diseases arise when this intricate system for the induction and maintenance of immune tolerance fails. These diseases result in cell and tissue destruction by antigen-specific CD8 cytotoxic T cells or autoantibodies (antibodies to self-proteins) and the accompanying inflammatory process. These mechanisms can lead to the destruction of the joints in rheumatoid arthritis, the destruction of the insulin-producing beta cells of the pancreas in type 1 diabetes, or damage to the kidneys in lupus. The reasons for the failure to induce or maintain tolerance are enigmatic. However, genetic factors, along with environmental and hormonal influences and certain infections, may contribute to tolerance and the development of autoimmune disease [4, 7].

HEMATOPOIETIC STEM CELL THERAPY FOR AUTOIMMUNE DISEASES

The current treatments for many autoimmune diseases include the systemic use of anti-inflammatory drugs and potent immunosuppressive and immunomodulatory agents (i.e., steroids and inhibitor proteins that block the action of inflammatory cytokines). However, despite their profound effect on immune responses, these therapies are unable to induce clinically significant remissions in certain patients. In recent years, researchers have contemplated the use of stem cells to treat autoimmune disorders. Discussed here is some of the rationale for this approach, with a focus on experimental stem cell therapies for lupus, rheumatoid arthritis, and type 1 diabetes.

The immune-mediated injury in autoimmune diseases can be organ-specific, such as type 1 diabetes which is the consequence of the destruction of the pancreatic beta islet cells or multiple sclerosis which results from the breakdown of the myelin covering of nerves. These autoimmune diseases are amenable to treatments involving the repair or replacement of damaged or destroyed cells or tissue (see Chapter 7. Stem Cells and Diabetes and Chapter 11. Use of Genetically Modified Stem Cells in Experimental Gene Therapies). In contrast, non-organ-specific autoimmune diseases, such as lupus, are characterized by widespread injury due to immune reactions against many different organs and tissues.

One approach is being evaluated in early clinical trials of patients with poorly responsive, life-threatening lupus. This is a severe disease affecting multiple organs in the body including muscles, skin, joints, and kidneys as well as the brain and nerves. Over 239,000 Americans, of which more than 90 percent are women, suffer from lupus. In addition, lupus disproportionately afflicts African-American and Hispanic women [11]. A major obstacle in the treatment of non-organ-specific autoimmune diseases such as lupus is the lack of a single specific target for the application of therapy.

The objective of hematopoietic stem cell therapy for lupus is to destroy the mature, long-lived, and auto-reactive immune cells and to generate a new, properly functioning immune system. In most of these trials, the patient's own stem cells have been used in a procedure known as autologous (from "one's self") hematopoietic stem cell transplantation. First, patients receive injections of a growth factor, which coaxes large numbers of hematopoietic stem cells to be released from the bone marrow into the blood stream. These cells are harvested from the blood, purified away from mature immune cells, and stored. After sufficient quantities of these cells are obtained, the patient undergoes a regimen of cytotoxic (cell-killing) drug and/or radiation therapy, which eliminates the mature immune cells. Then, the hematopoietic stem cells are returned to the patient via a blood transfusion into the circulation where they migrate to the bone marrow and begin to differentiate to become mature immune cells. The body's immune system is then restored. Nonetheless, the recovery phase, until the immune system is reconstituted represents a period of dramatically increased susceptibility to bacterial, fungal, and viral infection, making this a high-risk therapy.

Recent reports suggest that this replacement therapy may fundamentally alter the patient's immune system. Richard Burt and his colleagues [18] conducted a long-term follow-up (one to three years) of seven lupus patients who underwent this procedure and found that they remained free from active lupus and improved continuously after transplantation, without the need for immunosuppressive medications. One of the hallmarks of lupus is that during the natural progression of disease, the normally diverse repertoire of T cells become limited in the number of different antigens they recognize, suggesting that an increasing proportion of the patient's T cells are autoreactive. Burt and colleagues found that following hematopoietic stem cell transplantation, levels of T cell diversity were restored to those of healthy individuals. This finding provides evidence that stem cell replacement may be beneficial in reestablishing tolerance in T cells, thereby decreasing the likelihood of disease reoccurrence.

DEVELOPMENT OF HEMATOPOIETIC STEM CELL LINES FOR TRANSPLANTATION

The ability to generate and propagate unlimited numbers of hematopoietic stem cells outside the body—whether from adult, umbilical cord blood, fetal, or embryonic sources—would have a major impact on the safety, cost, and availability of stem cells for transplantation. The current approach of isolating hematopoietic stem cells from a patient's own peripheral blood places the patient at risk for a flare-up of their autoimmune disease. This is a potential consequence of repeated administration of the stem cell growth factors needed to mobilize hematopoietic stem cells from the bone marrow to the blood stream in numbers sufficient for transplantation. In addition, contamination of the purified hematopoietic stem cells with the patient's mature autoreactive T and B cells could affect the success of the treatment in some patients. Propagation of pure cell lines in the laboratory would avoid these potential drawbacks and increase the numbers of stem cells available to each patient, thus shortening the at-risk interval before full immune reconstitution.

Whether embryonic stem cells will provide advantages over stem cells derived from cord blood or adult bone marrow hematopoietic stem cells remains to be determined. However, hematopoietic stem cells, whether from umbilical cord blood or bone marrow, have a more limited potential for self-renewal than do pluripotent embryonic stem cells. Although new information will be needed to direct the differentiation of embryonic stem cells into hematopoietic stem cells, hematopoietic cells are present in differentiated cultures from human embryonic stem cells [9] and from human fetal-derived embryonic germ stem cells [17].

One potential advantage of using hematopoietic stem cell lines for transplantation in patients with autoimmune diseases is that these cells could be generated from unaffected individuals or, as predisposing genetic factors are defined, from embryonic stem cells lacking these genetic influences. In addition, use of genetically selected or genetically engineered cell types may further limit the possibility of disease progression or reemergence.

One risk of using nonself hematopoietic stem cells is of immune rejection of the transplanted cells. Immune rejection is caused by MHC protein differences between the donor and the patient (recipient). In this scenario, the transplanted hematopoietic stem cells and their progeny are rejected by the patient's own T cells, which are originating from the patient's surviving bone marrow hematopoietic stem cells. In this regard, embryonic stem cell-derived hematopoietic stem cells may offer distinct advantages over cord blood and bone marrow hematopoietic stem cell lines in avoiding rejection of the transplant. Theoretically, banks of embryonic stem cells expressing various combinations of the three most critical MHC proteins could be generated to allow close matching to the recipient's MHC composition.

Additionally, there is evidence that embryonic stem cells are considerably more receptive to genetic manipulation than are hematopoietic stem cells (see Chapter 11. Use of Genetically Modified Stem Cells in Experimental Gene Therapies).

This characteristic means that embryonic stem cells could be useful in strategies that could prevent their recognition by the patient's surviving immune cells. For example, it may be possible to introduce the recipient's MHC proteins into embryonic stem cells through targeted gene transfer. Alternatively, it is theoretically possible to generate a universal donor embryonic stem cell line by genetic alteration or removal of the MHC proteins. Researchers have accomplished this by genetically altering a mouse so that it has little or no surface expression of MHC molecules on any of the cells or tissues. There is no rejection of pancreatic beta islet cells from these genetically altered mice when the cells are transplanted into completely MHC-mismatched mice [13]. Additional research will be needed to determine the feasibility of these alternative strategies for prevention of graft rejection in humans [6].

Jon Odorico and colleagues have shown that expression of MHC proteins on mouse embryonic stem cells and differentiated embryonic stem cell progeny is either absent or greatly decreased compared with MHC expression on adult cells [8]. These preliminary findings raise the intriguing possibility that lines derived from embryonic stem cells may be inherently less susceptible to rejection by the recipient's immune system than lines derived from adult cells. This could have important implications for the transplantation of cells other than hematopoietic stem cells.

Another potential advantage of using pure populations of donor hematopoietic stem cells achieved through stem cell technologies would be a lower incidence and severity of graft-versus-host disease, a potentially fatal complication of bone marrow transplantation. Graft-versus-host disease results from the immune-mediated injury to recipient tissues that occurs when mature organ-donor T cells remain within the organ at the time of transplant. Such mature donor alloreactive T cells would be absent from pure populations of multipotent hematopoietic stem cells, and under ideal conditions of immune tolerance induction in the recipient's thymus, the donor-derived mature T cell population would be tolerant to the host.

GENE THERAPY AND STEM CELL APPROACHES FOR THE TREATMENT OF AUTOIMMUNE DISEASES

Gene therapy is the genetic modification of cells to produce a therapeutic effect (see Chapter 11. Use of Genetically Modified Stem Cells in Experimental Gene Therapies). In most investigational protocols, DNA containing the therapeutic gene is transferred into cultured cells, and these cells are subsequently administered to the animal or patient. DNA can also be injected directly, entering cells at the site of the injection or in the circulation. Under ideal conditions, cells take up the DNA and produce the therapeutic protein encoded by the gene.

Currently, there is an extensive amount of gene therapy research being conducted in animal models of autoimmune disease. The goal is to modify the aberrant, inflammatory immune response that is characteristic of autoimmune diseases [15, 19]. Researchers most often use one of two general strategies to modulate the immune system. The first strategy is to block the actions of an inflammatory cytokine (secreted by certain activated immune cells and inflamed tissues) by transferring a gene into cells that encodes a "decoy" receptor for that cytokine. Alternatively, a gene is transferred that encodes an anti-inflammatory cytokine, redirecting the auto-inflammatory immune response to a more "tolerant" state. In many animal studies, promising results have been achieved by using these approaches, and the

studies have advanced understanding of the disease processes and the particular inflammatory cytokines involved in disease progression [15, 19].

Serious obstacles to the development of effective gene therapies for humans remain, however. Foremost among these are the difficulty of reliably transferring genetic material into adult and slowly dividing cells (including hematopoietic stem cells) and of producing long-lasting expression of the intended protein at levels that can be tightly controlled in response to disease activity. Importantly, embryonic stem cells are substantially more permissive to gene transfer compared with adult cells, and embryonic cells sustain protein expression during extensive self-renewal. Whether adult-derived stem cells, other than hematopoietic stem cells, are similarly amenable to gene transfer has not yet been determined.

Ultimately, stem cell gene therapy should allow the development of novel methods for immune modulation in autoimmune diseases. One example is the genetic modification of hematopoietic stem cells or differentiated tissue cells with a "decoy" receptor for the inflammatory cytokine interferon gamma to treat lupus. For example, in a lupus mouse model, gene transfer of the decoy receptor, via DNA injection, arrested disease progression [12]. Other investigators have used a related but distinct approach in a mouse model of type 1 diabetes. Interleukin-12 (IL-12), an inflammatory cytokine, plays a prominent role in the development of diabetes in these mice. The investigators transferred the gene for a modified form of IL-12, which blocks the activity of the natural IL-12, into pancreatic beta islet cells (the target of autoimmune injury in type 1 diabetes). The islet cell gene therapy prevented the onset of diabetes in these mice [20]. Theoretically, embryonic stem cells or adult stem cells could be genetically modified before or during differentiation into pancreatic beta islet cells to be used for transplantation. The resulting immune-modulating islet cells might diminish the occurrence of ongoing autoimmunity, increase the likelihood of long-term function of the transplanted cells, and eliminate the need for immunosuppressive therapy following transplantation.

Researchers are exploring similar genetic approaches to prevent progressive joint destruction and loss of cartilage and to repair damaged joints in animal models of rheumatoid arthritis. Rheumatoid arthritis is a debilitating autoimmune disease characterized by acute and chronic inflammation, in which the immune system primarily attacks the joints of the body. In a recent study, investigators genetically transferred an anti-inflammatory cytokine, interleukin-4 (IL-4), into a specialized, highly efficient antigen-presenting cell called a dendritic cell, and then injected these IL-4-secreting cells into mice that can be induced to develop a form of arthritis similar to rheumatoid arthritis in humans. These IL-4-secreting dendritic cells are presumed to act on the CD4 helper T cells to reintroduce tolerance to self-proteins. Treated mice showed complete suppression of their disease and, in addition to its immune-modulatory properties, IL-4 blocked bone resorption (a serious complication of rheumatoid arthritis), making it a particularly attractive cytokine for this therapy [10]. However, one obstacle to this approach is that human dendritic cells are difficult to isolate in large numbers.

Investigators have also directed the differentiation of dendritic cells from mouse embryonic stem cells, indicating that a stem cell-based approach might work in patients with rheumatoid arthritis [5]. Longer-term follow-up and further characterization will be needed in animal models before researchers proceed with the development of such an approach in humans. In similar studies, using other inhibitors of inflammatory cytokines such as a decoy receptor for tumor necrosis factor–α (a prominent inflammatory cytokine in inflamed joints), an inhibitor of nuclear factor–κB (a protein within cells that turns on the production of many inflammatory cytokines), and interleukin-13 (an anti-inflammatory cytokine), researchers have shown promising results in animal models of rheumatoid arthritis [19]. Because of the complexity and redundancy of immune system signaling networks, it is likely that a multifaceted approach involving inhibitors of several different inflammatory cytokines will be successful, whereas approaches targeting single cytokines might fail or produce only short-lived responses. In addition, other cell types may prove to be even better vehicles for the delivery of gene therapy in this disease.

Chondrocytes, cells that build cartilage in joints, may provide another avenue for stem cell-based treatment of rheumatoid arthritis. These cells have been derived from human bone marrow stromal stem cells

derived from human bone marrow [14]. Little is known about the intermediate cells that ultimately differentiate into chondrocytes. In addition to adult bone marrow as a source for stromal stem cells, human embryonic stem cells can differentiate into precursor cells believed to lead ultimately to the stromal stem cells [16]. However, extensive research is needed to reliably achieve the directed derivation of the stromal stem cells from embryonic stem cells and, subsequently, the differentiation of chondrocytes from these stromal stem cells.

The ideal cell for optimum cartilage repair may be a more primitive cell than the chondrocyte, such as the stromal cell, or an intermediate cell in the pathway (e.g., a connective tissue precursor) leading to the chondrocyte. Stromal stem cells can generate new chondrocytes and facilitate cartilage repair in a rabbit model [3]. Such cells may also prove to be ideal targets for the delivery of immune-modulatory gene therapy. Like hematopoietic stem cells, stromal stem cells have been used in animal models for delivery of gene therapy [1]. For example, a recent study demonstrated that genetically engineered chondrocytes, expressing a growth factor, can enhance the function of transplanted chondrocytes [2].

Two obstacles to the use of adult stromal stem cells or chondrocytes are the limited numbers of these cells that can be harvested and the difficulties in propagating them in the laboratory. Embryonic stem cells, genetically modified and expanded before directed differentiation to a connective tissue stem cell, may be an attractive alternative.

Collectively, these results illustrate the tremendous potential these cells may offer for the treatment of rheumatoid arthritis and other autoimmune diseases.

CONCLUSION

Stem cell-based therapies offer many exciting possibilities for the development of novel treatments, and perhaps even cures, for autoimmune diseases. A challenging research effort remains to fully realize this potential and to address the many remaining questions, which include how best to direct the differentiation of specific cell types and determine which particular type of stem cell will be optimum for each therapeutic approach. Gene therapy with cytokines or their inhibitors is still in its infancy, but stem cells or their progeny may provide one of the better avenues for future delivery of immune-based therapies. Ultimately, the potential to alleviate these devastating chronic diseases with the use of stem cell-based technologies is enormous.

REFERENCES

1. Allay, J.A., Dennis, J.E., Haynesworth, S.E., Majumdar, M.K., Clapp, D.W., Shultz, L.D., Caplan, A.I., and Gerson, S.L. (1997). LacZ and interleukin-3 expression in vivo after retroviral transduction of marrow-derived human osteogenic mesenchymal progenitors. Hum. Gene Ther. 8, 1417-1427.

2. Brower-Toland, B.D., Saxer, R.A., Goodrich, L.R., Mi, Z., Robbins, P.D., Evans, C.H., and Nixon, A.J. (2001). Direct adenovirus-mediated insulin-like growth factor I gene transfer enhances transplant chondrocyte function. Hum. Gene Ther. 12, 117-129.

3. Caplan, A.I., Elyaderani, M., Mochizuki, Y., Wakitani, S., and Goldberg, V.M. (1997). Principles of cartilage repair and regeneration. Clin. Orthop. 342, 254-269.

4. Cooper, G.S., Dooley, M.A., Treadwell, E.L., St Clair, E.W., Parks, C.G., and Gilkeson, G.S. (1998). Hormonal, environmental, and infectious risk factors for developing systemic lupus erythematosus. Arthritis Rheum. 41, 1714-1724.

5. Fairchild, P.J., Brook, F.A., Gardner, R.L., Graca, L., Strong, V., Tone, Y., Tone, M., Nolan, K.F., and Waldmann, H. (2000). Directed differentiation of dendritic cells from mouse embryonic stem cells. Curr. Biol. 10, 1515-1518.

6. Gearhart, J. (1998). New potential for human embryonic stem cells. Science. 282, 1061-1062.

7. Grossman, J.M. and Tsao, B.P. (2000). Genetics and systemic lupus erythematosus. Curr. Rheumatol. Rep. 2, 13-18.

8. Harley, C.B., Gearhart, J., Jaenisch, R., Rossant, J., and Thomson, J. (2001). Keystone Symposia. Pluripotent stem cells: biology and applications. Durango, CO.

9. Itskovitz-Eldor, J., Schuldiner, M., Karsenti, D., Eden, A., Yanuka, O., Amit, M., Soreq, H., and Benvenisty, N. (2000). Differentiation of human embryonic stem cells into embryoid bodies comprising the three embryonic germ layers. Mol. Med. 6, 88-95.

10. Kim, S.H., Kim, S., Evans, C.H., Ghivizzani, S.C., Oligino, T., and Robbins, P.D. (2001). Effective treatment of established murine collagen-induced arthritis by systemic administration of dendritic cells genetically modified to express IL-4. J. Immunol. 166, 3499-3505.

11. Lawrence, R.C., Helmick, C.G., Arnett, F.C., Deyo, R.A., Felson, D.T., Giannini, E.H., Heyse, S.P., Hirsch, R., Hochberg, M.C., Hunder, G.G., Liang, M.H., Pillemer, S.R., Steen, V.D., and Wolfe, F. (1998). Estimates of the prevalence of arthritis and selected musculoskeletal disorders in the United States. Arthritis Rheum. 41, 778-799.

12. Lawson, B.R., Prud'homme, G.J., Chang, Y., Gardner, H.A., Kuan, J., Kono, D.H., and Theofilopoulos, A.N. (2000). Treatment of murine lupus with cDNA encoding IFN-gammaR/Fc. J. Clin. Invest. 106, 207-215.

13. Osorio, R.W., Ascher, N.L., Jaenisch, R., Freise, C.E., Roberts, J.P., and Stock, P.G. (1993). Major histocompatibility complex class I deficiency prolongs islet allograft survival. Diabetes. 42, 1520-1527.

14. Pittenger, M.F., Mackay, A.M., Beck, S.C., Jaiswal, R.K., Douglas, R., Mosca, J.D., Moorman, M.A., Simonetti, D.W., Craig, S., and Marshak, D.R. (1999). Multilineage potential of adult human mesenchymal stem cells. Science. 284, 143-147.

15. Prud'homme, G.J. (2000). Gene therapy of autoimmune diseases with vectors encoding regulatory cytokines or inflammatory cytokine inhibitors. J. Gene. Med. 2, 222-232.

16. Schuldiner, M., Yanuka, O., Itskovitz-Eldor, J., Melton, D., and Benvenisty, N. (2000). Effects of eight growth factors on the differentiation of cells derived from human embryonic stem cells. Proc. Natl. Acad. Sci. U. S. A. 97, 11307-11312.

17. Shamblott, M.J., Axelman, J., Littlefield, J.W., Blumenthal, P.D., Huggins, G.R., Cui, Y., Cheng, L., and Gearhart, J.D. (2000). Human embryonic germ cell derivatives express a broad range of developmentally distinct markers and proliferate extensively in vitro. Proc. Natl. Acad. Sci. U. S. A. 98, 113-118.

18. Traynor, A.E., Schroeder, J., Rosa, R.M., Cheng, D., Stefka, J., Mujais, S., Baker, S., and Burt, R.K. (2000). Treatment of severe systemic lupus erythematosus with high-dose chemotherapy and haemopoietic stem-cell transplantation: a phase I study. Lancet. 356, 701-707.

19. Tsokos, G.C. and Nepom, G.T. (2000). Gene therapy in the treatment of autoimmune diseases. J. Clin. Invest. 106, 181-183.

20. Yasuda, H., Nagata, M., Arisawa, K., Yoshida, R., Fujihira, K., Okamoto, N., Moriyama, H., Miki, M., Saito, I., Hamada, H., Yokono, K., and Kasuga, M. (1998). Local expression of immunoregulatory IL-12p40 gene prolonged syngeneic islet graft survival in diabetic NOD mice. J. Clin. Invest. 102, 1807-1814.

7. STEM CELLS AND DIABETES

Diabetes exacts its toll on many Americans, young and old. For years, researchers have painstakingly dissected this complicated disease caused by the destruction of insulin producing islet cells of the pancreas. Despite progress in understanding the underlying disease mechanisms for diabetes, there is still a paucity of effective therapies. For years investigators have been making slow, but steady, progress on experimental strategies for pancreatic transplantation and islet cell replacement. Now, researchers have turned their attention to adult stem cells that appear to be precursors to islet cells and embryonic stem cells that produce insulin.

INTRODUCTION

For decades, diabetes researchers have been searching for ways to replace the insulin-producing cells of the pancreas that are destroyed by a patient's own immune system. Now it appears that this may be possible. Each year, diabetes affects more people and causes more deaths than breast cancer and AIDS combined. Diabetes is the seventh leading cause of death in the United States today, with nearly 200,000 deaths reported each year. The American Diabetes Association estimates that nearly 16 million people, or 5.9 percent of the United States population, currently have diabetes.

Diabetes is actually a group of diseases characterized by abnormally high levels of the sugar glucose in the bloodstream. This excess glucose is responsible for most of the complications of diabetes, which include blindness, kidney failure, heart disease, stroke, neuropathy, and amputations. Type 1 diabetes, also known as juvenile-onset diabetes, typically affects children and young adults. Diabetes develops when the body's immune system sees its own cells as foreign and attacks and destroys them. As a result,

the islet cells of the pancreas, which normally produce insulin, are destroyed. In the absence of insulin, glucose cannot enter the cell and glucose accumulates in the blood. Type 2 diabetes, also called adult-onset diabetes, tends to affect older, sedentary, and overweight individuals with a family history of diabetes. Type 2 diabetes occurs when the body cannot use insulin effectively. This is called insulin resistance and the result is the same as with type 1 diabetes—a build up of glucose in the blood.

There is currently no cure for diabetes. People with type 1 diabetes must take insulin several times a day and test their blood glucose concentration three to four times a day throughout their entire lives. Frequent monitoring is important because patients who keep their blood glucose concentrations as close to normal as possible can significantly reduce many of the complications of diabetes, such as retinopathy (a disease of the small blood vessels of the eye which can lead to blindness) and heart disease, that tend to develop over time. People with type 2 diabetes can often control their blood glucose concentrations through a combination of diet, exercise, and oral medication. Type 2 diabetes often progresses to the point where only insulin therapy will control blood glucose concentrations.

Each year, approximately 1,300 people with type 1 diabetes receive whole-organ pancreas transplants. After a year, 83 percent of these patients, on average, have no symptoms of diabetes and do not have to take insulin to maintain normal glucose concentrations in the blood. However, the demand for transplantable pancreases outweighs their availability. To prevent the body from rejecting the transplanted pancreas, patients must take powerful drugs that suppress the immune system for their entire lives, a regimen that makes them susceptible to a host of other diseases. Many hospitals will not perform a pancreas transplant unless the patient also needs a kidney transplant. That is because the risk of infection due to immunosuppressant therapy can be a greater health threat than the diabetes itself. But if a patient is also receiving a new kidney and will require immuno-suppressant drugs anyway, many hospitals will perform the pancreas transplant.

Over the past several years, doctors have attempted to cure diabetes by injecting patients with pancreatic islet cells—the cells of the pancreas that secrete insulin and other hormones. However, the requirement for steroid immunosuppressant therapy to prevent rejection of the cells increases the metabolic demand on insulin-producing cells and eventually they may exhaust their capacity to produce insulin. The deleterious effect of steroids is greater for islet cell transplants than for whole-organ transplants. As a result, less than 8 percent of islet cell transplants performed before last year had been successful.

More recently, James Shapiro and his colleagues in Edmonton, Alberta, Canada, have developed an experimental protocol for transplanting islet cells that involves using a much larger amount of islet cells and a different type of immunosuppressant therapy. In a recent study, they report that [17], seven of seven patients who received islet cell transplants no longer needed to take insulin, and their blood glucose concentrations were normal a year after surgery. The success of the Edmonton protocol is now being tested at 10 centers around the world.

If the success of the Edmonton protocol can be duplicated, many hurdles still remain in using this approach on a wide scale to treat diabetes. First, donor tissue is not readily available. Islet cells used in transplants are obtained from cadavers, and the pro-cedure requires at least two cadavers per transplant. The islet cells must be immunologically compatible, and the tissue must be freshly obtained—within eight hours of death. Because of the shortage of organ donors, these requirements are difficult to meet and the waiting list is expected to far exceed available tissue, especially if the procedure becomes widely accepted and available. Further, islet cell transplant recipients face a lifetime of immunosuppressant therapy, which makes them susceptible to other serious infections and diseases.

DEVELOPMENT OF THE PANCREAS

Before discussing cell-based therapies for diabetes, it is important to understand how the pancreas develops. In mammals, the pancreas contains three classes of cell types: the ductal cells, the acinar cells, and the endocrine cells. The endocrine cells produce the hormones glucagon, somatostatin, pancreatic polypeptide (PP), and insulin, which are secreted into the blood stream and help the body regulate sugar metabolism. The acinar cells are part of the exocrine system, which manufactures digestive enzymes, and ductal cells from the pancreatic ducts, which connect the acinar cells to digestive organs.

In humans, the pancreas develops as an outgrowth of the duodenum, a part of the small intestine. The cells of both the exocrine system—the acinar cells—and of the endocrine system—the islet cells—seem to originate from the ductal cells during develop-ment. During development these endocrine cells emerge from the pancreatic ducts and form aggregates that eventually form what is known as Islets of Langerhans. In humans, there are four types of islet cells: the insulin-producing beta cells; the alpha cells, which produce glucagon; the delta cells, which secrete somatostatin; and the PP-cells, which produce pancreatic polypeptide. The hormones released from each type of islet cell have a role in regulating hormones released from other islet cells. In the human pancreas, 65 to 90 percent of islet cells are beta cells, 15 to 20 percent are alpha-cells, 3 to 10 percent are delta cells, and one percent is PP cells. Acinar cells form small lobules contiguous with the ducts (see Figure 7.1. Insulin Production in the Human Pancreas). The resulting pancreas is a combination of a lobulated, branched acinar gland that forms the exocrine pancreas, and, embedded in the acinar gland, the Islets of Langerhans, which constitute the endocrine pancreas.

During fetal development, new endocrine cells appear to arise from progenitor cells in the pancre-atic ducts. Many researchers maintain that some sort of islet stem cell can be found intermingled with ductal cells during fetal development and that these stem cells give rise to new endocrine cells as the fetus develops. Ductal cells can be distinguished from endocrine cells by their structure and by the genes they express. For example, ductal cells typically express a gene known as *cytokeratin-9*

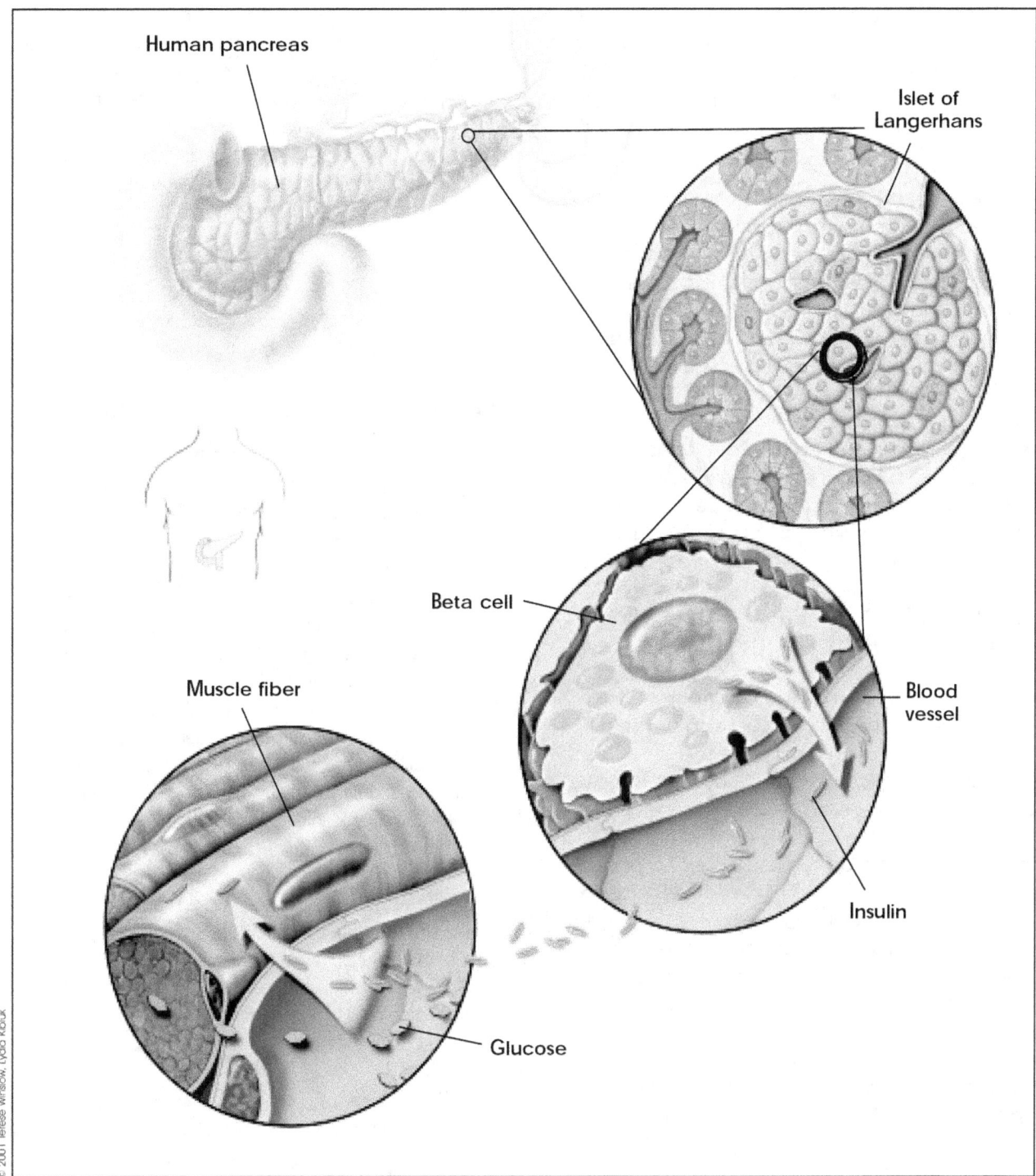

Figure 7.1. Insulin Production in the Human Pancreas.
The pancreas is located in the abdomen, adjacent to the duodenum (the first portion of the small intestine). A cross-section of the pancreas shows the islet of Langerhans which is the functional unit of the endocrine pancreas. Encircled is the beta cell that synthesizes and secretes insulin. Beta cells are located adjacent to blood vessels and can easily respond to changes in blood glucose concentration by adjusting insulin production. Insulin facilitates uptake of glucose, the main fuel source, into cells of tissues such as muscle.

(CK-9), which encodes a structural protein. Beta islet cells, on the other hand, express a gene called *PDX-1*, which encodes a protein that initiates transcription from the insulin gene. These genes, called cell markers, are useful in identifying particular cell types.

Following birth and into adulthood, the source of new islet cells is not clear, and some controversy exists over whether adult stem cells exist in the pancreas. Some researchers believe that islet stem cell-like cells can be found in the pancreatic ducts and even in the islets themselves. Others maintain that the ductal cells can differentiate into islet precursor cells, while others hold that new islet cells arise from stem cells in the blood. Researchers are using several approaches for isolating and cultivating stem cells or islet precursor cells from fetal and adult pancreatic tissue. In addition, several new promising studies indicate that insulin-producing cells can be cultivated from embryonic stem cell lines.

DEVELOPMENT OF CELL-BASED THERAPIES FOR DIABETES

In developing a potential therapy for patients with diabetes, researchers hope to develop a system that meets several criteria. Ideally, stem cells should be able to multiply in culture and reproduce themselves exactly. That is, the cells should be self-renewing. Stem cells should also be able to differentiate *in vivo* to produce the desired kind of cell. For diabetes therapy, it is not clear whether it will be desirable to produce only beta cells—the islet cells that manufacture insulin—or whether other types of pancreatic islet cells are also necessary. Studies by Bernat Soria and colleagues, for example, indicate that isolated beta cells—those cultured in the absence of the other types of islet cells—are less responsive to changes in glucose concentration than intact islet clusters made up of all islet cell types. Islet cell clusters typically respond to higher-than-normal concentrations of glucose by releasing insulin in two phases: a quick release of high concentrations of insulin and a slower release of lower concentrations of insulin. In this manner the beta cells can fine-tune their response to glucose. Extremely high concentrations of glucose may require that more insulin be released quickly, while intermediate concentrations of glucose can be handled by a balance of quickly and slowly released insulin.

Isolated beta cells, as well as islet clusters with lower-than-normal amounts of non-beta cells, do not release insulin in this biphasic manner. Instead insulin is released in an all-or-nothing manner, with no fine-tuning for intermediate concentrations of glucose in the blood [5, 18]. Therefore, many researchers believe that it will be preferable to develop a system in which stem or precursor cell types can be cultured to produce all the cells of the islet cluster in order to generate a population of cells that will be able to coordinate the release of the appropriate amount of insulin to the physiologically relevant concentrations of glucose in the blood.

FETAL TISSUE AS SOURCE FOR ISLET CELLS

Several groups of researchers are investigating the use of fetal tissue as a potential source of islet progenitor cells. For example, using mice, researchers have compared the insulin content of implants from several sources of stem cells—fresh human fetal pancreatic tissue, purified human islets, and cultured islet tissue [2]. They found that insulin content was initially higher in the fresh tissue and purified islets. However, with time, insulin concentration decreased in the whole tissue grafts, while it remained the same in the purified islet grafts. When cultured islets were implanted, however, their insulin content increased over the course of three months. The researchers concluded that precursor cells within the cultured islets were able to proliferate (continue to replicate) and differentiate (specialize) into functioning islet tissue, but that the purified islet cells (already differentiated) could not further proliferate when grafted. Importantly, the researchers found, however, that it was also difficult to expand cultures of fetal islet progenitor cells in culture [7].

ADULT TISSUE AS SOURCE FOR ISLET CELLS

Many researchers have focused on culturing islet cells from human adult cadavers for use in developing transplantable material. Although differentiated beta cells are difficult to proliferate and culture, some researchers have had success in engineering such cells to do this. For example, Fred Levine and his colleagues at the University of California, San Diego, have engineered islet cells isolated from human cadavers by adding to the cells' DNA special genes that stimulate cell proliferation. However, because once such cell lines that can proliferate in culture are established, they no longer produce insulin. The cell lines are further engineered to express the beta islet cell gene, *PDX-1*, which stimulates the expression of the insulin gene. Such cell lines have been shown to propagate in culture and can be induced to differentiate to cells, which produce insulin. When transplanted into immune-deficient mice, the cells secrete insulin in response to glucose. The researchers are currently investigating whether these cells will reverse diabetes in an experimental diabetes model in mice [6, 8].

These investigators report that these cells do not produce as much insulin as normal islets, but it is within an order of magnitude. The major problem in dealing with these cells is maintaining the delicate balance between growth and differentiation. Cells that proliferate well do not produce insulin efficiently, and those that do produce insulin do not proliferate well. According to the researchers, the major issue is developing the technology to be able to grow large numbers of these cells that will reproducibly produce normal amounts of insulin [9].

Another promising source of islet progenitor cells lies in the cells that line the pancreatic ducts. Some researchers believe that multipotent (capable of forming cells from more than one germ layer) stem cells are intermingled with mature, differentiated duct cells, while others believe that the duct cells themselves can undergo a differentiation, or a reversal to a less mature type of cell, which can then differentiate into an insulin-producing islet cell.

Susan Bonner-Weir and her colleagues reported last year that when ductal cells isolated from adult human pancreatic tissue were cultured, they could be induced to differentiate into clusters that contained both ductal and endocrine cells. Over the course of three to four weeks in culture, the cells secreted low amounts of insulin when exposed to low concentrations of glucose, and higher amounts of insulin when exposed to higher glucose concentrations. The researchers have determined by immunochemistry and ultrastructural analysis that these clusters contain all of the endocrine cells of the islet [4].

Bonner-Weir and her colleagues are working with primary cell cultures from duct cells and have not

established cells lines that can grow indefinitely. However the cells can be expanded. According to the researchers, it might be possible in principle to do a biopsy and remove duct cells from a patient and then proliferate the cells in culture and give the patient back his or her own islets. This would work with patients who have type 1 diabetes and who lack functioning beta cells, but their duct cells remain intact. However, the autoimmune destruction would still be a problem and potentially lead to destruction of these transplanted cells [3]. Type 2 diabetes patients might benefit from the transplantation of cells expanded from their own duct cells since they would not need any immunosuppression. However, many researchers believe that if there is a genetic component to the death of beta cells, then beta cells derived from ductal cells of the same individual would also be susceptible to autoimmune attack.

Some researchers question whether the ductal cells are indeed undergoing a dedifferentiation or whether a subset of stem-like or islet progenitors populate the pancreatic ducts and may be co-cultured along with the ductal cells. If ductal cells die off but islet precursors proliferate, it is possible that the islet precursor cells may overtake the ductal cells in culture and make it appear that the ductal cells are dedifferentiating into stem cells. According to Bonner-Weir, both dedifferentiated ductal cells and islet progenitor cells may occur in pancreatic ducts.

Ammon Peck of the University of Florida, Vijayakumar Ramiya of Ixion Biotechnology in Alachua, FL, and their colleagues [13, 14] have also cultured cells from the pancreatic ducts from both humans and mice. Last year, they reported that pancreatic ductal epithelial cells from adult mice could be cultured to yield islet-like structures similar to the cluster of cells found by Bonner-Weir. Using a host of islet-cell markers they identified cells that produced insulin, glucagon, somatostatin, and pancreatic polypeptide. When the cells were implanted into diabetic mice, the diabetes was reversed.

Joel Habener has also looked for islet-like stem cells from adult pancreatic tissue. He and his colleagues have discovered a population of stem-like cells within both the adult pancreas islets and pancreatic ducts. These cells do not express the marker typical of ductal cells, so they are unlikely to be ductal cells, according to Habener. Instead, they express a marker called nestin, which is typically found in developing neural cells. The nestin-positive cells do not express markers typically found in mature islet cells. However, depending upon the growth factors added, the cells can differentiate into different types of cells, including liver, neural, exocrine pancreas, and endocrine pancreas, judged by the markers they express, and can be maintained in culture for up to eight months [20].

EMBRYONIC STEM CELLS

The discovery of methods to isolate and grow human embryonic stem cells in 1998 renewed the hopes of doctors, researchers, and diabetes patients and their families that a cure for type 1 diabetes, and perhaps type 2 diabetes as well, may be within striking distance. In theory, embryonic stem cells could be cultivated and coaxed into developing into the insulin-producing islet cells of the pancreas. With a ready supply of cultured stem cells at hand, the theory is that a line of embryonic stem cells could be grown up as needed for anyone requiring a transplant. The cells could be engineered to avoid immune rejection. Before transplantation, they could be placed into nonimmunogenic material so that they would not be rejected and the patient would avoid the devastating effects of immunosuppressant drugs. There is also some evidence that differentiated cells derived from embryonic stem cells might be less likely to cause immune rejection (see Chapter 10. Assessing Human Stem Cell Safety). Although having a replenishable supply of insulin-producing cells for transplant into humans may be a long way off, researchers have been making remarkable progress in their quest for it. While some researchers have pursued the research on embryonic stem cells, other researchers have focused on insulin-producing precursor cells that occur naturally in adult and fetal tissues.

Since their discovery three years ago, several teams of researchers have been investigating the possibility that human embryonic stem cells could be developed as a therapy for treating diabetes. Recent studies in mice show that embryonic stem cells can be coaxed into differentiating into insulin-producing beta cells, and new reports indicate that this strategy may be possible using human embryonic cells as well.

Last year, researchers in Spain reported using mouse embryonic stem cells that were engineered to allow researchers to select for cells that were differentiating into insulin-producing cells [19]. Bernat Soria and his colleagues at the Universidad Miguel Hernandez in San Juan, Alicante, Spain, added DNA containing part of the insulin gene to embryonic cells from mice. The insulin gene was linked to another gene that rendered the mice resistant to an antibiotic drug. By growing the cells in the presence of an antibiotic, only those cells that were activating the insulin promoter were able to survive. The cells were cloned and then cultured under varying conditions. Cells cultured in the presence of low concentrations of glucose differentiated and were able to respond to changes in glucose concentration by increasing insulin secretion nearly sevenfold. The researchers then implanted the cells into the spleens of diabetic mice and found that symptoms of diabetes were reversed.

Manfred Ruediger of Cardion, Inc., in Erkrath, Germany, is using the approach developed by Soria and his colleagues to develop insulin-producing human cells derived from embryonic stem cells. By using this method, the non-insulin-producing cells will be killed off and only insulin-producing cells should survive. This is important in ensuring that undifferentiated cells are not implanted that could give rise to tumors [15]. However, some researchers believe that it will be important to engineer systems in which all the components of a functioning pancreatic islet are allowed to develop.

Recently Ron McKay and his colleagues described a series of experiments in which they induced mouse embryonic cells to differentiate into insulin-secreting structures that resembled pancreatic islets [10]. McKay and his colleagues started with embryonic stem cells and let them form embryoid bodies—an aggregate of cells containing all three embryonic germ layers. They then selected a population of cells from the embryoid bodies that expressed the neural marker nestin (see Appendix B. Mouse Embryonic Stem Cells). Using a sophisticated five-stage culturing technique, the researchers were able to induce the cells to form islet-like clusters that resembled those found in native pancreatic islets. The cells responded to normal glucose concentrations by secreting insulin, although insulin amounts were lower than those secreted by normal islet cells (see Figure 7.2. Development of Insulin-Secreting Pancreatic-Like Cells From Mouse Embryonic Stem Cells). When the cells were injected into diabetic mice, they

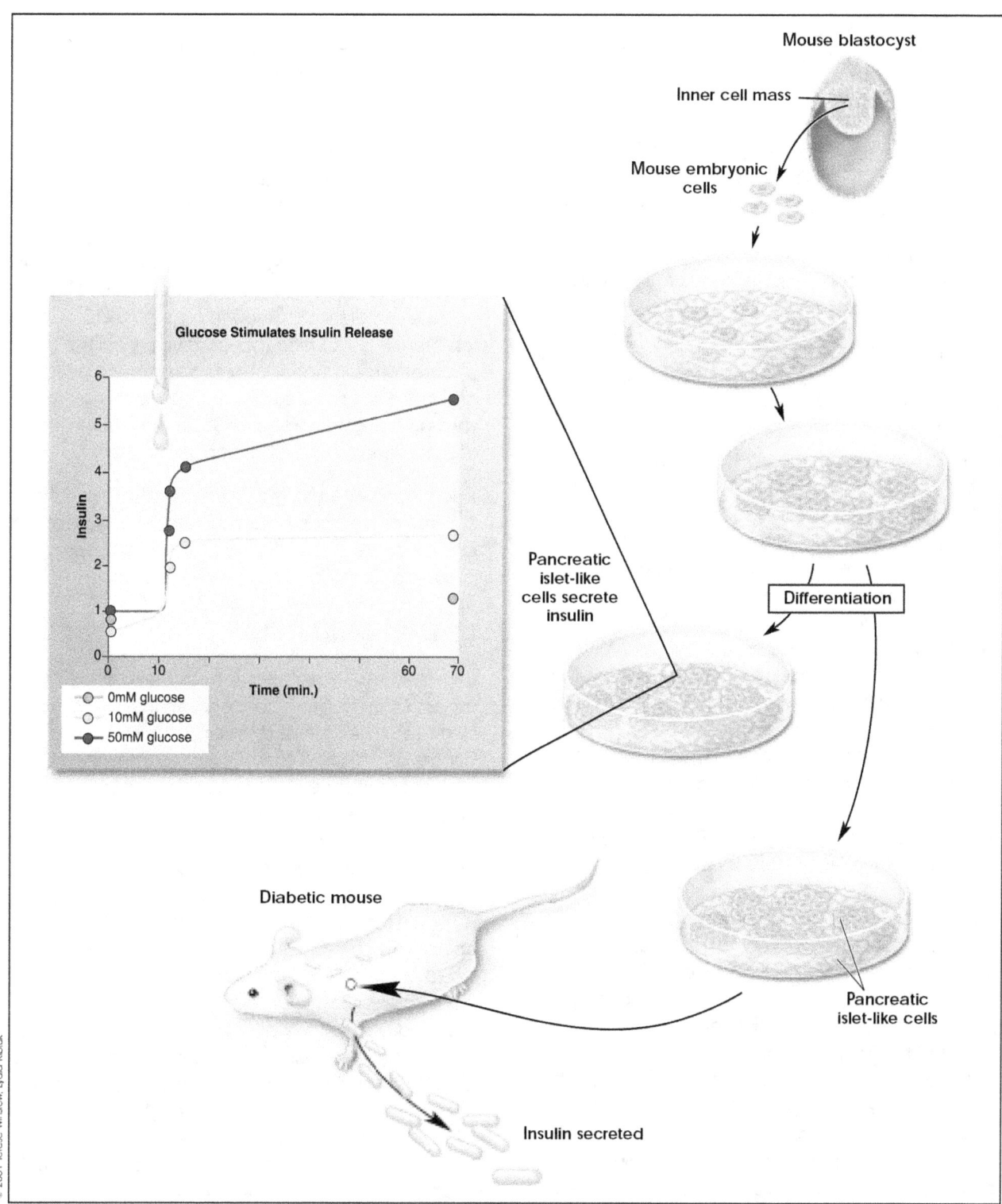

Figure 7.2. Development of Insulin-Secreting Pancreatic-Like Cells From Mouse Embryonic Stem Cells.
Mouse embryonic stem cells were derived from the inner cell mass of the early embryo (blastocyst) and cultured under specific conditions. The embryonic stem cells (in blue) were then expanded and differentiated. Cells with markers consistent with islet cells were selected for further differentiation and characterization. When these cells (in purple) were grown in culture, they spontaneously formed three-dimentional clusters similar in structure to normal pancreatic islets. The cells produced and secreted insulin. As depicted in the chart, the pancreatic islet-like cells showed an increase in release of insulin as the glucose concentration of the culture media was increased. When the pancreatic islet-like cells were implanted in the shoulder of diabetic mice, the cells became vascularized, synthesized insulin, and maintained physical characteristics similar to pancreatic islets.

survived, although they did not reverse the symptoms of diabetes.

According to McKay, this system is unique in that the embryonic cells form a functioning pancreatic islet, complete with all the major cell types. The cells assemble into islet-like structures that contain another layer, which contains neurons and is similar to intact islets from the pancreas [11]. Several research groups are trying to apply McKay's results with mice to induce human embryonic stem cells to differentiate into insulin-producing islets.

Recent research has also provided more evidence that human embryonic cells can develop into cells that can and do produce insulin. Last year, Melton, Nissim Benvinisty of the Hebrew University in Jerusalem, and Josef Itskovitz-Eldor of the Technion in Haifa, Israel, reported that human embryonic stem cells could be manipulated in culture to express the PDX-1 gene, a gene that controls insulin transcription [16]. In these experiments, researchers cultured human embryonic stem cells and allowed them to spontaneously form embryoid bodies (clumps of embryonic stem cells composed of many types of cells from all three germ layers). The embryoid bodies were then treated with various growth factors, including nerve growth factor. The researchers found that both untreated embryoid bodies and those treated with nerve growth factor expressed PDX-1. Embryonic stem cells prior to formation of the aggregated embryoid bodies did not express PDX-1. Because expression of the PDX-1 gene is associated with the formation of beta islet cells, these results suggest that beta islet cells may be one of the cell types that spontaneously differentiate in the embryoid bodies. The researchers now think that nerve growth factor may be one of the key signals for inducing the differentiation of beta islet cells and can be exploited to direct differentiation in the laboratory. Complementing these findings is work done by Jon Odorico of the University of Wisconsin in Madison using human embryonic cells of the same source. In preliminary findings, he has shown that human embryonic stem cells can differentiate and express the insulin gene [12].

More recently, Itskovitz-Eldor and his Technion colleagues further characterized insulin-producing cells in embryoid bodies [1]. The researchers found that embryonic stem cells that were allowed to spontaneously form embryoid bodies contained a significant percentage of cells that express insulin. Based on the binding of antibodies to the insulin protein, Itskovitz-Eldor estimates that 1 to 3 percent of the cells in embryoid bodies are insulin-producing beta-islet cells. The researchers also found that cells in the embryoid bodies express glut-2 and islet-specific glucokinase, genes important for beta cell function and insulin secretion. Although the researchers did not measure a time-dependent response to glucose, they did find that cells cultured in the presence of glucose secrete insulin into the culture medium. The researchers concluded that embryoid bodies contain a subset of cells that appear to function as beta cells and that the refining of culture conditions may soon yield a viable method for inducing the differentiation of beta cells and, possibly, pancreatic islets.

Taken together, these results indicate that the development of a human embryonic stem cell system that can be coaxed into differentiating into functioning insulin-producing islets may soon be possible.

FUTURE DIRECTIONS

Ultimately, type 1 diabetes may prove to be especially difficult to cure, because the cells are destroyed when the body's own immune system attacks and destroys them. This autoimmunity must be overcome if researchers hope to use transplanted cells to replace the damaged ones. Many researchers believe that at least initially, immunosuppressive therapy similar to that used in the Edmonton protocol will be beneficial. A potential advantage of embryonic cells is that, in theory, they could be engineered to express the appropriate genes that would allow them to escape or reduce detection by the immune system. Others have suggested that a technology should be developed to encapsulate or embed islet cells derived from islet stem or progenitor cells in a material that would allow small molecules such as insulin to pass through freely, but would not allow interactions between the islet cells and cells of the immune system. Such encapsulated cells could secrete insulin into the blood stream, but remain inaccessible to the immune system.

Before any cell-based therapy to treat diabetes makes it to the clinic, many safety issues must be addressed (see Chapter 10. Assessing Human Stem Cell Safety). A major consideration is whether any precursor or stem-like cells transplanted into the body might revert to a more pluripotent state and induce the formation of tumors. These risks would seemingly be lessened if fully differentiated cells are used in transplantation.

But before any kind of human islet-precursor cells can be used therapeutically, a renewable source of human stem cells must be developed. Although many progenitor cells have been identified in adult tissue, few of these cells can be cultured for multiple generations. Embryonic stem cells show the greatest promise for generating cell lines that will be free of contaminants and that can self renew. However, most researchers agree that until a therapeutically useful source of human islet cells is developed, all avenues of research should be exhaustively investigated, including both adult and embryonic sources of tissue.

REFERENCES

1. Assady, S., Maor, G., Amit, M., Itskovitz-Eldor, J., Skorecki, K.L., and Tzukerman, M. (2001). Insulin production by human embryonic stem cells. Diabetes. *50*. http://www.diabetes.org/Diabetes_Rapids/Suheir_Assady_06282001.pdf

2. Beattie, G.M., Otonkoski, T., Lopez, A.D., and Hayek, A. (1997). Functional beta-cell mass after transplantation of human fetal pancreatic cells: differentiation or proliferation? Diabetes. *46*, 244-248.

3. Bonner-Weir, S., personal communication.

4. Bonner-Weir, S., Taneja, M., Weir, G.C., Tatarkiewicz, K., Song, K.H., Sharma, A., and O'Neil, J.J. (2000). *In vitro* cultivation of human islets from expanded ductal tissue. Proc. Natl. Acad. Sci. U. S. A. *97*, 7999-8004.

5. Bosco, D. and Meda, P. (1997). Reconstructing Islet function *in vitro*. Adv. Exp. Med. Biol. *426*, 285-298.

6. Dufayet de la Tour, D., Halvorsen, T., Demeterco, C., Tyrberg, B., Itkin-Ansari, P., Loy, M., Yoo, S.J., Hao, S., Bossie, S., and Levine, F. (2001). b-cell differentiation from a human pancreatic cell line *in vitro* and *in vivo*. Mol. Endocrinol. *15*, 476-483.

7. Hayek, A., personal communication.

8. Itkin-Ansari, P., Demeterco, C., Bossie, S., Dufayet de la Tour, D., Beattie, G.M., Movassat, J., Mally, M.I., Hayek, A., and Levine, F. (2001). PDX-1 and cell-cell contact act in synergy to promote d-cell development in a human pancreatic endocrine precursor cell line. Mol. Endocrinol. *14*, 814-822.

9. Levine, F., personal communication.

10. Lumelsky, N., Blondel, O., Laeng, P., Velasco, I., Ravin, R., and McKay, R. (2001). Differentiation of Embryonic Stem Cells to Insulin-Secreting Structures Similiar to Pancreatic Islets. Science. *292*, 1389-1394.

11. McKay, R., personal communication

12. Odorico, J. S., personal communication.

13. Peck, A., personal communication.

14. Ramiya, V. K., personal communication.

15. Ruediger, M., personal communication.

16. Schuldiner, M., Yanuka, O., Itskovitz-Eldor, J., Melton, D., and Benvenisty, N. (2000). Effects of eight growth factors on the differentiation of cells derived from human embryonic stem cells. Proc. Natl. Acad. Sci. U. S. A. *97*, 11307-11312.

17. Shapiro, J., Lakey, J.R.T., Ryan, E.A., Korbutt, G.S., Toth, E., Warnock, G.L., Kneteman, N.M., and Rajotte, R.V. (2000). Islet transplantation in seven patients with type 1 diabetes mellitus using a glucocorticoid-free immunosuppressive regimen. N. Engl. J. Med. *343*, 230-238.

18. Soria, B., Martin, F., Andreu, E., Sanchez-Andrés, J.V., Nacher, V., and Montana, E. (1996). Diminished fraction of blockable ATP-sensitive K+ channels in islets transplanted into diabetic mice. Diabetes. *45*, 1755-1760.

19. Soria, B., Roche, E., Berná, G., Leon-Quinto, T., Reig, J.A., and Martin, F. (2000). Insulin-secreting cells derived from embryonic stem cells normalize glycemia in streptozotocin-induced diabetic mice. Diabetes. *49*, 157-162.

20. Zulewski, H., Abraham, E.J., Gerlach, M.J., Daniel, P.B., Moritz, W., Muller, B., Vallejo, M., Thomas, M.K., and Habener, J.F. (2001). Multipotential nestin-positive stem cells isolated from adult pancreatic islets differentiate ex vivo into pancreatic endocrine, exocrine, and hepatic phenotypes. Diabetes. *50*, 521-533.

This page intentionally left blank

8. REBUILDING THE NERVOUS SYSTEM WITH STEM CELLS

Today, most treatments for damage to the brain or spinal cord aim to relieve symptoms and limit further damage. But recent research into the regeneration mechanisms of the central nervous system, including the discovery of stem cells in the adult brain that can give rise to new neurons and neural support cells, has raised hopes that researchers can find ways to actually repair central nervous system damage. Research on stem cells in nervous system disorders is one of the few areas in which there is evidence that cell-replacement therapy can restore lost function.

STEM CELLS BRING NEW STRATEGIES FOR DEVELOPING REPLACEMENT NEURONS

Just a decade ago, neuroscience textbooks held that neurons in the adult human brain and spinal cord could not regenerate. Once dead, it was thought, central nervous system neurons were gone for good. Because rebuilding nervous tissue seemed out of the question, research focused almost entirely on therapeutic approaches to limiting further damage.

That dogma that brain tissue could not be regenerated is history. In the mid-1990s, neuroscientists learned that some parts of the adult human brain do, in fact, generate new neurons, at least under certain circumstances. Moreover, they found that the new neurons arise from "neural stem cells" in the fetal as well as the adult brain (see Chapter 4. The Adult Stem Cell). These undifferentiated cells resemble cells in a developing fetus that give rise to the brain and spinal cord. The researchers also found that these neural stem cells could generate many, if not all, types of cells found in the brain. This includes neurons—the main message carriers in the nervous system, which use long, thin projections called axons to transmit signals over long distances—as well as crucial neural-support cells called oligodendrocytes and astrocytes (see Figure 8.1. The Neuron).

The discovery of a regenerative capacity in the adult central nervous system holds out the promise that it may eventually be possible to repair damage from terrible degenerative diseases such as Parkinson's Disease and amyotrophic lateral sclerosis (ALS, also known as Lou Gehrig's disease), as well as from brain and spinal cord injuries resulting from stroke or trauma (see Box 8.1. Early Research Shows Stem Cells Can Improve Movement in Paralyzed Mice).

Researchers are pursuing two fundamental strategies to exploit this discovery. One is to grow differentiated cells in a laboratory dish that are suitable for implantation into a patient by starting with undifferentiated neural cells. The idea is either to treat the cells in culture to nudge them toward the desired differentiated neuronal cell type before implantation, or to implant them directly and rely on signals inside the body to direct their maturation into the right kind of brain cell. A variety of stem cells might be used for this task, including so-called "neural precursor cells" that are inwardly committed to differentiating into a particular cell type but are outwardly not yet changed or pluripotent embryonic stem cells—cells derived from a very early stage human embryo that retain the capacity to become any cell type in the body and that can be maintained in culture for a very long time without differentiating.

The other repair strategy relies on finding growth hormones and other "trophic factors"—growth factors, hormones, and other signaling molecules that help cells survive and grow—that can fire up a patient's own stem cells and endogenous repair mechanisms, to allow the body to cope with damage from disease or injury. Researchers are vigorously pursuing both strategies to find therapies for central nervous system disorders that involve cell death, but a great deal more basic research must be carried out before effective new therapies emerge.

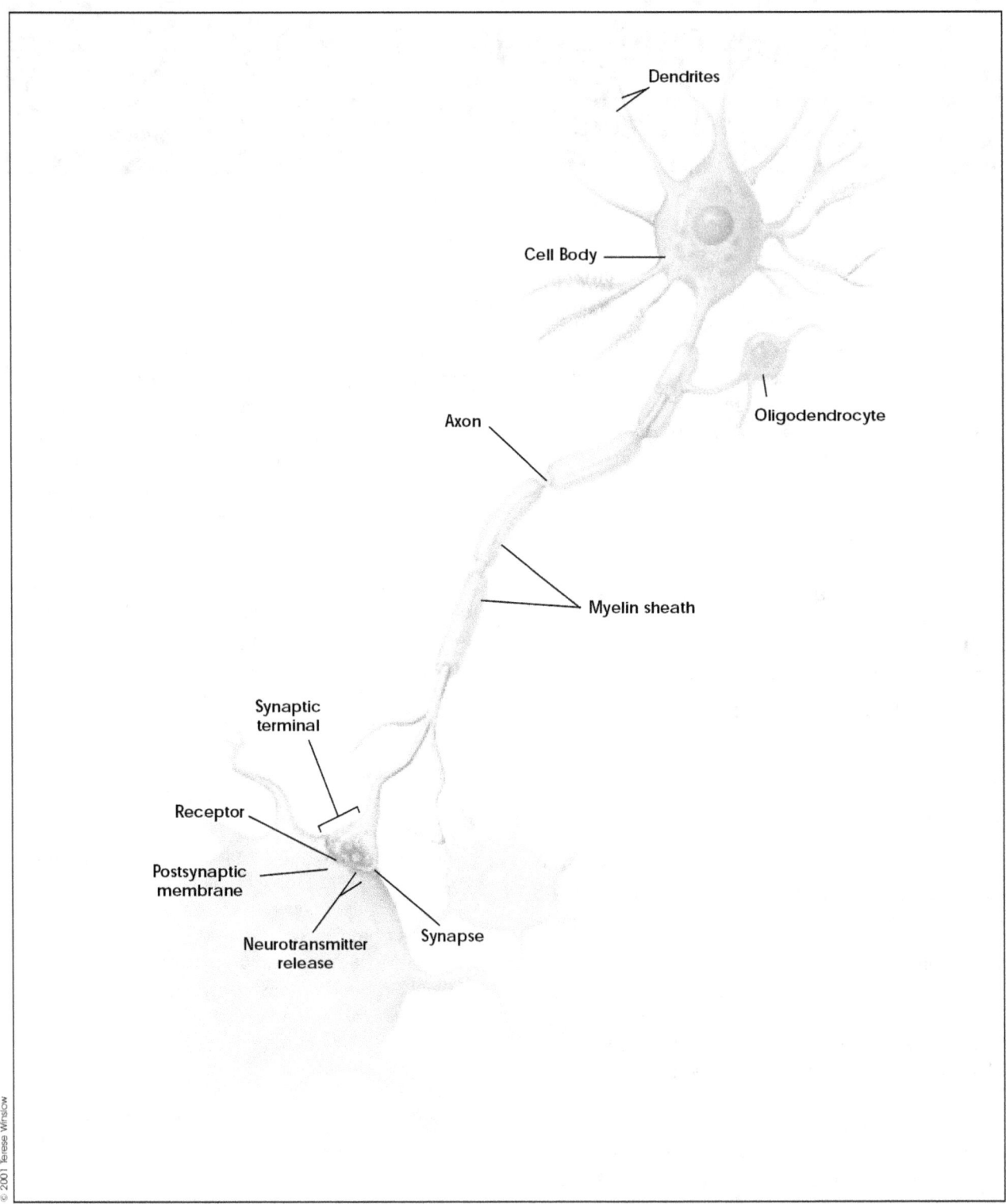

Figure 8.1. The Neuron.
When sufficient neurotransmitters cross synapses and bind receptors on the neuronal cell body and dendrites, the neuron sends an electrical signal down its axon to synaptic terminals, which in turn release neurotransmitters into the synapse that affects the following neuron. The brain neurons that die in Parkinson's Disease release the transmitter dopamine. Oligodendrocytes supply the axon with an insulating myelin sheath.

Box 8.1

Early Research Shows Stem Cells Can Improve Movement in Paralyzed Mice

Researchers at Johns Hopkins University recently reported preliminary evidence that cells derived from embryonic stem cells can restore movement in an animal model of amyotrophic lateral sclerosis (ALS) [1]. This degenerative disorder, also called as Lou Gehrig's disease, progressively destroys special nerves found in the spinal cord, known as motor neurons, that control movement. Patients with ALS develop increasing muscle weakness over months to years, which ultimately leads to paralysis and death. The cause is largely unknown, and there are no effective treatments.

In this new study, the researchers used a rat model of ALS to test for possible nerve cell- restoring properties of stem cells. The rats were exposed to Sindbis virus, which infects the central nervous system and destroys the motor neurons in the spinal cord. Rats that survive are left with paralyzed muscles in their hindquarters and weakened back limbs. Scientists assess the degree of impairment by measuring the rats' movement, quantifying electrical activity in the nerves serving the back limbs, and visually judging the extent of nerve damage through a microscope.

The researchers wanted to see whether stem cells could restore nerves and improve mobility in rats. Because scientists have had difficulty sustaining stem cell lines derived from rat embryos, the investigators conducted their experiments with embryonic germ cells that John Gearhart and colleagues isolated from human fetal tissue in 1998. These cells can produce unchanged copies of themselves when maintained in culture, and they form into clumps called embryoid bodies. Under certain conditions, research has shown that the cells in the embryoid bodies begin to look and function like neurons when subjected to specific laboratory conditions [2]. The researchers had an idea that these embryoid body cells in their nonspecialized state might become specialized as replacement neurons if placed into the area of the damaged spinal cord. So they carefully prepared cells from the embryoid bodies and injected them into the fluid surrounding the spinal cord of the paralyzed rats that had their motor neurons destroyed by the Sindbis virus.

To test this idea, the researchers selected from laboratory culture dishes barely differentiated embryonic germs cells that displayed the molecular markers of neural stem cells, including the proteins nestin and neuron specific enolase. They grew these cells in large quantities and injected them into the fluid surrounding the spinal cords of partially paralyzed, Sindbis-virus-treated rats.

The response was impressive. Three months after the injections, many of the treated rats were able to move their hind limbs and walk, albeit clumsily, while the rats that did not receive cell injections remained paralyzed. Moreover, at autopsy the researchers found that cells derived from human embryonic germ cells had migrated throughout the spinal fluid and continued to develop, displaying both the shape and molecular markers characteristic of mature motor neurons. The researchers are quick to caution that their results are preliminary, and that they do not know for certain whether the treatment helped the paralyzed rats because new neurons took the place of the old, or because trophic factors from the injected cells facilitated the recovery of the rats' remaining nerve cells and helped the rats improve in their ability to use their hind limbs. Nor do they know how well this strategy will translate into a therapy for human neurodegenerative diseases like ALS. And they emphasize that there are many hurdles to cross before the use of stem cells to repair damaged motor neurons in patients can be considered. Nevertheless, researchers are excited about these results, which, if confirmed, would represent a major step toward using specialized stem cells from embryonic and fetal tissue sources to restore nervous system function.

REFERENCES

1. Kerr, D.A., Llado, J., Shamblott, M., Maragakis, N., Irani, D.N., Dike, S., Sappington, A., Gearhart, J., and Rothstein, J. (2001). Human embryonic germ cell derivatives facilitate motor recovery of rats with diffuse motor neuron injury.

2. Shamblott, M.J., Axelman, J., Wang, S., Bugg, E.M., Littlefield, J.W., Donovan, P.J., Blumenthal, P.D., Huggins, G.R., and Gearhart, J.D. (1998). Derivation of pluripotent stem cells from cultured human primordial germ cells. Proc. Natl. Acad. Sci. U. S. A. 95, 13726-13731.

MULTIPLE APPROACHES FOR USING STEM CELLS IN PARKINSON'S DISEASE RESEARCH

Efforts to develop stem cell based therapies for Parkinson's Disease provide a good example of research aimed at rebuilding the central nervous system. As is the case with other disorders, both the cell-implantation and the trophic-factor strategies are under active development. Both approaches are promising. This is especially true of cell implantation, which involves using primary tissue transplanted directly form developing fetal brain tissue. Parkinson's is a progressive movement disorder that usually strikes after age 50. Symptoms often begin with an uncontrollable hand tremor, followed by increasing rigidity, difficulty walking, and trouble initiating voluntary movement. The symptoms result from the death of a particular set of neurons deep in the brain.

The neurons that die in Parkinson's Disease connect a structure in the brain called the substantia nigra to another structure called the striatum, composed of the caudate nucleus and the putamen

(see Figure 8.2. Neuronal Pathways that Degenerate in Parkinson's Disease). These "nigro-striatal" neurons release the chemical transmitter dopamine onto their target neurons in the striatum. One of dopamine's major roles is to regulate the nerves that control body movement. As these cells die, there is less dopamine produced, leading to the movement difficulties characteristic of Parkinson's. At this point, no one knows for certain why the neurons die.

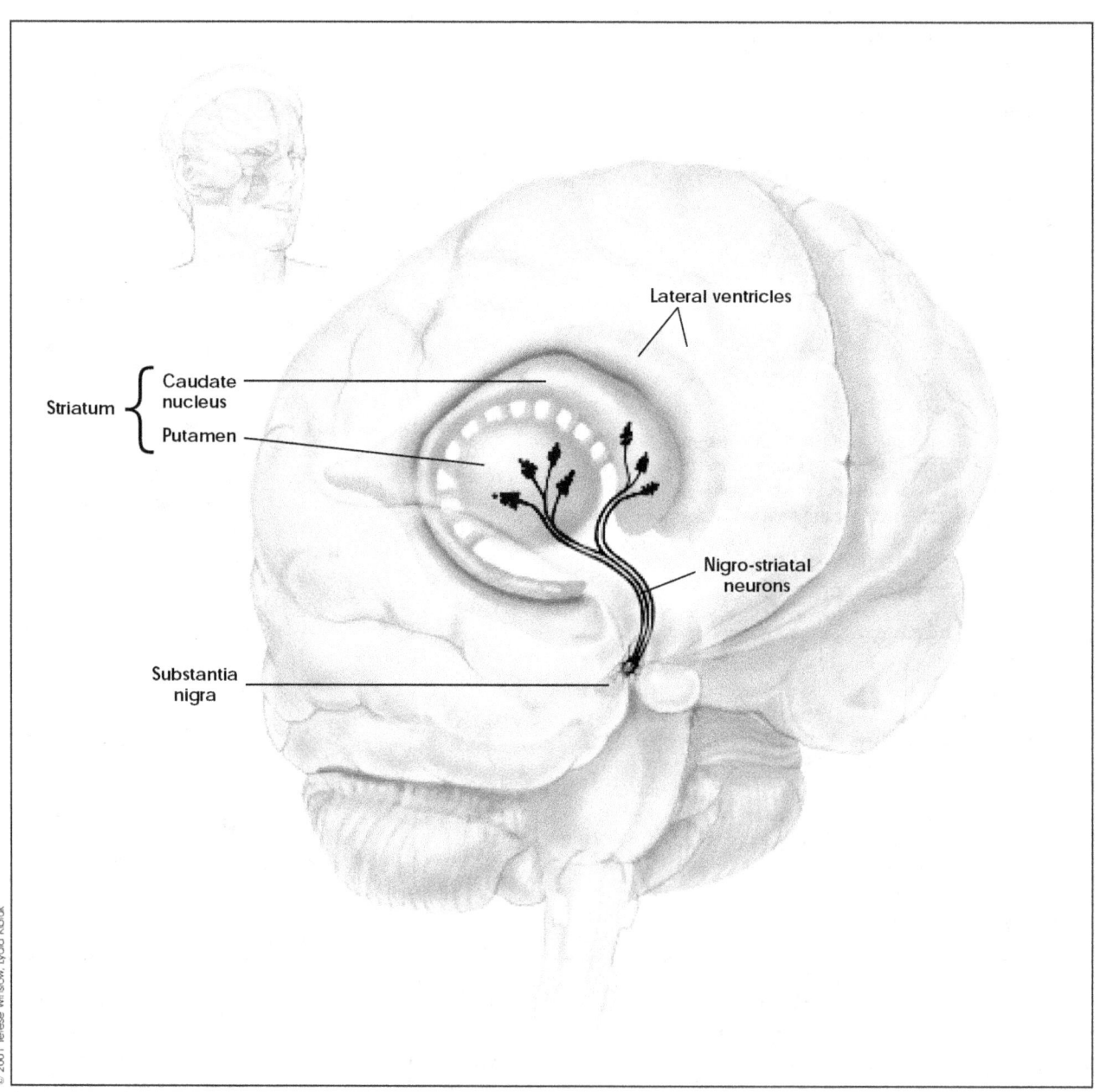

Figure 8.2. Neuronal Pathways that Degenerate in Parkinson's Disease.
Signals that control body movements travel along neurons that project from the substantia nigra to the caudate nucleus and putamen (collectively called the striatum). These "nigro-striatal" neurons release dopamine at their stargets in the striatum. In Parkinson's patients, dopamine neurons in the nigro-striatal pathway degenerate for unknown reasons.

Most patients suffering from Parkinson's Disease are treated with a drug called levodopa, which the brain converts into dopamine. It initially helps most patients, but unfortunately, side effects of the drug increase over time and its effectiveness wanes. This leaves Parkinson's patients and their doctors fighting a long, uphill battle to balance medication with side effects to maintain function. In the end, many patients are utterly helpless.

FETAL TISSUE TRANSPLANTS IN PARKINSON'S DISEASE RESEARCH

The idea of growing dopamine cells in the laboratory to treat Parkinson's is the most recent step in the long history of cell or tissue transplantation to reverse this devastating disease. The concept was, and still is, straightforward: implant cells into the brain that can replace the lost dopamine-releasing neurons. Although conceptually straightforward, this is not an easy task. Fully developed and differentiated dopamine neurons do not survive transplantation, so direct transplantation of fully developed brain tissue from cadavers, for example, is not an option. Moreover, full functional recovery depends on more than cell survival and dopamine release; transplanted cells must also make appropriate connections with their normal target neurons in the striatum.

One of the first attempts at using cell transplantation in humans was tried in the 1980s. This surgical approach involved the transplantation of dopamine-producing cells found in the adrenal glands, which sit atop the kidneys in the abdomen. Neurosurgeons in Mexico reported that they had achieved dramatic improvement in Parkinson's patients by transplanting dopamine-producing chromaffin cells from several patients' own adrenal glands to the nigro-striatal area of their brains. Surgeons in the United States, however, observed only very modest and inconsistent improvement in their patients' symptoms, and any gains disappeared within a year after surgery. Furthermore, it became clear that the risks associated with the procedure—which required both brain and abdominal surgery on patients who are often frail and elderly—outweigh the benefits [13].

Another strategy, based on transplanting developing dopamine neurons from fetal brain tissue, has fared better, however. Lars Olsen and his colleagues showed in the early 1970s that fetal tissue

transplanted directly from the developing nigro-striatal pathways of embryonic mice into the anterior chamber of an adult rat's eye continues to mature into fully developed dopamine neurons [3]. By the early 1980s Anders Bjorkland and others had shown that transplantation of fetal tissue into the damaged areas of the brains of rats and monkeys used as models of the disease could reverse their Parkinson's-like symptoms. Subsequently, researchers refined their surgical techniques and showed that functional recovery depends on the implanted neurons growing and making functional connections at the appropriate brain locations—essentially finishing their maturation by integrating into the adult host brain [3].

The promising animal results led to human trials in several centers worldwide, starting in the mid-1980s. Using tissue removed from a fetus electively aborted seven to nine weeks after conception, these early human transplantation studies showed encouraging, but inconsistent, benefit to patients. Although not all patients improved, in the best cases patients receiving fetal tissue transplants showed a clear reduction in the severity of their symptoms. Also, researchers could measure an increase in dopamine neuron function in the striatum of these patients by using a brain-imaging method called positron emission tomography (PET) (see Figure 8.3. Positron Emission Tomography [PET] images from a Parkinson's patient before and after fetal tissue transplantation). Also, autopsies done on the few patients who died from causes unrelated to either Parkinson's or the surgery revealed a robust survival of the grafted neurons. Moreover, the grafted neurons sent outgrowths from the cell body that integrated well into the normal target areas in the striatum.

A major weakness in these initial studies was that they were all done "open label," meaning that both researchers and patients knew which patients received the transplanted tissue. When appropriate, the best test of a new therapy is a placebo controlled, double-blind trial, in which neither researcher nor patient knows who has received the experimental treatment. In the mid-1990s, NIH approved funding for two rigorous clinical trials of fetal tissue transplantation for Parkinson's patients. Both studies provided for placebo control, in the form of sham surgery conducted on half the study patients, and they were done double blind—neither the

Dopamine-Neuron Transplantation

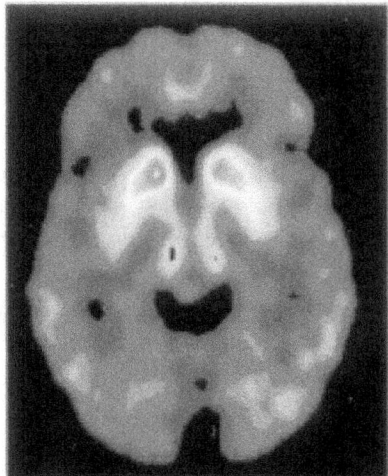

Before Surgery

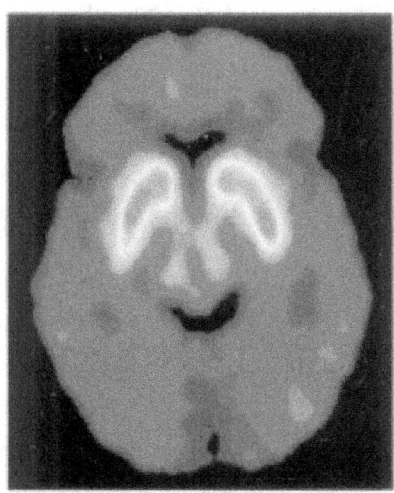

After Surgery

Figure 8.3. Positron Emission Tomography (PET) images from a Parkinson's patient before and after fetal tissue transplantation. The image taken before surgery (left) shows uptake of a radioactive form of dopamine (red) only in the caudate nucleus, indicating that dopamine neurons have degenerated. Twelve months after surgery, an image from the same patient (right) reveals increased dopamine function, especially in the putamen. (Reprinted with permission from N Eng J Med 2001;344 (10) p. 710.)

researchers evaluating the effects of the surgery nor the patients themselves knew who got tissue implants.

The results of one of these trials, led by Curt Freed, were published recently [5]. Compared with control, patients who received the fetal-tissue transplant showed no significant benefit in a subjective assessment of the patient's quality of life, which was the study's primary endpoint. Moreover, two years after surgery, 5 out of 33 treated patients developed persistent dyskinesia—uncontrolled flailing movements—that had not been observed in the open-label work described above.

The Freed study results, nonetheless, provide important information about the ability of dopamine neurons to survive in humans. Moreover, PET-scanning data from the treated patients, as well as autopsies of two patients who died of unrelated causes several months after the surgery, showed that many of the dopamine neurons survived and grew. Researchers are now awaiting the results of the second NIH-sponsored double-blind trial, led by Warren Olanow [12]. The procedures used in this study differ substantially from those of Freed and his colleagues—including the tissue-handling method, the number of cells implanted, the use of immunosuppressive drugs

to limit rejection of the implanted tissue, and the tests used to assess patient response—and are closer to those used in the most successful of the early open-label experiments.

Most Parkinson's researchers are still hopeful that the cell-implantation approach will one day lead to a useful and widely used therapy for Parkinson's Disease. At the same time, however, most researchers are also convinced they must find a different source of cells for transplant. The logistical and technical problems involved in recovering enough developing dopamine neurons from fetal tissue are very great. Moreover, it is virtually impossible to standardize the tissue collected from different fetuses and to fully characterize the cells implanted. This absence of tissue standardization makes it very difficult to determine the most important factors that lead to a good patient response and may add risk (see Chapter 10. Assessing Human Stem Cell Safety).

One alternative to cell implantation with human fetal tissue is to use fetal cells and tissues from animals. Researchers at Diacrin and Genzyme, two biotechnology companies, recently announced preliminary results from a clinical trial in which 10 Parkinson's patients received neural cells from the brains of fetal pigs. Eighteen months after the surgery, treated patients did not improve enough to show a statistically significant difference from eight control patients who received a sham immunosuppression regimen and underwent sham surgery. Autopsy of one treated patient who died of a pulmonary embolism eight months after surgery revealed that a small portion of the transplanted pig cells had survived [2], but PET studies looking for improvement in dopamine uptake in all treated patients did not show clear improvement. The researchers are still analyzing their data [15].

RAISING NEURONS FOR REPLACEMENT IN PATIENTS WITH PARKINSON'S DISEASE

What Parkinson's researchers ultimately want is a renewable source of cells that can differentiate into functional dopamine neurons when placed in the striatum. Laboratory-grown cells derived from a stem cell may be the best potential alternative source for transplantable material. One way to get these is to find the right combination of growth factors and cell-culture conditions to bring undifferentiated cells along in a culture dish to a point where they are committed to becoming dopamine neurons, then implant them to finish growth and differentiation in the host brain. Another possibility is to put less-committed cells into a damaged brain and rely on "environmental" signals in the brain to guide them into becoming the right kind of replacement cell. These developmental signals may be expressed in the brain transiently following neural degeneration or acute damage.

Whether the cells ultimately implanted are half-differentiated or completely immature, however, researchers need a reliable source. To that end, they have identified a whole host of different immature cells that may have the potential to become, among other things, dopamine neurons, and they are now in the process of sorting out how best to make them do so. Neural stem cells isolated from animals and humans cannot be grown efficiently in the lab without changing them in some way, such as by engineering them to express a gene normally turned on only early in development. Embryonic stem cells—derived from the inner cell mass of an embryo at the blastocyst stage, when only a few hundred cells are present—can be kept in culture in a completely undifferentiated state. They are still capable of

becoming not just nervous system cells but every cell type in the body. If researchers want to be able to implant cells derived from undifferentiated embryonic stem cells, they must take care that no cells in the mix give rise to unwanted cell types, such as muscle or bone, within the nervous system. Stem cells from other tissues—including umbilical cord blood and human bone marrow—can also be coaxed to display many of the surface-protein "markers" characteristic of nervous system cells. It is not yet clear, however, whether these cells are capable of giving rise to fully functional neurons.

A great deal of basic research remains to be done to find which of these cells provides the best way to get a workable therapy for Parkinson's Disease. For example, although researchers have shown for certain that both primary human fetal cells and mouse embryonic stem cells can become fully functional dopamine neurons, they do not yet know if adult neural stem cells have the same potential. Also, no one has yet published evidence that cells from any renewable source that are laboratory-directed to differentiate into dopamine neurons can eliminate symptoms in animal models of Parkinson's when implanted.

Researchers are making rapid progress, however. For example, Ron McKay and his colleagues at NIH reported in 1998 that they were able to expand a population of neurons from embryonic mouse brain in culture, and that these cells relieved Parkinson's-like symptoms in a rat model [16]. And last year, McKay's lab also described a procedure for efficiently converting mouse pluripotent embryonic stem cells into neurons that have all the characteristics of dopamine neurons, including the ability to form synapses [17]. McKay and other researchers say they have encouraging unpublished results that dopamine precursors derived from mouse embryonic stem cells can eliminate symptoms in rat models of Parkinson's Disease [7, 10].

Privately funded researchers are following an analogous path using pluripotent human embryonic stem cells. Thomas Okarma of Geron Corporation confirms that his company is testing the potential of human embryonic stem cells in animal models of Parkinson's Disease, but the results are not yet complete [11]. In abstracts presented at a recent conference, Geron reports having succeeded in directing human embryonic stem cells to become mature neural cells in laboratory culture, including cells that have the structural and chemical characteristics of dopamine neurons [6].

TURNING ON THE BRAIN'S OWN STEM CELLS AS A REPAIR MECHANISM

Parkinson's researchers are also looking for ways to spark the repair mechanisms already in a patient's brain to fix damage that these mechanisms could not otherwise manage. This strategy is less developed than cell implantation, but it also holds promise [1]. In the future, researchers may use stem cells from embryonic or adult sources not to replace lost cells directly, but rather to turn on the body's own repair mechanisms. Alternatively, researchers may find effective drug treatments that help a patient's own stem cells and repair mechanisms work more effectively.

Stem cells in the adult primate brain occur in two locations. One, the subventricular zone, is an area under fluid-filled spaces called ventricles. The other is the dentate gyrus of the hippocampus. In primates, very few new neurons normally appear in either place, which is why the phenomenon escaped notice until recently. Researchers showed in the mid-1990s that when the brain is injured, stem cells in these two areas proliferate and migrate toward the site of the damage. The researchers are now trying to discover how far this kind of response can go toward ameliorating certain kinds of damage.

Recent research shows the direction that this may be heading for Parkinson's Disease. James Fallon and colleagues studied the effects on rat brain of a protein called transforming growth factor alpha (TGFα)—a natural peptide found in the body from the very earliest stages of embryonic development onward that is important in activating normal repair processes in several organs, including liver and skin. Fallon's studies suggest that the brain's normal repair process may never be adequately triggered in a slowly developing degenerative disease like Parkinson's and that providing more TGFα can turn it on. Specifically, Fallon found that TGFα injected into healthy rat brain causes stem cells in the subventricular zone to proliferate for several days, after which they disappear. But if the researchers make similar injections into rats in which they first damage the nigro-striatal neurons with

a toxin called 6-hydroxydopamine—a frequently used animal model for Parkinson's Disease—two things happen. After several days of cell proliferation, Fallon observes what he calls a "wave of migration" of the stem cells to the damaged areas, where they differentiate into dopamine neurons. Most importantly, the treated rats do not show the behavioral abnormalities associated with the loss of the neurons. Whether the beneficial effect on symptoms is the result of the newly formed cells or some other trophic effect is not yet entirely clear [4].

STEM CELLS' FUTURE ROLE IN SPINAL CORD INJURY REPAIR

Parkinson's Disease is only one of many nervous system disorders that researchers are trying to solve by regenerating damaged tissue. But Parkinson's, difficult as it is to reverse, is a relatively easy target because a regenerative therapy need only replace one particular cell type in one part of the brain.

Therapies for other disorders face much bigger hurdles. Complete restoration after severe spinal cord injury, for example, is probably far in the future, if it can ever be done at all. Many cell types are destroyed in these injuries, including neurons that carry messages between the brain and the rest of the body. Getting these neurons to grow past an injury site and connect appropriately with their targets is extraordinarily difficult. But spinal cord injury patients would benefit greatly from an even limited restoration of lost functions—gaining partial use of a limb instead of none, or restoring bladder control, or being freed from pain. Such limited restoration of part of a patient's lost functions is, for some less severe types of injury, perhaps a more achievable goal.

In many spinal injuries, the spinal cord is not actually cut and at least some of the signal-carrying neuronal axons are intact. But the surviving axons no longer carry messages because cells called oligodendrocytes, which make the axons' insulating myelin sheath, are lost. Researchers have recently made the first steps in learning to replace these lost myelin-producing cells [14]. For example, researchers have shown that stem cells can aid remyelination in rodents [8, 9]. Specifically, they found that injection of oligodendrocytes derived from mouse embryonic stem cells could remyelinate axons in chemically demyelinated rat spinal cord and that the treated rats regained limited use of their hind limbs compared with the controls. They are not certain, however, whether the limited increase in function they observed in rats is actually due to the remyelination or an unidentified trophic effect of the treatment.

Spinal injury researchers emphasize that much more basic and preclinical research must be done before attempting human trials using stem cell therapies to repair the damaged nervous system. Despite the fact that there is much basic work left to do and many fundamental questions still to be answered, researchers are hopeful that effective repair for once-hopeless nervous system damage may eventually be achieved. Whether through developing replacement cells or activating the body's own stem cells *in vivo*, research on the use of stem cells for nervous system disorders is a rapidly advancing field. This research promises to answer key questions about how to repair nervous system damage and how to restore key body functions damaged by disease or disability.

REFERENCES

1. Bjorklund, A. and Lindvall, O. (2000). Self-repair in the brain. Nature. *405*, 892-895.

2. Deacon, T., Schumacher, J., Dinsmore, J., Thomas, C., Palmer, P., Kott, S., Edge, A., Penney, D., Kassissieh, S., Dempsey, P., and Isacson, O. (1997). Histological evidence of fetal pig neural cell survival after transplantation into a patient with Parkinson's disease. Nat. Med. *3*, 350-353.

3. Dunnett, S.B., Bjorklund, A., and Lindvall, O. (2001). Cell therapy in Parkinson's disease—stop or go? Nat. Rev. Neurosci. *2*, 365-369.

4. Fallon, J., Reid, S., Kinyamu, R., Opole, I., Opole, R., Baratta, J., Korc, M., Endo, T.L., Duong, A., Nguyen, G., Karkehabadhi, M., Twardzik, D., and Loughlin, S. (2000). *In vivo* induction of massive proliferation, directed migration, and differentiation of neural cells in the adult mammalian brain. Proc. Natl. Acad. Sci. U. S. A. *97*, 14686-14691.

5. Freed, C.R., Greene, P.E., Breeze, R.E., Tsai, W.Y., DuMouchel, W., Kao, R., Dillon, S., Winfield, H., Culver, S., Trojanowski, J.Q., Eidelberg, D., and Fahn, S. (2001). Transplantation of embryonic dopamine neurons for severe Parkinson's disease. N. Engl. J. Med. *344*, 710-719.

6. Harley, C.B., Gearhart, J., Jaenisch, R., Rossant, J., and Thomson, J. (2001). Pluripotent stem cells: biology and applications. Durango, CO.

7. Isacson, O., personal communication.

8. Liu, S., Qu, Y., Stewart, T.J., Howard, M.J., Chakrabortty, S., Holekamp, T.F., and McDonald, J.W. (2000). Embryonic stem cells differentiate into oligodendrocytes and myelinate in culture and after spinal cord transplantation. Proc. Natl. Acad. Sci. U. S. A. *97*, 6126-6131.

9. McDonald, J.W., Liu, X.Z., Qu, Y., Liu, S., Mickey, S.K., Turetsky, D., Gottlieb, D.I., and Choi, D.W. (1999). Transplanted embryonic stem cells survive, differentiate and promote recovery in injured rat spinal cord. Nat. Med. *5*, 1410-1412.

10. McKay, R., personal communication.

11. Okarma, T., personal communication.

12. Olanow, C. W., personal communication.

13. Quinn, N.P. (1990). The clinical application of cell grafting techniques in patients with Parkinson's disease. Prog. Brain Res. *82*, 619-625.

14. Raisman, G. (2001). Olfactory ensheathing cells—another miracle cure for spinal cord injury? Nat. Rev. Neurosci. *2*, 369-374.

15. Schumacher, J.M., Ellias, S.A., Palmer, E.P., Kott, H.S., Dinsmore, J., Dempsey, P.K., Fischman, A.J., Thomas, C., Feldman, R.G., Kassissieh, S., Raineri, R., Manhart, C., Penney, D., Fink, J.S., and Isacson, O. (2000). Transplantation of embryonic porcine mesencephalic tissue in patients with PD. Neurology. *54*, 1042-1050.

16. Studer, L., Csete, M., Lee, S.H., Kabbani, N., Walikonis, J., Wold, B., and McKay, R. (2000). Enhanced proliferation, survival, and dopaminergic differentiation of CNS precursors in lowered oxygen. J. Neurosci. *20*, 7377-7383.

17. Studer, L., Tabar, V., and McKay, R.D. (1998). Transplantation of expanded mesencephalic precursors leads to recovery in parkinsonian rats. Nat. Neurosci. *1*, 290-295.

This page intentionally left blank

9. CAN STEM CELLS REPAIR A DAMAGED HEART?

Heart attacks and congestive heart failure remain among the Nation's most prominent health challenges despite many breakthroughs in cardiovascular medicine. In fact, despite successful approaches to prevent or limit cardiovascular disease, the restoration of function to the damaged heart remains a formidable challenge. Recent research is providing early evidence that adult and embryonic stem cells may be able to replace damaged heart muscle cells and establish new blood vessels to supply them. Discussed here are some of the recent discoveries that feature stem cell replacement and muscle regeneration strategies for repairing the damaged heart.

INTRODUCTION

For those suffering from common, but deadly, heart diseases, stem cell biology represents a new medical frontier. Researchers are working toward using stem cells to replace damaged heart cells and literally restore cardiac function.

Today in the United States, congestive heart failure—the ineffective pumping of the heart caused by the loss or dysfunction of heart muscle cells—afflicts 4.8 million people, with 400,000 new cases each year. One of the major contributors to the development of this condition is a heart attack, known medically as a myocardial infarction, which occurs in nearly 1.1 million Americans each year. It is easy to recognize that impairments of the heart and circulatory system represent a major cause of death and disability in the United States [5].

What leads to these devastating effects? The destruction of heart muscle cells, known as cardiomyocytes, can be the result of hypertension, chronic insufficiency in the blood supply to the heart muscle caused by coronary artery disease, or a heart attack, the sudden closing of a blood vessel supplying oxygen to the heart. Despite advances in surgical procedures, mechanical assistance devices, drug therapy, and organ transplantation, more than half of patients with congestive heart failure die within five years of initial diagnosis. Research has shown that therapies such as clot-busting medications can reestablish blood flow to the damaged regions of the heart and limit the death of cardiomyocytes. Researchers are now exploring ways to save additional lives by using replacement cells for dead or impaired cells so that the weakened heart muscle can regain its pumping power.

How might stem cells play a part in repairing the heart? To answer this question, researchers are building their knowledge base about how stem cells are directed to become specialized cells. One important type of cell that can be developed is the cardiomyocyte, the heart muscle cell that contracts to eject the blood out of the heart's main pumping chamber (the ventricle). Two other cell types are important to a properly functioning heart are the vascular endothelial cell, which forms the inner lining of new blood vessels, and the smooth muscle cell, which forms the wall of blood vessels. The heart has a large demand for blood flow, and these specialized cells are important for developing a new network of arteries to bring nutrients and oxygen to the cardiomyocytes after a heart has been damaged. The potential capability of both embryonic and adult stem cells to develop into these cells types in the damaged heart is now being explored as part of a strategy to restore heart function to people who have had heart attacks or have congestive heart failure. It is important that work with stem cells is not confused with recent reports that human cardiac myocytes may undergo cell division after myocardial infarction [1]. This work suggests that injured heart cells can shift from a quiescent state into active cell division. This is not different from the

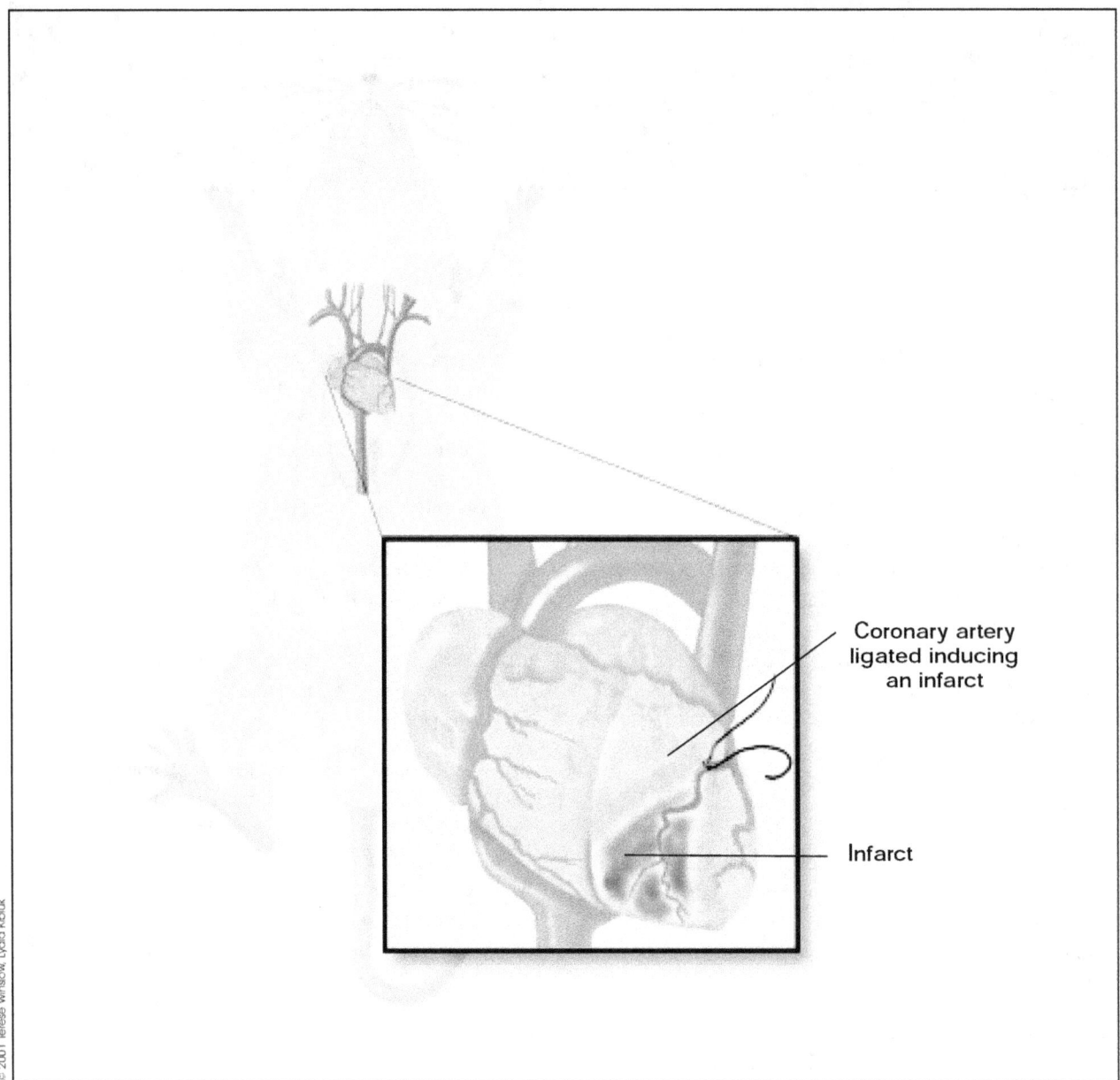

Figure 9.1. Rodent Model of Myocardial Infarction.

ability of a host of other cells in the body that begin to divide after injury. There is still no evidence that there are true stem cells in the heart which can proliferate and differentiate.

Researchers now know that under highly specific growth conditions in laboratory culture dishes, stem cells can be coaxed into developing as new cardiomyocytes and vascular endothelial cells. Scientists are interested in exploiting this ability to provide replacement tissue for the damaged heart. This

approach has immense advantages over heart transplant, particularly in light of the paucity of donor hearts available to meet current transplantation needs.

What is the evidence that such an approach to restoring cardiac function might work? In the research laboratory, investigators often use a mouse or rat model of a heart attack to study new therapies (see Figure 9.1. Rodent Model of Myocardial Infarction). To create a heart attack in a mouse or rat, a ligature is placed around a major blood vessel serving the heart muscle, thereby depriving the cardiomyocytes of their oxygen and nutrient supplies. During the past year, researchers using such models have made several key discoveries that kindled interest in the application of adult stem cells to heart muscle repair in animal models of heart disease.

Recently, Orlic and colleagues [9] reported on an experimental application of hematopoietic stem cells for the regeneration of the tissues in the heart. In this study, a heart attack was induced in mice by tying off a major blood vessel, the left main coronary artery. Through the identification of unique cellular surface markers, the investigators then isolated a select group of adult primitive bone marrow cells with a high capacity to develop into cells of multiple types. When injected into the damaged wall of the ventricle, these cells led to the formation of new cardiomyocytes, vascular endothelium, and smooth muscle cells, thus generating de novo myocardium, including coronary arteries, arterioles, and capillaries. The newly formed myocardium occupied 68 percent of the damaged portion of the ventricle nine days after the bone marrow cells were transplanted, in effect replacing the dead myocardium with living, functioning tissue. The researchers found that mice that received the transplanted cells survived in greater numbers than mice with heart attacks that did not receive the mouse stem cells. Follow-up experiments are now being conducted to extend the posttransplantation analysis time to determine the longer-range effects of such therapy [8]. The partial repair of the damaged heart muscle suggests that the transplanted mouse hematopoietic stem cells responded to signals in the environment near the injured myocardium. The cells migrated to the damaged region of the ventricle, where they multiplied and became "specialized" cells that appeared to be cardiomyocytes.

A second study, by Jackson et al. [3], demonstrated that cardiac tissue can be regenerated in the mouse heart attack model through the introduction of adult stem cells from mouse bone marrow. In this model, investigators purified a "side population" of hematopoietic stem cells from a genetically altered mouse strain. These cells were then transplanted into the marrow of lethally irradiated mice approximately 10 weeks before the recipient mice were subjected to heart attack via the tying off of a different major heart blood vessel, the left anterior descending (LAD) coronary artery. At two to four weeks after the

induced cardiac injury, the survival rate was 26 percent. As with the study by Orlic et al., analysis of the region surrounding the damaged tissue in surviving mice showed the presence of donor-derived cardiomyocytes and endothelial cells. Thus, the mouse hematopoietic stem cells transplanted into the bone marrow had responded to signals in the injured heart, migrated to the border region of the damaged area, and differentiated into several types of tissue needed for cardiac repair. This study suggests that mouse hematopoietic stem cells may be delivered to the heart through bone marrow transplantation as well as through direct injection into the cardiac tissue, thus providing another possible therapeutic strategy for regenerating injured cardiac tissue.

More evidence for potential stem cell-based therapies for heart disease is provided by a study that showed that human adult stem cells taken from the bone marrow are capable of giving rise to vascular endothelial cells when transplanted into rats [6]. As in the Jackson study, these researchers induced a heart attack by tying off the LAD coronary artery. They took great care to identify a population of human hematopoietic stem cells that give rise to new blood vessels. These stem cells demonstrate plasticity meaning that they become cell types that they would not normally be. The cells were used to form new blood vessels in the damaged area of the rats' hearts and to encourage proliferation of preexisting vasculature following the experimental heart attack.

Like the mouse stem cells, these human hematopoietic stem cells can be induced under the appropriate culture conditions to differentiate into numerous tissue types, including cardiac muscle [10] (see Figure 9.2. Heart Muscle Repair with Adult Stem Cells). When injected into the bloodstream leading to the damaged rat heart, these cells prevented the death of hypertrophied or thickened but otherwise viable myocardial cells and reduced progressive formation of collagen fibers and scars. Control rats that underwent surgery with an intact LAD coronary artery, as well as LAD-ligated rats injected with saline or control cells, did not demonstrate an increase in the number of blood vessels. Furthermore, the hematopoietic cells could be identified on the basis of highly specific cell markers that differentiate them from cardiomyocyte precursor cells, enabling the cells to be used alone or in conjunction with myocyte-regeneration strategies or pharmacological therapies. (For more

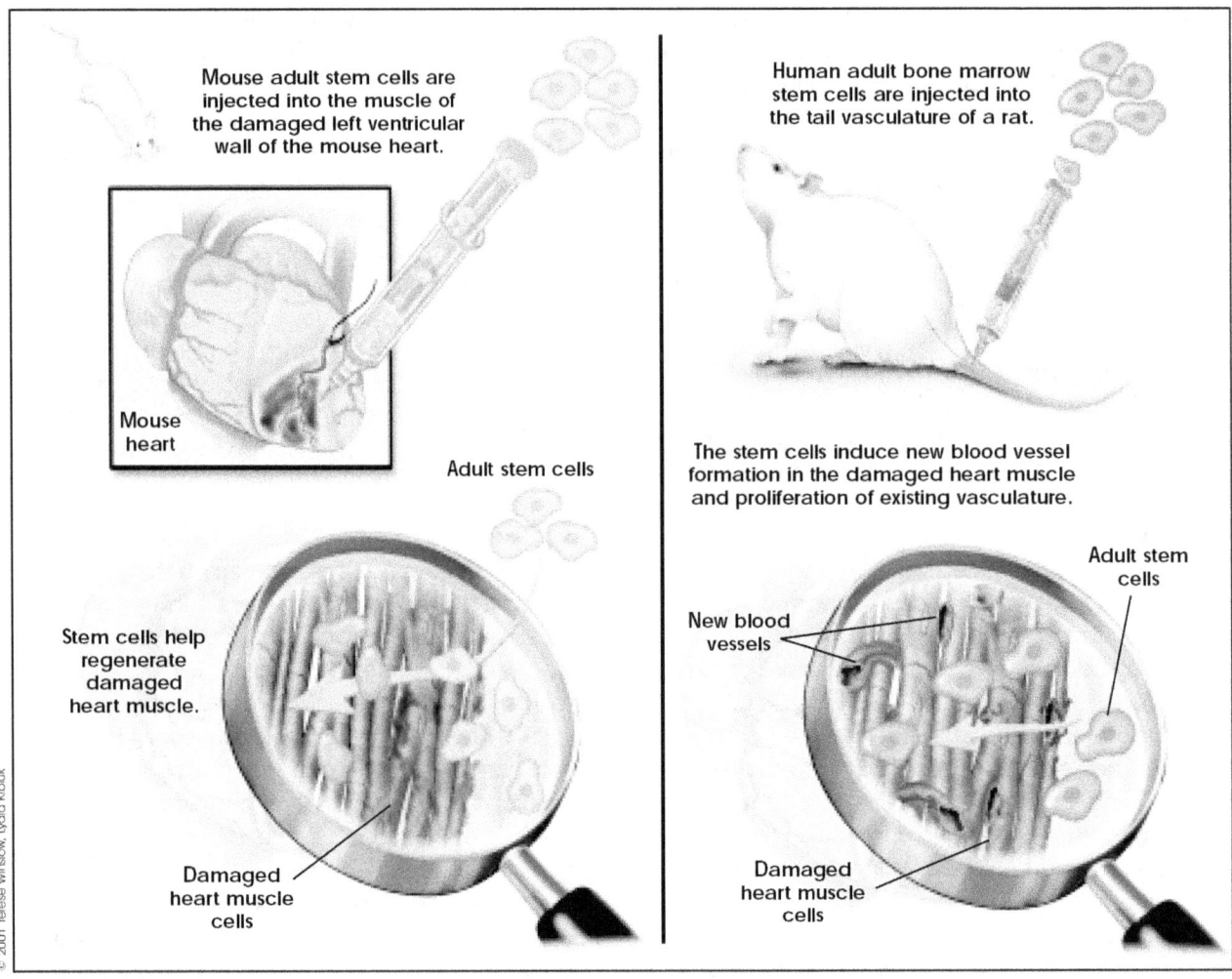

Mouse adult stem cells are injected into the muscle of the damaged left ventricular wall of the mouse heart.

Mouse heart

Adult stem cells

Stem cells help regenerate damaged heart muscle.

Damaged heart muscle cells

Human adult bone marrow stem cells are injected into the tail vasculature of a rat.

The stem cells induce new blood vessel formation in the damaged heart muscle and proliferation of existing vasculature.

Adult stem cells

New blood vessels

Damaged heart muscle cells

© 2001 Terese Winslow, Lydia Kibiuk

Figure 9.2. Heart Muscle Repair with Adult Stem Cells.

about stem cell markers see Appendix E.i. How Do Researchers Use Markers to Identify Stem Cells?)

Exciting new advances in cardiomyocyte regeneration are being made in human embryonic stem cell research. Because of their ability to differentiate into any cell type in the adult body, embryonic stem cells are another possible source population for cardiac-repair cells. The first step in this application was taken by Itskovitz-Eldor et al. [2] who demonstrated that human embryonic stem cells can reproducibly differentiate in culture into embryoid bodies made up of cell types from the body's three embryonic germ layers. Among the various cell types noted were cells that had the physical appearance of cardiomyocytes, showed cellular markers consistent with heart cells, and demonstrated contractile activity similar to cardiomyocytes when observed under the microscope.

In a continuation of this early work, Kehat et al. [4] displayed structural and functional properties of early stage cardiomyocytes in the cells that develop from the embryoid bodies. The cells that have spontaneously contracting activity are positively identified by using markers with antibodies to myosin heavy chain, alpha-actinin, desmin, antinaturietic protein, and cardiac troponin—all proteins found in heart tissue. These investigators have done genetic analysis of these cells and found that the transcription-factor genes expressed are consistent with early stage cardiomyocytes. Electrical recordings from these cells, changes in calcium-ion movement within the cells, and contractile responsiveness to catecholamine hormone stimulation by the cells were similar to the recordings, changes, and responsiveness seen in early cardiomyocytes observed during mammalian development. A next step in this research is to see whether the experimental evidence of improvement in outcome from heart attack in rodents can be reproduced using embryonic stem cells.

These breakthrough discoveries in rodent models present new opportunities for using stem cells to repair damaged heart muscle. The results of the studies discussed above are growing evidence that adult stem cells may develop into more cell types than first thought. In those studies, hematopoietic stem cells appear to be able to develop not only into blood, but also into cardiac muscle and endothelial tissue. This capacity of adult stem cells, increasingly referred to as "plasticity," may make such adult stem cells a viable candidate for heart repair. But this evidence is not complete; the mouse hematopoietic stem cell populations that give rise to these replacement cells are not homogenous. Rather, they are enriched for the cells of interest through specific and selective stimulating factors that promote cell growth. Thus, the originating cell population for these injected cells has not been identified, and the possibility exists for inclusion of other cell populations that could cause the recipient to reject the transplanted cells. This is a major issue to contend with in clinical applications, but it is not as relevant in the experimental models described here because the rodents have been bred to be genetically similar.

What are the implications for extending the research on differentiated growth of replacement tissues for damaged hearts? There are some practical aspects of producing a sufficient number of cells for clinical application. The repair of one damaged human heart would likely require millions of cells. The unique capacity for embryonic stem cells to replicate in culture may give them an advantage over adult stem cells by providing large numbers of replacement cells in tissue culture for transplantation purposes. Given the current state of the science, it is unclear how adult stem cells could be used to generate sufficient heart muscle outside the body to meet patients' demand [7].

Although there is much excitement because researchers now know that adult and embryonic stem cells can repair damaged heart tissue, many questions remain to be answered before clinical applications can be made. For example, how long will the replacement cells continue to function? Do the rodent research models accurately reflect human heart conditions and transplantation responses? Do these new replacement cardiomyocytes derived from stem cells have the electrical-signal-conducting capabilities of native cardiac muscle cells?

Stem cells may well serve as the foundation upon which a future form of "cellular therapy" is constructed. In the current animal models, the time between the injury to the heart and the application of stem cells affects the degree to which regeneration takes place, and this has real implications for the patient who is rushed unprepared to the emergency room in the wake of a heart attack. In the future, could the patient's cells be harvested and expanded for use in an efficient manner? Alternatively, can at-risk patients donate their cells in advance, thus minimizing the preparation necessary for the cells' administration? Moreover, can these stem cells be genetically "programmed" to migrate directly to the site of injury and to synthesize immediately the heart proteins necessary for the regeneration process? Investigators are currently using stem cells from all sources to address these questions, thus providing a promising future for therapies for repairing or replacing the damaged heart and addressing the Nation's leading causes of death.

REFERENCES

1. Beltrami, A.P., Urbanek, K., Kajstura, J., Yan, S.M., Finato, N., Bussani, R., Nadal-Ginard, B., Silvestri, F., Leri, A., Beltrami, C.A., and Anversa, P. (2001). Evidence that human cardiac myocytes divide after myocardial infarction. N. Engl. J. Med. *344*, 1750-1757.

2. Itskovitz-Eldor, J., Schuldiner, M., Karsenti, D., Eden, A., Yanuka, O., Amit, M., Soreq, H., and Benvenisty, N. (2000). Differentiation of human embryonic stem cells into embryoid bodies comprising the three embryonic germ layers. Mol. Med. *6*, 88-95.

3. Jackson, K.A., Majka, S.M., Wang, H., Pocius, J., Hartley, C.J., Majesky, M.W., Entman, M.L., Michael, L.H., Hirschi, K.K., and Goodell, M.A. (2001). Regeneration of ischemic cardiac muscle and vascular endothelium by adult stem cells. J. Clin. Invest. *107*, 1-8.

4. Kehat, I., Kenyagin-Karsenti, D., Druckmann, M., Segev, H., Amit, M., Gepstein, A., Livne, E., Binah, O., Itskovitz-Eldor, J., and Gepstein, L. (2001). Human embryonic stem cells can differentiate into myocytes portraying cardiomyocytic structural and functional properties. J. Clin. Invest. (in press)

5. Kessler, P.D. and Byrne, B.J. (1999). Myoblast cell grafting into heart muscle: cellular biology and potential applications. Annu. Rev. Physiol. *61*, 219-242.

6. Kocher, A.A., Schuster, M.D., Szabolcs, M.J., Takuma, S., Burkhoff, D., Wang, J., Homma, S., Edwards, N.M., and Itescu, S. (2001). Neovascularization of ischemic myocardium by human bone-marrow-derived angioblasts prevents cardiomyocyte apoptosis, reduces remodeling and improves cardiac function. Nat. Med. *7*, 430-436.

7. Lanza, R., personal communication.

8. Orlic, D., personal communication.

9. Orlic, D., Kajstura, J., Chimenti, S., Jakoniuk, I., Anderson, S.M., Li, B., Pickel, J., McKay, R., Nadal-Ginard, B., Bodine, D.M., Leri, A., and Anversa, P. (2001). Bone marrow cells regenerate infarcted myocardium. Nature. *410*, 701-705.

10. Pittenger, M.F., Mackay, A.M., Beck, S.C., Jaiswal, R.K., Douglas, R., Mosca, J.D., Moorman, M.A., Simonetti, D.W., Craig, S., and Marshak, D.R. (1999). Multilineage potential of adult human mesenchymal stem cells. Science. *284*, 143-147.

10. ASSESSING HUMAN STEM CELL SAFETY

The isolation of human stem cells offers the promise of a remarkable array of novel therapeutics. Biologic therapies derived from such cells—through tissue regeneration and repair as well as through the targeted delivery of genetic material—are expected to be effective in the treatment of a wide range of medical conditions. Efforts to analyze and assess the safety of using human stem cells in the clinical setting are vitally important to this endeavor.

Transplanted human stem cells are dynamic biological entities that interact intimately with—and are influenced by—the physiology of the recipient. Before they are transplanted, cultured human stem cells are maintained under conditions that promote either the self-renewing expansion of undifferentiated progenitors or the acquisition of differentiated properties indicative of the phenotype the cells will assume. After incompletely differentiated human stem cells are transplanted, additional fine-tuning occurs as a consequence of instructions received from the cells' physiologic microenvironments within the recipient. The capabilities to self-renew and differentiate that are inherent to human stem cells point simultaneously to their perceived therapeutic potential and to the challenge of assessing their safety.

Assessing human stem cell safety requires the implementation of a comprehensive strategy. Each step in the human stem cell development process—beginning with identifying and evaluating suitable human stem cell sources—must be carefully scrutinized. Included in this global assessment are the derivation, expansion, manipulation, and characterization of human stem cell lines, as well as preclinical efficacy and toxicity testing in appropriate animal models. Being able to trace back from the cell population prepared for transplantation to the source of the founder human stem cells also allows each safety checkpoint to be connected, one to the other.

WEAVING A STEM CELL SAFETY NET

A diversity of opinion exists among researchers about the feasibility of initiating pilot clinical studies using human stem cells. Some are of the view that it is reasonable to expect within the next five years that human stem cells will be used in transplantation settings to replace dead or dying cells within organs such as the failing heart or that genetically modified human stem cells will be created for delivery of therapeutic genes. Others argue that a good deal more information about the basic biology of human stem cells needs to be accumulated before their therapeutic potential in humans can be assessed.

Clinical studies involving the transplantation of blood-restoring, or hematopoietic, stem cells have been under way for a number of years. Reconstituting the blood and immune systems through stem cell transplantation is an established practice for treating hematological malignancies such as leukemia and lymphoma. Transplanting hematopoietic stem cells resident in the bone marrow or isolated from cord blood or circulating peripheral blood is used to counter the destruction of certain bone marrow cells caused by high-intensity chemotherapeutic regimens used to battle various solid tumors. Moreover, clinical trials are being conducted to assess the safety and efficacy of using hematopoietic stem cell transplantation to treat various autoimmune conditions including multiple sclerosis, lupus, and rheumatoid arthritis.

Although precedents exist for the clinical use of human stem cells, there is considerable reluctance to proceed with clinical trials involving human stem cells derived from embryonic and fetal sources. This hesitancy extends to adult human stem cells of non-hematopoietic origin, even though, by contrast, their plasticity is generally considered to be lower than that of their embryo- and fetus-derived counterparts. For human stem cells to advance to the stage of clinical investigation, a virtual safety net composed of a core set of safeguards is required (see Table 10.1. Safeguards for clinical applications of human stem cells, by source of cell).

Safety Assurance Begins with Adequate Donor Screening

Whether human stem cells are of embryonic, fetal, or adult origin, donor sources must be carefully screened. Routine testing should be done to guard against the inadvertent transmission of infectious diseases. Additionally, pedigree assessment and molecular genetic testing appear to be warranted. This is arguably the case when human stem cells

intended for transplantation are derived from an allogeneic donor—that is, someone other that the recipient—and especially if the cells are obtained from a master cell bank that has been established using human embryonic stem or human embryonic germ cells.

The purpose of pedigree evaluation and/or genetic testing is to establish whether the human stem cells in question are suitable for use in the context of a particular clinical situation. For example, embryos derived from a donor with a family history of cardio-vascular diseases may not be the best suited for the derivation of cardiac muscle cells intended to repair damaged heart tissue. Similarly, the use of molecular

Table 10.1. Safeguards for clinical applications of human stem cells, by source of cell*

Safeguard	Embryo	Fetus	Adult: Autologous (self)	Adult: Allogeneic (nonself)
Screen donors • Infectious-agent testing • Pedigree assessment • Molecular genetic testing	++	++	+	++
Use controlled, standardized practices and procedures for establishing stem cell lines	++	++	++	++
Develop alternatives to culturing on cell-feeder layer	++	++	NA	NA
Perform detailed characterization of tem cell lines • Morphology • Cell-surface antigens • Biochemical markers • Gene expression • Karyotype analysis • Biologic activity	++	++	++	++

Conduct preclinical animal testing
• Proof of concept: disease models
  – Cell integration
  – Cell migration
• Comprehensive toxicity
• Proliferative potential
	++
	
	++
	++
		++
		
		++
		++
			++
			
			++
			+
				++
				
				++
				+

Monitor patient and do long-term follow-up	++	++	++	++

++= more important; +=less important; NA=not applicable.

genetic analysis could detect a mutation in the gene for alpha-synuclein. This gene is known to be responsible for the rare occurrence of early onset Parkinson's Disease. Detecting such a genetic abnormality in neuronal progenitor cells derived from an established embryonic germ cell line could block the use of those cells as a treatment for a number of neurodegenerative conditions, including Parkinson's Disease.

The number of genes known to be directly responsible for causing disease or anomalous physiologic function is relatively small. Advances in techniques for identifying, isolating, and analyzing genes, coupled with the wealth of information destined to become available as one outcome of the human genome sequencing projects, will raise this number. Considerably more will also be learned about how multiple gene products, each contributing an incremental quantity to the overall sum, predispose an individual to develop particular diseases. Clearly, it will eventually not be possible, or even necessary, to screen every source of human stem cells for the entire panoply of disease-associated genes. The screening of targeted genes will be conducted within the context of the relevant clinical population.

Using Controlled, Standardized Practices and Procedures for Establishing Cultured Human Stem Cell Lines Enhances Safety

To ensure the integrity, uniformity, and reliability of human stem cell preparations intended for clinical use, it is essential to demonstrate that rigorously controlled, standardized practices and procedures are being followed in establishing and maintaining human stem cell lines in culture.

Human stem cells from virtually every source other than blood-derived hematopoietic stem cells are maintained in tissue culture for some defined period of time. This is necessary to obtain a sufficient number of cells for use in clinical studies involving transplantation. Culturing human stem cells requires the use of formulated liquid media supplemented with growth factors and other chemical substances that promote cellular replication and govern the differentiation of the cultured human stem cells. Since human stem cells are a dynamic, biological entity, failure to standardize procedures for maintaining and expanding cells in culture could result in unintended alterations in the intrinsic properties of the cells. The initial seeding density of the cells, the frequency with which the culture medium is replenished, and the density

cells are permitted to achieve before subdividing will all affect the characteristics of human stem cells maintained in culture. Altering the concentrations of supplemental growth factors and chemical substances, even switching from one supplier to another, may lead to changes in cell growth rate, expression of defining cell markers, and differentiation potential. Alterations in stem cell properties caused by the use of nonstandardized culture practices are likely to affect the behavior and effectiveness of the cells once transplanted.

One particular concern is how safe it is to use serum derived from cows as a supplement to culture media. Due to the outbreak of bovine spongiform encephalopathy (BSE) in cattle herds, primarily those raised in the United Kingdom, only serum produced from cows reared in countries certified to be free of BSE should be used. Consumption of beef contaminated with the agent responsible for causing BSE has lead to the limited emergence of new variant Creutzfeldt-Jakob disease (nvCJD) in humans. This disease results in the relentless destruction of brain tissue and is invariably fatal. Placing neural stem cells contaminated with the BSE infectious agent in a patient's nervous system to investigate cellular-replacement therapies for neurological disorders would be both irresponsible and devastating. Researchers are engaged in a vigorous effort to develop serum-free, chemically defined media that obviate risks associated with the use of bovine serum.

Alternatives to Culturing on a Feeder Layer of Animal Cells Improve Safety

An issue unique to the culturing of human embryonic stem and embryonic germ cells involves the use of mouse embryonic fibroblast feeder cells to keep the embryonic cells in a proliferating, undifferentiated condition. Human embryonic stem and embryonic germ cells are seeded directly onto a bed of irradiated mouse feeder cells. Transplanting into humans stem cell preparations derived from founder cells that have been in direct, intimate contact with nonhuman animal cells constitutes xenotransplantation—the use of organs, tissues, and cells derived from animals to treat human disease. The principal concern of xenotransplantation is the unintended transfer of animal viruses into humans.

Researchers are devoting considerable attention to developing culture conditions that do not use mouse feeder cells. In February of this year, scientists from

Geron Corporation, a biotech company focusing on the development of embryonic stem cell technology for treating disease, presented findings at a scientific conference demonstrating that human embryonic stem cells can be maintained without mouse feeder cells. Human embryonic stem cells seeded on a commercially available basement membrane matrix in media conditioned by feeder cells retain their proliferative potential and capacity to form all three embryonic germ layers (mesoderm, endoderm, and ectoderm). This suggests that human embryonic stem cells maintained in the absence of direct culture on a mouse feeder cell layer are comparable to human embryonic stem cells co-cultured with mouse feeder cells.

Detailed Characterization of Human Stem Cell Populations Reinforces the Safety Net

Detailed characterization of cell preparations intended for transplantation is critical to the development of human stem cells for clinical use. Identifying the cells that make up an human stem cell population intended for clinical study requires identifying cells exhibiting the desired phenotype within the preparation, as well as those that do not. This poses considerable challenges because human embryonic stem and embryonic germ cells have the capacity to give rise to all differentiated cell types, while adult human stem cells, though generally more restricted in their plasticity, are capable of generating all cell types that make up the tissue from which they were derived.

On the basis of the complex biological properties of human stem cells, including their potential to differentiate along multiple lineages and give rise to a variety of cell types, it is expected that the characterization of stem cell preparations will require a panel of orthogonal assessments. Parameters that will prove useful in establishing identity include 1) cell morphology (visual microscopic inspection of cells to assess their appearance), 2) expression of unique cell-surface antigens (as is the case for CD34$^+$ hematopoietic stem cells), 3) characterization of biochemical markers such as a tissue-specific enzymatic activity (e.g., enzymes that produce neurotransmitters for nerve cells), and 4) expression of genes that are unique to a particular cell type. Further, analysis of the nuclear chromosomal karyotype may be used to assess genetic stability of established human embryonic stem and embryonic germ cell lines maintained

in culture for extended periods of time. Continued development and standardization of DNA microarray analysis (simultaneous screening for many genes) and proteomics (protein profiling) technologies will significantly enhance stem cell characterization.

Rigorous and quantitative identification of cell types within a heterogeneous population of differentiating human stem cells provides the means to gauge purity of a cellular preparation. In turn, this permits evaluation of the extent to which purity of a human stem cell preparation predicts efficacy after transplantation. It is not necessarily the case that homogenous populations composed of a single cell type will be more effective as a cell-replacement therapy than mixed populations of cells. It is conceivable that the reason differentiation of cultured stem cells obtained from the brain leads to formation of all the cell types found within the nervous system (namely, neurons, astrocytes, and oligodendrocytes) is that their coincidental presence is required to ensure maximum survival and functional capability. The interaction of various phenotypic cell types within a preparation of progenitor cells obtained after the controlled differentiation of cultured human embryonic stem cells is being actively investigated.

Once the purity profile has been established for a population of human stem cells generated using standardized procedures, deviations that occur outside what is expected due to normal biologic variation serve as a harbinger that significant, and possibly deleterious, changes may have occurred. Such alterations could reflect the introduction of genetic mutations as a consequence of culture conditions used to promote expansion and to induce differentiation of the progenitor cell population.

Before clinical studies involving human stem cell transplantation can be done, it is essential to demonstrate that human stem cell preparations possess relevant biological activity. The bioassay provides a quantitative measure of the potency of a cell preparation and ensures that cells destined for transplantation are not inert. Assays may be based on a biologic activity such as insulin release from pancreatic islet-like cells, glycogen storage by cells intended for regeneration of liver tissue, or synchronous contraction in the case of stem cell-derived cardiomyocytes to be used for repairing damaged heart muscle. When cells that have not acquired fully differentiated functionality are to be transplanted, it may be appropriate to use surrogate markers that predict the acquisition of the intended biologic activity upon further differentiation. (For example, counting tyrosine hydroxylase-expressing neural progenitor cells in a mixed population of cells intended to provide dopaminergic neurons for treating Parkinson's Disease could predict the acquisition of relevant biologic activity after transplantation.)

Proof of Concept, Toxicity Testing, and Evaluation of Proliferative Potential in Animal Models Are Important to the Assessment of Human Stem Cell Safety

A critical element of the safety net is the transplantation of human stem cells into animals to demonstrate that the therapy does what it is supposed to do ("proof of concept") and to assess toxicity. Admittedly, animal models of human disease are imperfect because most human maladies do not spontaneously occur in animals. Chemical, surgical, and immunologic methods are used to damage neurons; induce diabetes; simulate heart attacks, stroke, and hypertension; or compromise organ function. In situations when focal genetic lesions are known to cause disease, the creation of transgenic mouse colonies in which the culpable gene is either eliminated or overexpressed results in disease models that are capable of faithfully reproducing human-disease-specific pathologies.

Human stem cells must be transplanted into animal models of human disease. Transplantation of neural stem cells should demonstrate measurable evidence of efficacy in models of neurodegenerative disease, such as Parkinson's Disease, Huntington's disease, and amyotrophic lateral sclerosis (ALS), Alzheimer's disease, as well as spinal cord injury and stroke. Improved liver function after transplantation of hepatocyte precursors should be observed in an animal model of hepatic failure. Normalization of blood insulin concentrations and amelioration of diabetic disease symptoms should result from the transplantation of pancreatic islet progenitors in a mouse model of diabetes. It is likely that in all cases, immunosuppression will be required due to immunologic incompatibility between humans and the animal model species (usually mouse or rat).

In addition to efficacy, evidence for anatomic and functional integration of transplanted human stem cells should be assessed. human stem cells destined for transplantation may be tagged with a marker, such as green fluorescent protein, that allows transplanted cells to be readily identified upon histological examination. A similar approach should be used to evaluate the migration of transplanted human stem cells from the site of injection into adjacent and more distant tissues. The migration of transplanted human stem cells to a nontarget site and subsequent differentiation into a tissue type that is inappropriate for that anatomic location could be problematic.

Questions about the use of embryonic compared with adult stem cells with respect to robustness and durability should be addressed in animal-transplantation models. Similarly, the issue of whether less-differentiated cells will be more effective than more-differentiated cells following transplantation should be investigated. Continued advancements in noninvasive imaging technologies, such as magnetic resonance imaging (MRI) and positron emission tomography (PET scanning), will allow these events to be observed in real time with reasonable resolution and without having to use large numbers of animals.

From the perspective of toxicology, the proliferative potential of undifferentiated human embryonic and embryonic germ cells evokes the greatest level of concern. A characteristic of human embryonic stem cells is their capacity to generate teratomas when transplanted into immunologically incompetent strains of mice. Undifferentiated embryonic stem cells are not considered as suitable for transplantation due to the risk of unregulated growth. The question that remains is, at what point during differentiation does this risk become insignificant, if ever? Identifying the stage at which the risk for tumor formation is minimized will depend on whether the process of stem cell differentiation occurs only in a forward direction or is reversible. Before clinical trials are begun in humans, the issue of unregulated growth potential and its relationship to stem cell differentiation must be evaluated. It is essential that careful toxicology studies are performed that are of the appropriate duration and that involve transplantation into immunocompromised animals of undifferentiated or partially differentiated embryonic stem cells, as well as adult stem cells.

This page intentionally left blank

11. USE OF GENETICALLY MODIFIED STEM CELLS IN EXPERIMENTAL GENE THERAPIES

To date, only nonembryonic human stem cells have been used in cell-based gene therapy studies. The inherent limitations of these stem cells, as discussed below, have prompted scientists to ponder and explore whether human embryonic stem cells might overcome the current barriers to the clinical success of cell-based gene therapies.

PRINCIPLES AND PROMISE OF GENE THERAPY

Gene therapy is a relatively recent, and still highly experimental, approach to treating human disease. While traditional drug therapies involve the adminis-tration of chemicals that have been manufactured outside the body, gene therapy takes a very different approach: directing a patient's own cells to produce and deliver a therapeutic agent. The instructions for this are contained in the therapeutic transgene (the new genetic material introduced into the patient). Gene therapy uses genetic engineering—the intro-duction or elimination of specific genes by using molecular biology techniques to physically mani-pulate genetic material—to alter or supplement the function of an abnormal gene by providing a copy of a normal gene, to directly repair such a gene, or to provide a gene that adds new functions or regulates the activity of other genes.

Clinical efforts to apply genetic engineering tech-nology to the treatment of human diseases date to 1989. Initially, gene therapy clinical trials focused on cancer, infectious diseases, or disorders in which only a single gene is abnormal, such as cystic fibrosis. Increasingly however, efforts are being directed toward complex, chronic diseases that involve more than one gene. Prominent examples include heart disease, inadequate blood flow to the limbs, arthritis, and Alzheimer's disease.

The potential success of gene therapy technology depends not only on the delivery of the therapeutic transgene into the appropriate human target cells, but also on the ability of the gene to function properly in the cell. Both requirements pose considerable technical challenges.

Gene therapy researchers have employed two major strategies for delivering therapeutic transgenes into human recipients (see Figure 11.1. Strategies for Delivering Therapeutic Transgenes into Patients). The first is to "directly" infuse the gene into a person. Viruses that have been altered to prevent them from causing disease are often used as the vehicle for delivering the gene into certain human cell types, in much the same way as ordinary viruses infect cells. This delivery method is fairly imprecise and limited to the specific types of human cells that the viral vehicle can infect. For example, some viruses commonly used as gene-delivery vehicles can only infect cells that are actively dividing. This limits their usefulness in treating diseases of the heart or brain, because these organs are largely composed of nondividing cells. Nonviral vehicles for directly delivering genes into cells are also being explored, including the use of plain DNA and DNA wrapped in a coat of fatty molecules known as liposomes.

The second strategy involves the use of living cells to deliver therapeutic transgenes into the body. In this method, the delivery cells—often a type of stem cell, a lymphocyte, or a fibroblast—are removed from the body, and the therapeutic transgene is introduced into them via the same vehicles used in the pre-viously described direct-gene-transfer method. While still in the laboratory, the genetically modified cells are tested and then allowed to grow and multiply and, finally, are infused back into the patient.

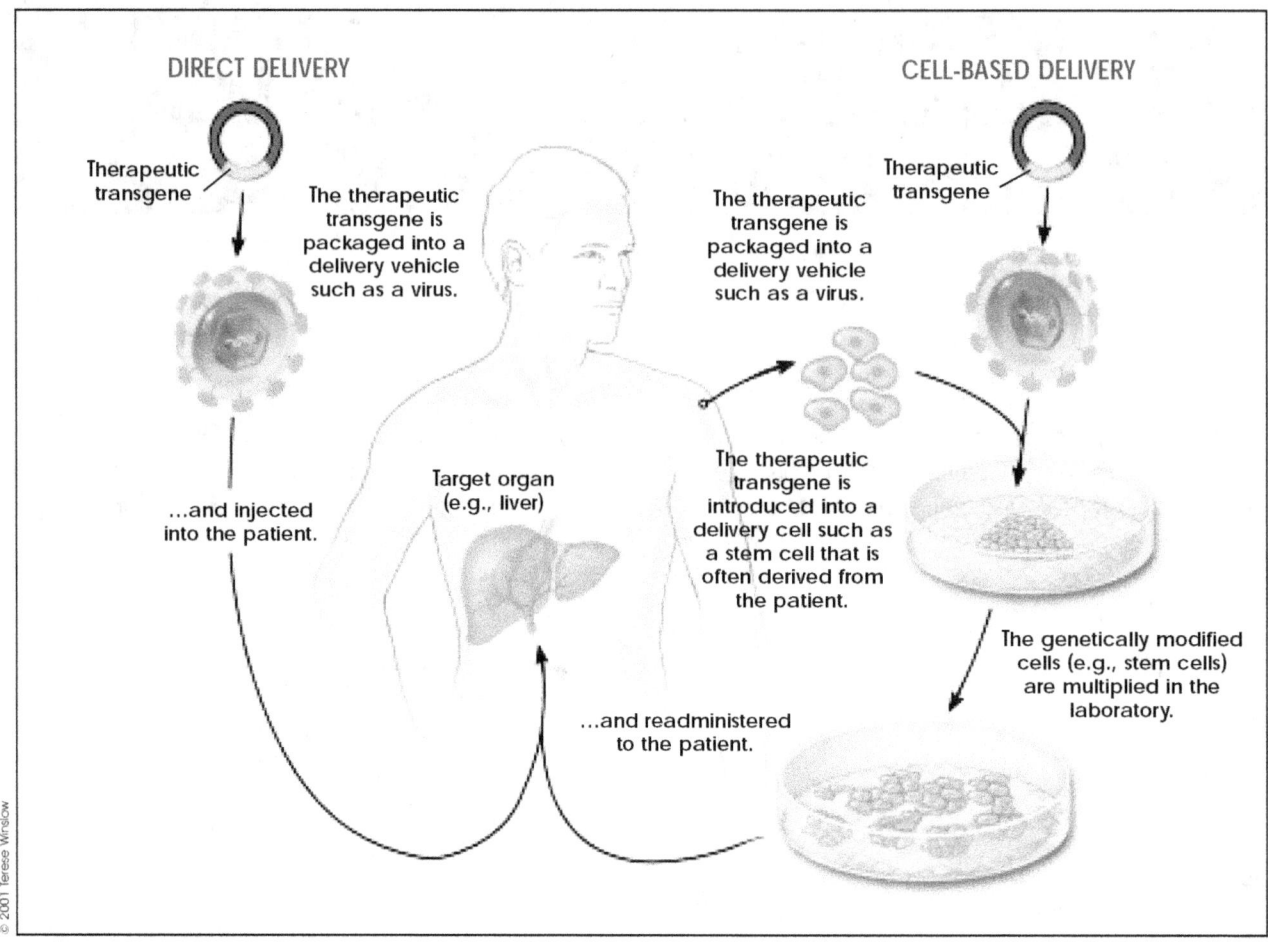

Figure 11.1. Strategies for Delivering Therapeutic Transgenes into Patients.

Gene therapy using genetically modified cells offers several unique advantages over direct gene transfer into the body and over cell therapy, which involves administration of cells that have not been genetically modified. First, the addition of the therapeutic transgene to the delivery cells takes place outside the patient, which allows researchers an important measure of control because they can select and work only with those cells that both contain the transgene and produce the therapeutic agent in sufficient quantity. Second, investigators can genetically engineer, or "program," the cells' level and rate of production of the therapeutic agent. Cells can be programmed to steadily churn out a given amount of the therapeutic product. In some cases, it is desirable to program the cells to make large amounts of the therapeutic agent so that the chances that sufficient quantities are secreted and reach the diseased tissue in the patient are high. In other cases, it may be desirable to program the cells to produce the therapeutic

agent in a regulated fashion. In this case, the therapeutic transgene would be active only in response to certain signals, such as drugs administered to the patient to turn the therapeutic transgene on and off.

WHY STEM CELLS ARE USED IN SOME CELL-BASED GENE THERAPIES

To date, about 40 percent of the more than 450 gene therapy clinical trials conducted in the United States have been cell-based. Of these, approximately 30 percent have used human stem cells—specifically, blood-forming, or hematopoietic, stem cells—as the means for delivering transgenes into patients.

Several of the early gene therapy studies using these stem cells were carried out not for therapeutic purposes per se, but to track the cells' fate after they were infused back into the patient. The studies aimed to determine where the stem cells ended up and whether they were indeed producing the desired gene product, and if so, in what quantities and for what length of time. Of the stem cell-based gene therapy trials that have had a therapeutic goal, approximately one-third have focused on cancers (e.g., ovarian, brain, breast, myeloma, leukemia, and lymphoma), one-third on human immunodeficiency virus disease (HIV-1), and one-third on so-called single-gene diseases (e.g., Gaucher's disease, severe combined immune deficiency (SCID), Fanconi anemia, Fabry disease, and leukocyte adherence deficiency).

But why use stem cells for this method of gene therapy, and why hematopoietic stem cells in particular? The major reason for using stem cells in cell-based gene therapies is that they are a self-renewing population of cells and thus may reduce or eliminate the need for repeated administrations of the gene therapy.

Since the advent of gene therapy research, hematopoietic stem cells have been a delivery cell of choice for several reasons. First, although small in number, they are readily removed from the body via the circulating blood or bone marrow of adults or the umbilical cord blood of newborn infants. In addition, they are easily identified and manipulated in the laboratory and can be returned to patients relatively easily by injection.

The ability of hematopoietic stem cells to give rise to many different types of blood cells means that once the engineered stem cells differentiate, the therapeutic transgene will reside in cells such as T and B lymphocytes, natural killer cells, monocytes, macrophages, granulocytes, eosinophils, basophils, and megakaryocytes. The clinical applications of hematopoietic stem cell-based gene therapies are thus also diverse, extending to organ transplantation, blood and bone marrow disorders, and immune system disorders.

In addition, hematopoietic stem cells "home," or migrate, to a number of different spots in the body—primarily the bone marrow, but also the liver, spleen, and lymph nodes. These may be strategic locations for localized delivery of therapeutic agents for disorders unrelated to the blood system, such as liver diseases and metabolic disorders such as Gaucher's disease.

The only type of human stem cell used in gene therapy trials so far is the hematopoietic stem cell. However, several other types of stem cells are being studied as gene-delivery-vehicle candidates. They include muscle-forming stem cells known as myoblasts, bone-forming stem cells called osteoblasts, and neural stem cells.

Myoblasts appear to be good candidates for use in gene therapy because of an unusual and advantageous biological property: when injected into muscle, they fuse with nearby muscle fibers and become an integral part of the muscle tissue. Moreover, since muscle tissue is generally well supplied with nerves and blood, the therapeutic agents produced by the transgene are also accessible to nerves and the circulatory system. Thus, myoblasts may not only be useful for treating muscle disorders such as muscular dystrophy, but also possibly nonmuscle disorders such as neurodegenerative diseases, inherited hormone deficiencies, hemophilia, and cancers.

Several promising animal studies of myoblast-mediated gene therapy have been reported [17]. For instance, this approach was successful in correcting liver and spleen abnormalities associated with a lysosomal storage disease in mice. Investigators have also achieved stable production of the human clotting factor IX deficient in hemophilia at therapeutic concentrations in mice for at least eight months. Myoblasts engineered to secrete erythropoietin (a hormone that stimulates red blood cell production) were successful in reversing a type of anemia associated with end-stage renal disease in a mouse model of renal failure.

Another animal study of myoblast-mediated gene transfer involved a mouse model of familial amyotrophic lateral sclerosis (ALS, also known as Lou Gehrig's disease), a fatal disorder characterized by progressive degeneration of the brain and spinal cord nerves that control muscle activity. Investigators injected myoblasts containing the transgene for a human nerve growth factor into the muscles of the ALS mice before the onset of disease symptoms and motor neuron degeneration. The transgene remained active in the muscle for up to 12 weeks, and, most importantly, the gene therapy successfully delayed the onset of disease symptoms, slowed muscle atrophy, and delayed the deterioration of motor skills [16].

In a series of experiments in rodents, a team of investigators has been testing neural stem cells as vehicles for cell-based gene therapy for brain tumors known as gliomas. Gliomas are virtually impossible to treat because the tumor cells readily invade the surrounding tissue and migrate extensively into the normal brain. The researchers genetically modified human neural stem cells to produce a protein—cytosine deaminase—that converts a nontoxic precursor drug into an active form that kills cancer cells. The engineered neural stem cells were then injected into the brains of mice with human-derived gliomas. Within two weeks of the gene therapy and systemic treatment with the precursor drug, the tumors had shrunk by 80 percent. The animal studies also revealed that neural stem cells were able to quickly and accurately "find" glioma cells, regardless of whether the stem cells were implanted directly into the tumors, implanted far from the tumors (but still within the brain), or injected into circulating blood outside the brain [1].

Another cell-based gene therapy system under investigation involves the use of osteoblasts, or bone-forming stem cells. In a recent preliminary study examining a gene therapy approach to bone repair and regeneration, researchers genetically engineered osteoblasts to produce a bone growth factor. The osteoblasts were added to a biodegradable matrix that could act as a "scaffold" for new bone formation. Within a month after the cell-impregnated scaffold was implanted into mice, new bone formation was detectable. Although this work is in the very early stages, it offers hope of an effective alternative to conventional bone-grafting techniques [14].

HOW EMBRYONIC STEM CELLS MIGHT PLAY A ROLE IN GENE THERAPY RESEARCH

With one notable exception, no therapeutic effects have been achieved in gene therapy trials to date. The first successful gene therapy occurred in a recent French study in which a therapeutic transgene for correcting X-linked severe combined immune deficiency was introduced into the bone marrow cells of children, resulting in improved function of their immune systems and correction of the disease [5]. This encouraging success aside, the generally disappointing results are due, in part, to the inherent limitations of adult and cord blood stem cells. In principle at least, the use of human embryonic stem cells

might overcome some of these limitations, but further research will be needed to determine whether embryonic stem cells are better suited to meet the needs of gene therapy applications than are adult stem cells.

One important feature of the optimal cell for delivering a therapeutic transgene would be its ability to retain the therapeutic transgene even as it proliferates or differentiates into specialized cells. Most of the cell-based gene therapies attempted so far have used viral vehicles to introduce the transgene into the hematopoietic stem cell. One way to accomplish this is to insert the therapeutic transgene into the one of the chromosomes of the stem cell. Retroviruses are able to do this, and for this reason, they are often used as the vehicle for infecting the stem cell and introducing the therapeutic transgene into the chromosomal DNA. However, mouse retroviruses are only efficient at infecting cells that are actively dividing. Unfortunately, hematopoietic stem cells are quiescent and seldom divide. The percentage of stem cells that actually receive the therapeutic transgene has usually been too low to attain a therapeutic effect. Because of this problem, investigators have been exploring the use of viral vehicles that can infect nondividing cells, such as lentiviruses (e.g., HIV) or adeno-associated viruses. This approach has not been entirely successful, however, because of problems relating to the fact that the cells themselves are not in an active state [13, 19].

One approach to improving the introduction of transgenes into hematopoietic stem cells has been to stimulate the cells to divide so that the viral vehicles can infect them and insert the therapeutic transgene. Inder Verma of the Salk Institute has noted, however, that this manipulation can change other important properties of the hematopoietic stem cells, such as plasticity, self-renewal, and the ability to survive and grow when introduced into the patient [23]. This possibility might be overcome with the use of embryonic stem cells if they require less manipulation. And in fact, some preliminary data suggest that retroviral vectors may work more efficiently with embryonic stem cells than with the more mature adult stem cells. For example, researchers have noted that retroviral vectors introduce transgenes into human fetal cord blood stem cells more efficiently than into cord blood stem cells from newborns, and that the fetal cord blood stem cells also had a higher proliferative capacity (i.e., they underwent more subsequent cell divisions). This suggests that fetal cord blood stem cells might be useful in cell-based in utero gene therapy to correct hematopoietic disorders before birth [15, 21].

In some cases—such as a treatment of a chronic disease—achieving continued production of the therapeutic transgene over the life of the patient will be very important. Generally, however, gene therapies using hematopoietic stem cells have encountered a phenomenon known as "gene silencing," where, over time, the therapeutic transgene gets "turned off" due to cellular mechanisms that alter the structure of the area of the chromosome where the therapeutic gene has been inserted [6, 7, 11, 22, 24]. Whether the use of embryonic stem cells in gene therapy could overcome this problem is unknown, although preliminary evidence suggests that this phenomenon may occur in these cells as well [8, 18].

Persistence of the cell containing the therapeutic transgene is equally important for ensuring continued availability of the therapeutic agent. Verma noted that the optimal cells for cell-mediated gene transfer would be cells that will persist for "the rest of the patient's life; they can proliferate and they would make the missing protein constantly and forever" [23]. Persistence, or longevity, of the cells can come about in two ways: a long life span for an individual cell, or a self-renewal process whereby a short-lived cell undergoes successive cell divisions while maintaining the therapeutic transgene. Ideally, then, the genetically modified cell for use in cell-based gene therapy should be able to self-renew (in a controlled manner so tumors are not formed) so that the therapeutic agent is available on a long-term basis. This is one of the reasons why stem cells are used, but adult stem cells seem to be much more limited in the number of times they can divide compared with embryonic stem cells. The difference between the ability of adult and embryonic stem cells to self-renew has been documented in the mouse, where embryonic stems cells were shown to have a much higher proliferative capacity than do adult hematopoietic stem cells [25].

Researchers are beginning to understand the biological basis of the difference in proliferative capacity between adult and embryonic stem cells. Persistence of cells and the ability to undergo successive cell divisions are in part, at least, a function of the length of structures at the tips of chromosomes called telomeres. Telomere length is, in turn, maintained by an enzyme known as telomerase. Low levels of telomerase activity result in short telomeres and, thus, fewer rounds of cell division—in other words, shorter longevity. Higher levels of telomerase activity result in longer telomeres, more possible cell divisions, and overall longer persistence. Mouse embryonic stem cells have been found to have longer telomeres and higher levels of telomerase activity compared with adult stem cells and other more specialized cells in the body. As mouse embryonic stem cells give rise to hematopoietic stem cells, telomerase activity levels drop, suggesting a decrease in the self-renewing potential of the hematopoietic stem cells [3, 4]. (For more detailed information regarding telomeres and telomerase, see Figure C.2. Telomeres and Telomerase.)

Human embryonic stem cells have also been shown to maintain pluripotency (the ability to give rise to other, more specialized cell types) and the ability to proliferate for long periods in cell culture in the laboratory [2]. Adult stem cells appear capable of only a limited number of cell divisions, which would prevent long-term expression of the therapeutic gene needed to correct chronic diseases. "Embryonic stem cells can be maintained in culture, whereas that is nearly impossible with cord blood stem cells," says Robert Hawley of the American Red Cross Jerome H. Holland Laboratory for Biomedical Sciences, who is developing gene therapy vectors for insertion into human hematopoietic cells [12]. "So with embryonic stem cells, you have the possibility of long-term maintenance and expansion of cell lines, which has not been possible with hematopoietic stem cells."

The patient's immune system response can be another significant challenge in gene therapy. Most cells have specific proteins on their surface that allow the immune system to recognize them as either "self" or "nonself." These proteins are known as major histocompatibility proteins, or MHC proteins. If adult stem cells for use in gene therapy cannot be isolated from the patient, donor cells can be used. But because of the differences in MHC proteins among individuals, the donor stem cells may be recognized as nonself by the patient's immune system and be rejected.

John Gearhart of Johns Hopkins University and Peter Rathjen at the University of Adelaide speculate that embryonic stem cells may be useful for avoiding such immune reactions [10, 20]. For instance, it may be possible to establish an extensive "bank" of embryonic stem cell lines, each with a different set of MHC genes. Then, an embryonic stem cell that is immunologically compatible for a patient could be selected, genetically modified, and triggered to develop into the appropriate type of adult stem cell that could be administered to the patient. By genetically modifying the MHC genes of an embryonic stem cell, it may also be possible to create a "universal" cell that would be compatible with all patients. Another approach might be to "customize" embryonic stem cells such that cells derived from them have a patient's specific MHC proteins on their surface and then to genetically modify them for use in gene therapy. Such approaches are hypothetical at this point, however, and research is needed to assess their feasibility.

Ironically, the very qualities that make embryonic stem cells potential candidates for gene therapy (i.e., pluripotency and unlimited proliferative capacity) also raise safety concerns. In particular, undifferentiated embryonic stem cells can give rise to teratomas, tumors composed of a number of different tissue types (see Chapter 10. Assessing Human Stem Cell Safety). It may thus be preferable to use a differentiated derivative of genetically modified embryonic stem cells that can still give rise to a limited number of cell types (akin to an adult stem cell). Cautions Esmail Zanjani of the University of Nevada, "We could differentiate embryonic stem cells into, say, liver cells, and then use them, but I don't see how we can take embryonic stem cells per se and put genes into them to use therapeutically" [26].

Further research is needed to determine whether the differentiated stem cells retain the advantages, such as longer life span, of the embryonic stem cells from which they were derived. Because of the difficulty in isolating and purifying many of the types of adult stem cells, embryonic stem cells may still be better targets for gene transfer. The versatile embryonic stem cell could be genetically modified, and then, in theory, it could be induced to give rise to all varieties of adult stem cells. Also, since the genetically modified stem cells can be easily expanded, large, pure populations of the differentiated cells could be produced and saved. Even if the differentiated cells were not as long-lived as the embryonic stem cells, there would still be sufficient genetically modified cells to give to the patient whenever the need arises again.

Achieving clinical success with cell-based gene therapy will require new knowledge and advances in several key areas, including the design of viral and nonviral vehicles for introducing transgenes into cells, the ability to direct where in a cell the transgene is introduced, the ability to direct the genetically modified stem cells or the secreted therapeutic agent to diseased tissues, optimization and regulation of the production of the therapeutic agent within the stem cell, and management of immune reactions to the gene therapy process. The ability of embryonic stem cells to generate a wide variety of specialized cell types and being able to maintain them in the laboratory would make embryonic stem cells a promising model for exploring critical questions in many of these areas.

"There are possibilities of long-term maintenance and expansion of embryonic stem cells and of differentiation along specific lineages that have not been possible with hematopoietic stem cells," Zanjani says. "And if they [embryonic stem cells] could be used [in the laboratory] as a model for differentiation, you could evaluate ... vectors for gene delivery and get an idea of how genes are translated in patients." Cynthia Dunbar, a gene therapy researcher at the National Institutes of Health, similarly notes that embryonic stem cells could be useful not only in screening new viral and nonviral vectors designed to introduce therapeutic transgenes into cells, but especially for testing levels of production of the therapeutic agent after the embryonic stem cells differentiate in culture [9]. Explains Dunbar, "These behaviors are hard to predict for human cells based on animal studies ... so this would be a very useful laboratory tool." Indeed, the major contribution of embryonic stem cells to gene therapy may be to advance the general scientific knowledge needed to overcome many of the current technical hurdles to successful therapeutic gene transfer.

REFERENCES

1. Aboody, K.S., Brown, A., Rainov, N.G., Bower, K.A., Liu, S., Yang, W., Small, J.E., Herrlinger, U., Ourednik, V., Black, P.M., Breakefield, X.O., and Snyder, E.Y. (2000). Neural stem cells display extensive tropism for pathology in adult brain: evidence from intracranial gliomas. Proc. Natl. Acad. Sci. U. S. A. 97, 12846-12851.

2. Amit, M., Carpenter, M.K., Inokuma, M.S., Chiu, C.P., Harris, C.P., Waknitz, M.A., Itskovitz-Eldor, J., and Thomson, J.A. (2000). Clonally derived human embryonic stem cell lines maintain pluripotency and proliferative potential for prolonged periods of culture. Dev. Biol. *227*, 271-278.

3. Armstrong, L., Lako, M., Lincoln, J., Cairns, P.M., and Hole, N. (2000). mTert expression correlates with telomerase activity during the differentiation of murine embryonic stem cells. Mech. Dev. *97*, 109-116.

4. Betts, D.H., Bordignon, V., Hill, J.R., Winger, Q., Westhusin, M.E., Smith, L.C., and King, W.A. (2001). Reprogramming of telomerase activity and rebuilding of telomere length in cloned cattle. Proc. Natl. Acad. Sci. U. S. A. *98*, 1077-1082.

5. Cavazzana-Calvo, M., Hacein-Bey, S., de Saint, B.G., Gross, F., Yvon, E., Nusbaum, P., Selz, F., Hue, C., Certain, S., Casanova, J.L., Bousso, P., Deist, F.L., and Fischer, A. (2000). Gene therapy of human severe combined immuno-deficiency (SCID)-X1 disease. Science. *288*, 669-672.

6. Challita, P.M. and Kohn, D.B. (1994). Lack of expression from a retroviral vector after transduction of murine hemato-poietic stem cells is associated with methylation *in vivo*. Proc. Natl. Acad. Sci. U. S. A. *91*, 2567-2571.

7. Chen, W.Y. and Townes, T.M. (2000). Molecular mechanism for silencing virally transduced genes involves histone deacetylation and chromatin condensation. Proc. Natl. Acad. Sci. U. S. A. *97*, 377-382.

8. Cherry, S.R., Biniszkiewicz, D., van Parijs, L., Baltimore, D., and Jaenisch, R. (2000). Retroviral expression in embryonic stem cells and hematopoietic stem cells. Mol. Cell. Biol. *20*, 7419-7426.

9. Dunbar, C., personal communication.

10. Gearhart, J. (1998). New potential for human embryonic stem cells. Science. *282*, 1061-1062.

11. Halene, S. and Kohn, D.B. (2000). Gene therapy using hematopoietic stem cells: Sisyphus approaches the crest. Hum. Gene Ther. *11*, 1259-1267.

12. Hawley, R., personal communication.

13. Korin, Y.D. and Zack, J.A. (1998). Progression to the G(1)b phase of the cell cycle is required for completion of human immunodeficiency virus type 1 reverse transcription in T cells. J. Virol. *72*, 3161-3168.

14. Laurencin, C.T., Attawia, M.A., Lu, L.Q., Borden, M.D., Lu, H.H., Gorum, W.J., and Lieberman, J.R. (2001). Poly(lactide-co-glycolide)/hydroxyapatite delivery of BMP-2-producing cells: a regional gene therapy approach to bone regeneration. Biomaterials. *22*, 1271-1277.

15. Luther-Wyrsch, A., Costello, E., Thali, M., Buetti, E., Nissen, C., Surbek, D., Holzgreve, W., Gratwohl, A., Tichelli, A., and Wodnar-Filipowicz, A. (2001). Stable transduction with lenti-viral vectors and amplification of immature hematopoietic progenitors from cord blood of preterm human fetuses. Hum. Gene. Ther. *12*, 377-389.

16. Mohajeri, M.H., Figlewicz, D.A., and Bohn, M.C. (1999). Intramuscular grafts of myoblasts genetically modified to secrete glial cell line-derived neurotrophic factor prevent motoneuron loss and disease progression in a mouse model of familial amyotrophic lateral sclerosis. Hum. Gene Ther. *10*, 1853-1866.

17. Ozawa, C.R., Springer, M.L., and Blau, H.M. (2000). A novel means of drug delivery: myoblast-mediated gene therapy and regulatable retroviral vectors. Annu. Rev. Pharmacol. Toxicol. *40*, 295-317.

18. Pannell, D., Osborne, C.S., Yao, S., Sukonnik, T., Pasceri, P., Karaiskakis, A., Okano, M., Li, E., Lipshitz, H.D., and Ellis, J. (2000). Retrovirus vector silencing is de novo methylase independent and marked by a repressive histone code. EMBO J. *19*, 5884-5894.

19. Park, F., Ohashi, K., Chiu, W., Naldini, L., and Kay, M.A. (2000). Efficient lentiviral transduction of liver requires cell cycling *in vivo*. Nat. Genet. *24*, 49-52.

20. Rathjen, P.D., Lake, J., Whyatt, L.M., Bettess, M.D., and Rathjen, J. (1998). Properties and uses of embryonic stem cells: prospects for application to human biology and gene therapy. Reprod. Fertil. Dev. *10*, 31-47.

21. Shields, L.E., Kiem, H.P., and Andrews, R.G. (2000). Highly efficient gene transfer into preterm CD34+ hematopoietic progenitor cells. Am. J. Obstet. Gynecol. *183*, 732-737.

22. Struhl, K. (1998). Histone acetylation and transcriptional regulatory mechanisms. Genes. Dev. *12*, 599-606.

23. Verma, I., personal communication.

24. Wade, P.A., Pruss, D., and Wolffe, A.P. (1997). Histone acetylation: chromatin in action. Trends Biochem. Sci. *22*, 128-132.

25. Yoder, M.C. and Hiatt, K. (1999). Murine yolk sac and bone marrow hematopoietic cells with high proliferative potential display different capacities for producing colony-forming cells ex vivo. J. Hemato. Stem Cell Res. *8*, 421-430.

26. Zanjani, E., personal communication.

This page intentionally left blank

APPENDIX A:

EARLY DEVELOPMENT

How does a single cell—the fertilized egg—give rise to a complex, multicellular organism? The question reflects one of the greatest mysteries of life, and represents a fundamental challenge in developmental biology. As yet, knowledge about the processes by which a fertilized egg divides (cleavage), forms a ball of cells (morula), develops a cavity (blastocyst stage), forms the three primary germ layers of cells that will ultimately give rise to all the cell types of the body (gastrula stage), and ultimately generates all the specialized tissues and organs of a mature organism is far from complete. Little is known about the specific genes that regulate these early events or how interactions among cells or how cellular interactions with other factors in the three-dimensional environment of the early embryo affect development. The processes by which a fertilized egg becomes an embryo, called embryogenesis, include coordinated cell division, cell specialization, cell migration, and genetically programmed cell death [24, 35].

A description of the stages of early embryogenesis in humans and mice follows. It includes an explanation of some of the more technical terms and concepts that are used throughout the document. It also includes a selective discussion of some of the genes, molecules, signaling pathways, and other influences on early embryonic development in the living organism (in vivo) that are used in experiments with stem cells maintained in the laboratory (in vitro).

EXPERIMENTAL SYSTEMS USED TO UNDERSTAND EMBRYOGENESIS

Many kinds of experimental systems have been used to understand how a fertilized egg produces a blastocyst, the first structure in which any cell specialization occurs, and a gastrula, in which the three embryonic germ layers—endoderm, mesoderm, and ectoderm—first appear. They include experiments with yeast cells; invertebrates such as tiny, jellyfish-like hydra, the microscopic roundworm Caenorhabditis elegans, and the fruit fly Drosophila melanogaster; and vertebrates such as amphibians, chick embryos and more recently, zebrafish Danio rerio, which are transparent as embryos and allow the detailed monitoring of cell differentiation and migration during development. The vast majority of studies on embryogenesis in mammals has been conducted in mice. For obvious ethical reasons, detailed research on human embryos has been limited. But the study of embryogenesis in all of these systems yields as many questions as answers.

For example, what signals the earliest cell differentiation events in the embryo? What regulates the activity of genes that are important for embryonic development? How and when are the axes of the embryo's body—anterior-posterior (head-tail), dorsal-ventral (back-belly), left-right—determined? What role does genetically controlled cell death, also known as apoptosis, play in embryogenesis? What influences the cell cycle, the controlled series of molecular events that leads to cell division or the cessation of cell division?

Much of the information about human embryonic development comes from studies of embryogenesis in the mouse. Like mammalian embryonic development in general, many aspects of embryogenesis in mice resembles that of humans, but development in mice also differs in several important respects from human development. For example, embryonic and fetal development in mice takes 18 to 20 days; in humans, the process takes nine months. The placenta forms and functions differently in the two species. In humans, an embryonic disk develops after the embryo implants in the uterine wall, whereas in mice an egg cylinder forms. The yolk sac of a mouse embryo persists and functions throughout gestation; in humans, the yolk sac functions only in early embryogenesis [28]. The primary roles of the human embryonic yolk sac are to initiate hematopoiesis and help in the formation of the primary germ cells, which will ultimately differentiate into eggs and sperm in the adult. And even for mice, knowledge about the genes, factors, and signal-transduction pathways that control embryonic development is limited. Signal transduction is a series of molecular events triggered by a signal at the surface of the cell and leading to a response by the cell—the secretion of a hormone, or a change in the activity of a particular gene, for instance [20].

Other sources of information about human development include studies of human embryonal carcinoma (EC) cells maintained *in vitro* and of histological sections of human embryos. (EC cells are derived from unusual tumors called teratocarcinomas, which may form spontaneously in the human testis or ovary.) Also, within the past 20 years, clinics and research institutes in many countries have developed *in vitro* conditions that allow fertilization and blastocyst formation. Thus, the study of methods to improve pregnancy rates following *in vitro* fertilization (IVF) has yielded important information about early human embryogenesis.

A FERTILIZED EGG FORMS A BLASTOCYST

Prior to fertilization in humans and mice, the egg (oocyte) enlarges, divides by meiosis, and matures in its ovarian follicle until it reaches a stage of meiotic division called metaphase II (see Figure A.1. Cell Cycle). At this point, the follicle releases the oocyte into the oviduct, one of two tube-like structures that lead from the ovaries to the uterus. The mature oocyte, a haploid cell that contains half the normal number of chromosomes, is surrounded by a protective coat of noncellular material (made of extracellular matrix and glycoproteins), called the zona pellucida. For fertilization to occur, a haploid sperm cell must bind to and penetrate the zona pellucida, fuse with the cell membrane of the oocyte, enter the oocyte cytoplasm, and fuse its pronucleus with the oocyte pronucleus. Fusion of the sperm and egg pronuclei restores the number of chromosomes that is typical of a given species. In humans, the normal diploid number of chromosomes for all the cells of the body (somatic cells) is 46 (23 pairs of chromosomes). Mature sperm and egg cells (germ cells)

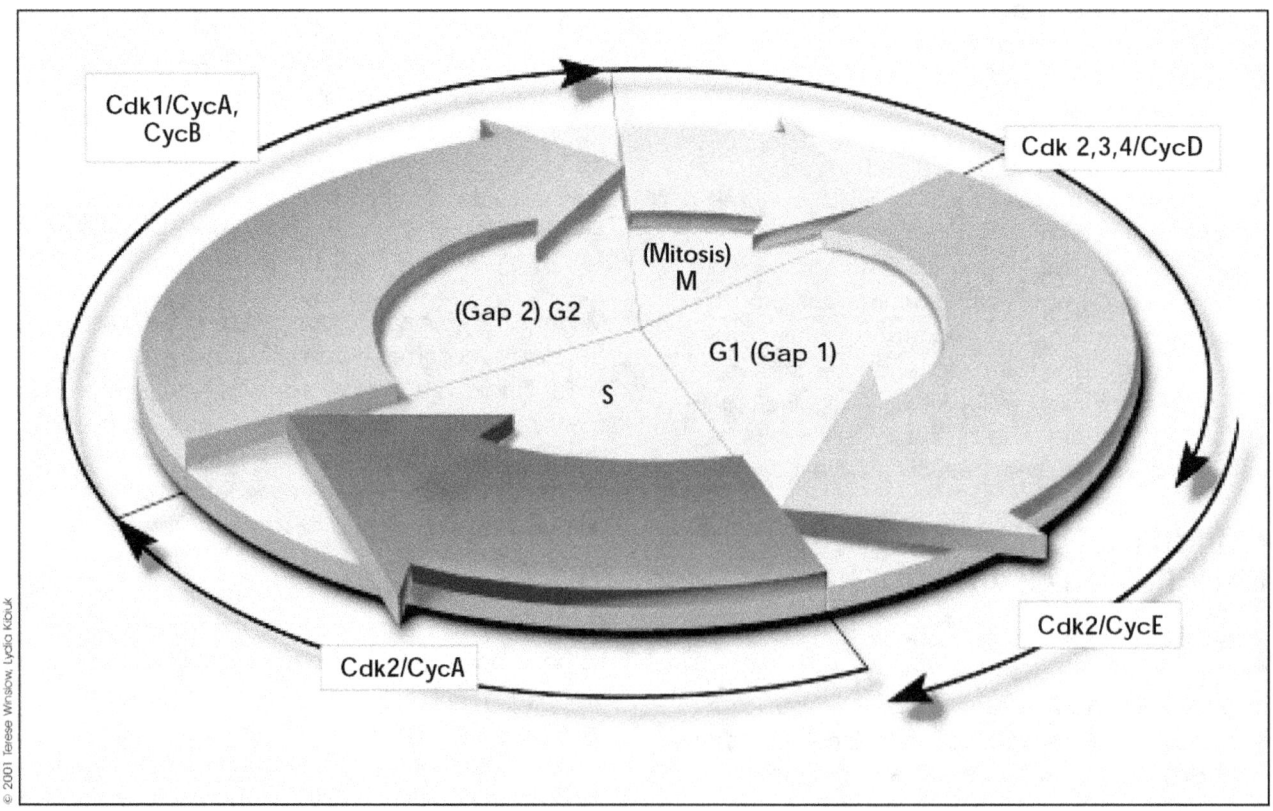

Figure A.1. Cell Cycle.

in contrast, carry only 23 chromosomes, the haploid number [1].

Under normal conditions, fertilization of the human oocyte occurs in the oviduct, near the ovary. A human egg is many times larger than a sperm cell, which means the oocyte contributes most of the cytoplasm of the zygote, another name for the fertilized egg. As a result, any maternal gene products in the zygote cytoplasm influence its first few divisions, called cleavages. Within several days, and after several cleavages, the genome (all the DNA or hereditary information in the cell's chromosomes) of the zygote becomes activated and controls subsequent embryonic development [19, 28]. Also, during these initial cleavages, the resulting daughter cells do not increase in size. Rather, as early cell division proceeds, the amount of cytoplasm of each daughter cell is reduced by half, and the total volume of the early embryo remains unchanged from that of the fertilized egg [30, 35].

After fertilization, the zygote makes its way to the uterus, a journey that takes three to four days in mice and five to seven days in humans. As it travels, the zygote divides. The first cleavage produces two identical cells and then divides again to produce four cells. If these cells separate, genetically identical embryos result, the basis of identical twinning. Usually, however, the cells remain together, dividing asynchronously to produce 8 cells, 16 cells, and so on [19]. Each early round of cell division takes approximately 36 hours, according to information gleaned from the study of human embryos in vitro [34]. In humans and mice, at about the eight-cell stage, the embryo compacts, meaning that the formerly "loose" ball of cells comes together in a tight array that is interconnected by gap junctions. These specialized membrane structures consist of an array of six protein molecules called connexins, which form a pore that allows the exchange of ions and small molecules between cells [27].

Recent information from studies of mouse embryos indicates that even at this early stage of embryogenesis, the anterior-posterior axis of the embryo has been established, a point of some concern for in vitro fertilization techniques, which disrupt early patterning events. The establishment of the anterior-posterior axis is critical to normal fetal development, because it helps determine the overall body plan of the embryo [3, 15, 18].

By the 16-cell stage, the compacted embryo is termed a morula. In mice, the first evidence that cells have become specialized occurs when the outer cells of the 16-cell morula divide to produce an outer rim of cells—the trophectoderm—and an inner core of cells, the inner cell mass [19]. Although the signals within the 16-cell morula that regulate the differentiation of the trophectoderm are largely unknown, it is clear that the outer cells of the morula are polarized. That is, one side of the cell differs from the other side. Thus, in the first differentiation event of embryogenesis, the outer, polar cells give rise to trophectoderm and the inner, apolar cells become the inner cell mass. This suggests that individual cells of the early embryo exhibit more intrinsic polarity than had been thought [27].

Ultimately, the cells of the inner cell mass will give rise to all the tissues of the embryo's body, as well as to the nontrophoblast tissues that support the developing embryo. The latter are referred to as extraembryonic tissues and include the yolk sac, allantois, and amnion. The trophectoderm, in turn, will generate the trophoblast cells of the chorion, the embryo's contribution to the extraembryonic tissue known as the placenta [19, 28].

The cells of the inner cell mass and trophectoderm continue to divide. Information gained from the study of mouse embryos suggests that the two tissues need to interact; the inner cell mass helps maintain the ability of trophectoderm cells to divide, and the trophectoderm appears to support the continued development of the inner cell mass [32]. Secreted paracrine factors (molecular signals that affect other cell types), including fibroblast growth factor-4 (FGF-4), which is released from inner cell mass cells [46], help direct embryogenesis at this stage. FGF-4 signaling also helps regulate the division and differentiation of trophectoderm cells [29].

By embryonic day 3 (E3.0) in the mouse and days 5 to 6 in human development [14], the embryo develops a cavity called the blastocoel. It fills with a watery fluid secreted by trophectodermal cells and transported in from the exterior. As a result of cavitation and the physical separation and differentiation of the trophectoderm from the inner cell mass, the morula becomes a blastocyst. Its chief structural features are the outer sphere of flattened trophectoderm cells (which become the trophoblast), the small, round

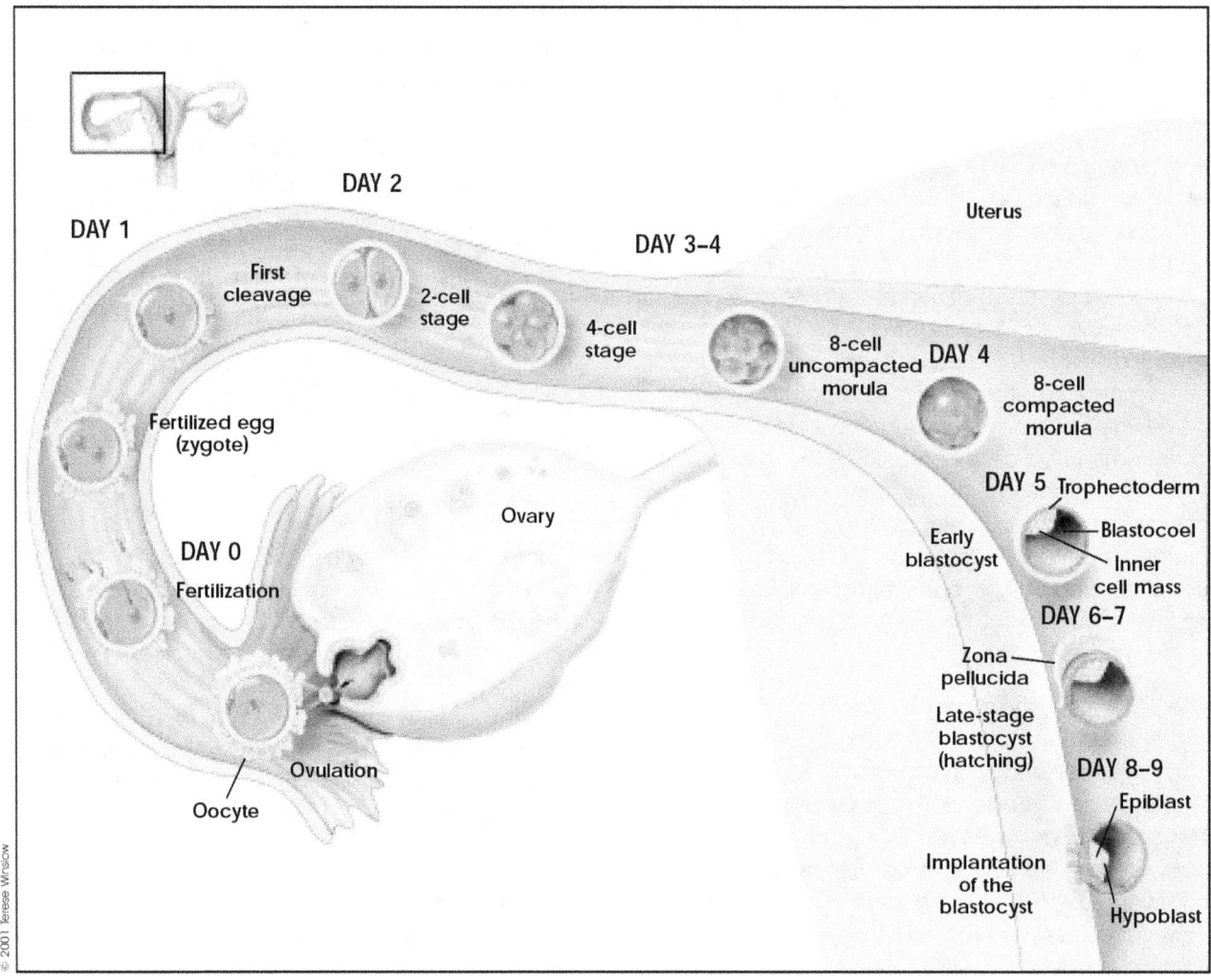

Figure A.2. Development of the Preimplantation Blastocyst in Humans.

cells of the inner cell mass, and the fluid-filled blastocoel [3, 19].

By E4.0 in mice, and between 5 to 7 days post-fertilization in humans, the blastocyst reaches the uterus. It has not yet implanted into the uterine wall and is therefore still a pre-implantation embryo. When it arrives in the uterus, the blastocyst "hatches" out of the zona pellucida, the structure that originally surrounded the oocyte and that also prevented the implantation of the blastocyst into the wall of the oviduct [19]. (An embryo that does implant in the oviduct results in a tubal pregnancy, which can result in severe hemorrhaging.)

The nutritional requirements of the embryo change markedly during the time from zygote formation to the compaction of the morula, to the development of the blastocyst. Also, the physiology and biochem-istry of the cells change as they increase in number and begin to differentiate. For example, the primary sources of energy for the cleavage-stage embryo are pyruvate, lactate, and amino acids—simple molecules that play important roles in various meta-bolic pathways. But after compaction of the morula, glucose is taken up by the embryo and used as a primary source of energy [15]. Indeed, mammalian blastocysts may have a unique transporter molecule, GLUT8, that ferries glucose into the blastocyst. GLUT8 appears in the blastocyst at the same time as the receptor for insulin-like growth factor-1 (IGF-1). Thus, the blastocyst, which requires a great deal of energy at this stage of development, is equipped to respond to insulin by taking up glucose [7].

These and other observations about the preimplan-tation blastocyst have led to recommendations

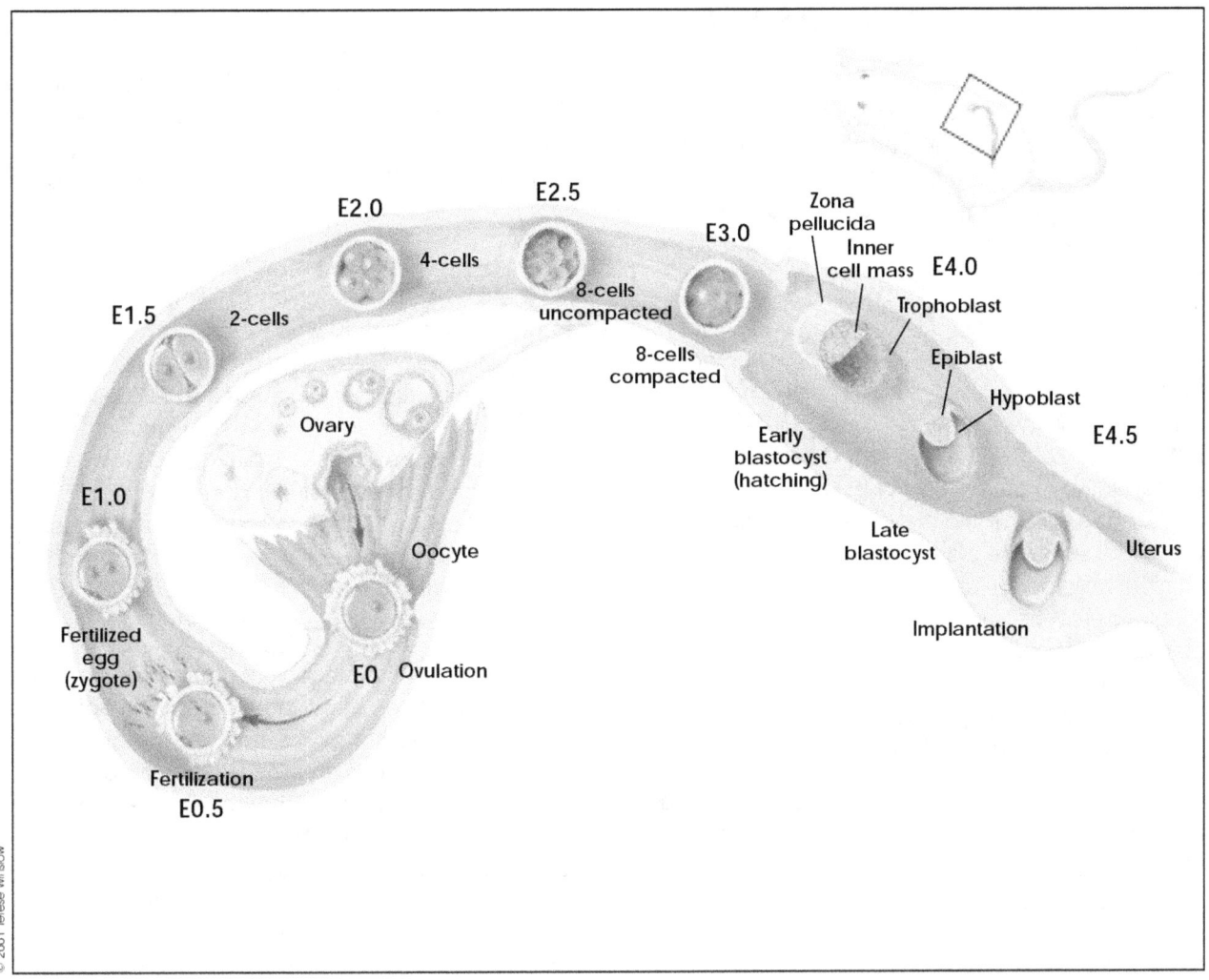

© 2001 Terese Winslow

Figure A.3. Development of the Preimplantation Blastocyst in Mice from Embryonic Day 0 (E0) Through Day 5 (E5.0).

about the importance of adapting the culture conditions to accommodate the changing nutritional requirements of the embryo when animal embryos are grown in the laboratory [16].

It is at this stage of embryogenesis—near the end of the first week of development in humans and about E4.0 in mice—that embryonic stem (ES) cells can be derived from the inner cell mass of the blastocyst. Human ES cells are derived from embryos generated through *in vitro* fertilization procedures and donated for research. An embryo at this stage of development *in vivo* would not yet be physically connected to the uterine wall; it would still be a preimplantation embryo.

ES cells, per se, may be an *in vitro* phenomenon. Some scientists argue that the apparent immortality

of ES cells occurs only in a laboratory culture dish [41]. ES cells that are grown in the laboratory most closely resemble cells of the epiblast [5], but ES cells are not identical to epiblast cells [42]. The term epiblast refers to all the pluripotent cell populations that follow the formation of the primitive endoderm and precede the formation of the gastrula [23]. Like the epiblast cells of the embryo, ES cells in culture have the potential to give rise to all the cell types of the body. However, unlike the epiblast cells of the embryo, ES cells *in vitro* cannot give rise to a complete organism. They do not have the three-dimensional environment that is essential for embryonic development *in vivo*, and they lack the trophectoderm and other tissues that support fetal development *in vivo* (see Chapter 2. The Embryonic Stem Cell).

THE BLASTOCYST IMPLANTS IN THE UTERINE WALL

Many of the molecular and cellular events that occur during the second week of human embryonic development, and at the end of the first week of embryogenesis in the mouse, help establish the placenta. The placenta connects the fetal and maternal bloodstreams and provides nutrients to the embryo throughout the remainder of gestation.

On or about postfertilization days 8 to 9 in humans (and E4.5 in the mouse), the ball-shaped embryo implants into in the uterine wall (see Figure A.2. Development of the Preimplantation Blastocyst in Humans). The inner cell mass of the human embryo at this stage has split into layers. One is the hypoblast, which lies next to the blastocoel and gives rise to the primitive endoderm. (Later, the primitive endoderm will give rise to the outer layer of the yolk sac, a curious reminder of reptilian ancestry in mammalian embryos.) The other cell layer that develops from the inner cell mass is the epiblast. It will give rise to all the cells of the embryo's body [19, 23].

The epiblast can be thought of as the group of cells that succeeds the inner cell mass. Pluripotent cells are defined differently in scientific articles and text books. In general, however, pluripotent cells are capable of giving rise to all the kinds of cells that occur in the mature organism. So at this stage of embryogenesis, the only pluripotent cells are the undifferentiated cells of the epiblast.

By E6.0 in the mouse, three differentiated cell types exist: the trophoblast, the epiblast (also called the embryonic ectoderm or primitive ectoderm at this stage), and the primitive endoderm (see Figure A.3. Development of the Preimplantation Blastocyst in Mice). During the next major phase of development, termed gastrulation, the embryonic ectoderm will differentiate into the three primary germ layers—endoderm, mesoderm, and ectoderm. Thus, the embryonic ectoderm has succeeded the epiblast as the tissue that will generate the body of the embryo. The primitive endoderm differentiates into parietal and visceral endoderm, the anterior region of which will help regulate the development of the body plan during gastrulation [23].

Prior to gastrulation, the majority of cells (approximately 75 percent) in the preimplantation blastocyst comprise the trophectoderm and the primitive endoderm. The preimplantation mouse embryo consists of approximately 200 cells, approximately 20 to 25 of which are inner cell mass or epiblast cells [20, 23]. The day 5, preimplantation human embryo contains 200 to 250 cells, only 30 to 34 of which are inner cell mass cells [4].

The extraembryonic cells of both species differentiate into the tissues that will convey nutrients to the embryo and remove its waste products. For example, some of the trophoblast cells invade the epithelial lining of the uterus (also known as the decidua), and form a multinucleated tissue called a syncitium. This syncytiotrophoblast, as it is called, then develops lacunae (cavities). By postfertilization day 10 to 11 in humans, the syncytiotrophoblast becomes supplied with maternal blood vessels. The fusion of the embryonic chorion and the maternal decidua and vascular tissue generates the placenta [19, 29].

The formation of the placenta is a critical process in human embryogenesis. Without a healthy placenta, the embryo does not survive; its malformation can trigger a spontaneous abortion [49]. The placenta anchors the developing embryo to the uterine wall and connects it to the maternal bloodstream, thus supplying the embryo with ions and metabolites and providing a waste-removal mechanism for the embryo [10, 26]. Later, the umbilical cord connects the embryo to the chorion portion of the placenta. The cord contains the fetal arteries and veins. Usually, the maternal and fetal blood do not mix directly. Instead, soluble substances pass through fingerlike projections called villi that have embedded in the uterine wall, and that have also developed from the trophoblast of the embryo [19].

In mice, some of the genes that regulate the development of the placenta have been identified. One is the *Mash2* gene, which is expressed in the trophoblast cells of the embryo after it implants into the uterine wall. If *Mash2* is inactivated, the placenta does not form and the embryo dies (at E10.5 in the mouse) [21, 45]. However, it is not known whether the same genes that regulate placenta formation in the mouse act in humans.

Meanwhile, during postfertilization days 7 to 14 of human development, the epiblast splits to form the amnionic cavity. The cavity fills with fluid and cushions the embryo throughout gestation.

THE BLASTOCYST BECOMES A GASTRULA

At the start of the third week of human development, and about E6.0 in the mouse (the egg-cylinder stage), the cells of the epiblast begin to differentiate. By the end of the third week, they will have generated the three primary germ layers of the embryo—endoderm, mesoderm, and ectoderm. A detailed description of all the events of this critical stage of differentiation—known as gastrulation—is beyond the scope of this report. However, the onset of gastrulation is triggered at the posterior end of the embryo with the formation of a structure called the node (from Hensen's node in chick embryogenesis). The node, together with another important signaling center, the anterior visceral endoderm (AVE), helps regulate the formation of the pattern of the embryo's body at this stage of development [19].

The process of gastrulation begins between days 14 and 16 of human development and at about E6.5 in the mouse. At that time, a primitive streak forms in a specific region of the epiblast along the posterior axis of the embryo. Little is known about the signals that regulate the generation of the primitive streak, although the genes goosecoid, T, Evx-1, and follistatin are expressed [23]. Nevertheless, the forward migration of the posterior epiblast cells occurs as their cell-cell contacts break down, and they release enzymes that digest the basement membrane that lies underneath. This allows the epiblast cells to migrate into the space between the epiblast and the visceral endoderm [6].

The forward-moving epiblast cells also spread laterally, a migration that induces the formation of the mesoderm and the notochord. The notochord is a temporary, rod-like structure that develops along the dorsal surface of the embryo and will ultimately connect the anterior visceral endoderm (AVE) and the node. Cells at the anterior end of the notochord will eventually underlie the forebrain [19].

At the anterior end of the primitive streak is the node, a two-layered structure and important signaling center in the embryo. The ventral layer of cells in the node comes from the epiblast and generates the notochordal plate, which then forms the notochord. Endoderm, which will give rise to the gut, also develops near the node, along the sides of the notochord.

Meanwhile, the anterior region of the mesoderm that develops from the primitive streak is preparing to give rise to the heart. The anterior epiblast is generating the neuroectoderm and the ectoderm that covers the surface of the embryo. The ectodermal tissue that lies dorsal to the notochord will generate the neural plate, which will round up to form the neural tube, the precursor to the central nervous system (brain and spinal cord) [23].

Thus, by the end of the third week of embryonic development in humans, and by E8.0 in the mouse, the primitive ectoderm of the postimplantation blastocyst has generated the ectoderm, mesoderm, and endoderm of the gastrula (see Figure A.4. Development of Human Embryonic Tissues). These and other complex processes result in the formation of the tissues and organs that occur in an adult mammal (see Figure 1.1. Differentiation of Human Tissues). They require the activation and inactivation of specific genes at specific times, highly integrated cell-cell interactions, and interactions between cells and their noncellular environment, the extracellular matrix [3, 19].

In general, the embryonic "outer" layer, or ectoderm, gives rise to the following tissues: central nervous system (brain and spinal cord) and peripheral nervous system; outer surface or skin of the organism; cornea and lens of the eye; epithelium that lines the mouth and nasal cavities and the anal canal; epithelium of the pineal gland, pituitary gland, and adrenal medulla; and cells of the neural crest (which gives rise to various facial structures, pigmented skin cells called melanocytes, and dorsal root ganglia, clusters of nerve cells along the spinal cord). The embryonic "middle" layer, or mesoderm, gives rise to skeletal, smooth, and cardiac muscle; structures of the urogenital system (kidneys, ureters, gonads, and reproductive ducts); bone marrow and blood; fat; bone, and cartilage; other connective tissues; and the lining of the body cavity. The embryonic "inner" layer, or endoderm, gives rise to the epithelium of the entire digestive tract (excluding the mouth and anal canal); epithelium of the respiratory tract; structures associated with the digestive tract (liver and pancreas); thyroid, parathyroid, and thymus glands; epithelium of the reproductive ducts and glands; epithelium of the urethra and bladder [19].

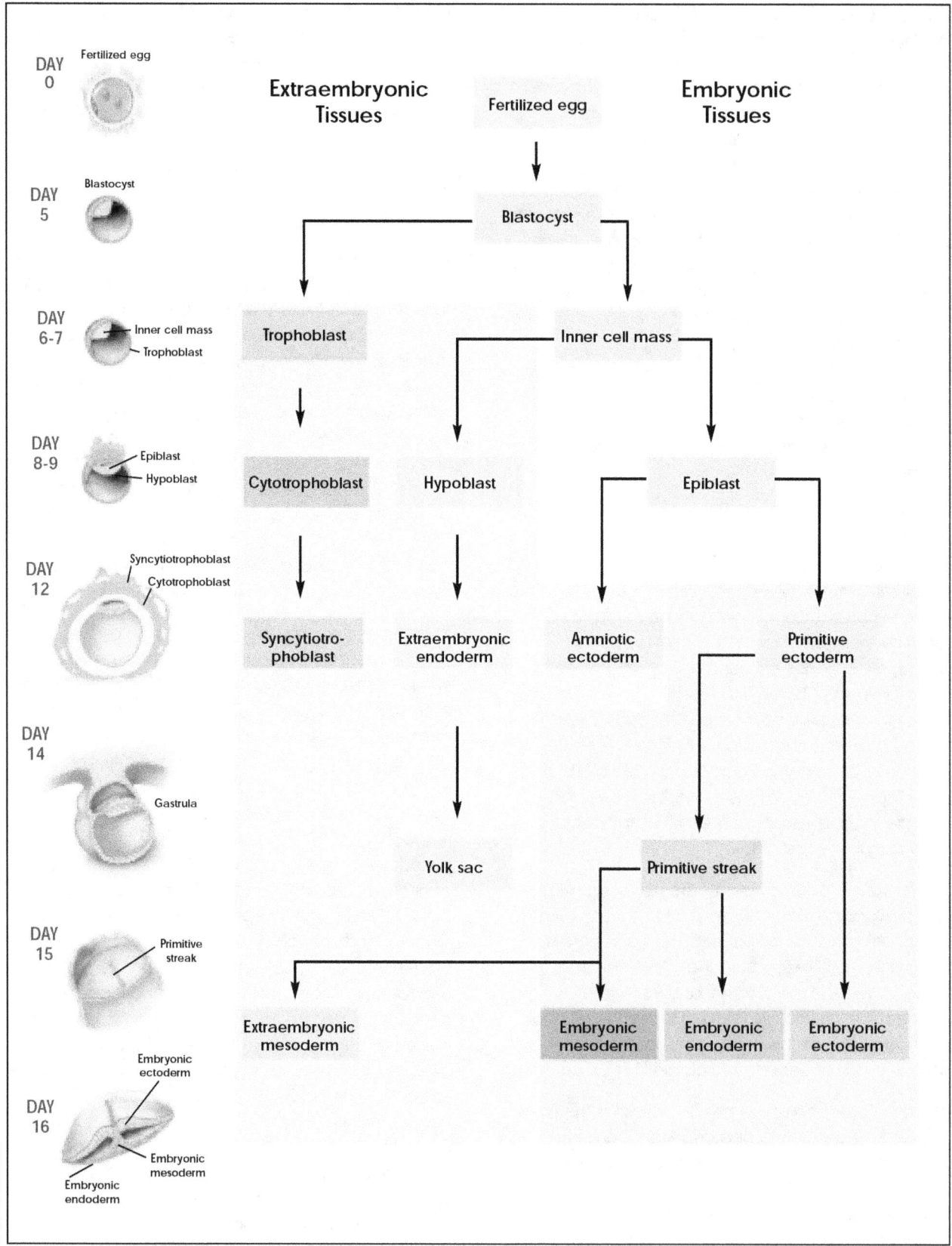

Figure A.4. Development of Human Embryonic Tissues.

PRIMORDIAL GERM CELLS ARE THE PRECURSORS TO EGGS AND SPERM

Not to be forgotten in this developmental scheme are the primordial germ (PG) cells, which will give rise to eggs and sperm in the adult organism (see Figure A.5. Development of Mouse Embryonic Primordial Germ Cells). Prior to gastrulation, at about the time of primitive streak formation, these precursor cells split off from the proximal region of the epiblast and migrate into the extraembryonic mesoderm (which generates the yolk sac and allantois). It is not until the proximal epiblast cells reach the extraembryonic mesoderm that they are committed to becoming PG cells. Their location in this tissue—which is remote from the rest of the embryo's body, or somatic, cells—may allow PG cells to avoid some of the events that drive somatic cells through the process of differentiation. One such event is DNA methylation, a means of silencing genes inherited from one parent—a process termed genomic imprinting (discussed below).

Another feature that distinguishes primordial germ cells from somatic cells is their continuous expression of Oct-4, a transcription factor produced by proliferating, unspecialized cells. Thus, the regulation of PG cell fate in the mammalian embryo is a result of the local environment of the cells, a recurring theme in mammalian embryogenesis, and the expression of genes in the PG cells [37]. Later in development, the PG cells embark in another migration and ultimately come to rest in the genital ridge, the tissue that will give rise to the gonads: testes in males and ovaries in females [35]. In the testis, the PG cells give rise to spermatagonial stem cells that reside in the testis throughout the life of the male. They continuously renew themselves and differentiate through the process of spermatogenesis into mature, functional sperm cells. There is no evidence, however, that they have pluripotential properties [39].

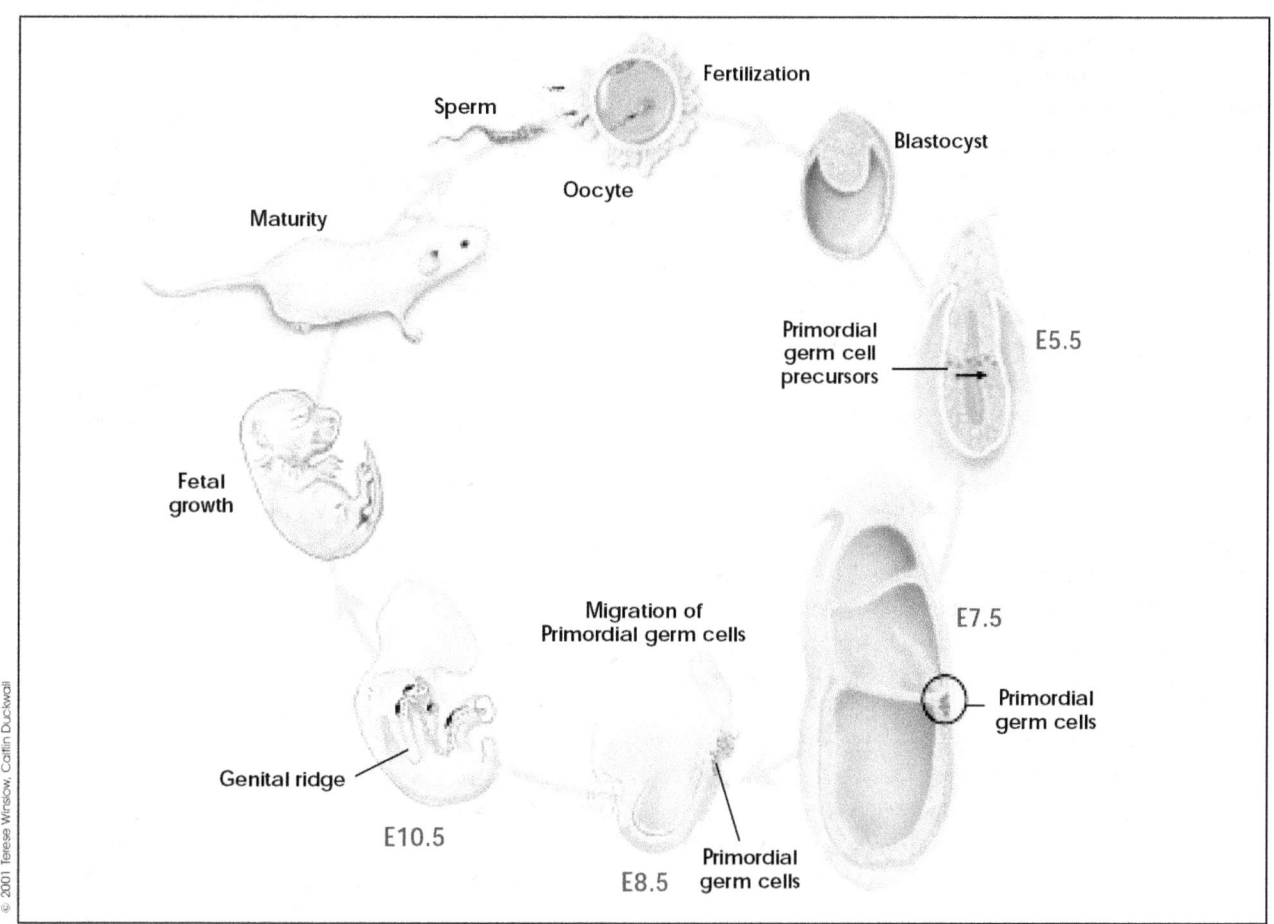

Figure A.5. Development of Mouse Embryonic Primordial Germ Cells.

GENES, MOLECULES, AND OTHER SIGNALS ARE IMPORTANT IN EARLY EMBRYOGENESIS

This overview of the processes of blastocyst formation, implantation, and gastrulation has ignored most of the crucial signals that direct embryonic development. These signals include genes expressed by cells at different stages of development, molecular factors secreted by cells, complex molecular signaling systems that allow cells to respond to secreted factors, specialized membrane junctions that connect cells and allow them to communicate, components of the noncellular environment (known as the extracellular matrix), and genomic imprinting. These signals—as well as their origins and effects—are the least understood elements of embryonic development in any organism.

GENE TRANSCRIPTION, TRANS-LATION, AND PROTEIN SYNTHESIS

A gene is a linear segment of a DNA molecule that encodes one or more proteins. The process occurs in three major steps (see Figure A.6. Gene Transcription, Translation, and Protein Synthesis). The DNA, which is double-stranded, unwinds and copies its triplet code (varying sequences of the four nitrogen bases adenine (A), thymine (T), cytosine (C), and guanine (G)) into a messenger RNA (mRNA) molecule. In RNA, uracil (U) is substituted for T. The process is called transcription because the triplet code of a DNA molecule is transcribed into the triplet code of an mRNA molecule. A gene that makes an mRNA transcript is active; the gene is said to be expressed.

The process of initiating transcription is complex. It requires the binding of certain proteins, called transcription factors, to regions of the DNA near the site where transcription begins. Transcription factors bind at sequences of DNA called the promoter enhancer region. The factors can activate or repress transcription. Although some transcription factors bind directly to the DNA molecule, many bind to other transcription factors. Thus, protein-DNA interactions and protein-protein interactions regulate gene activity. Their interactions then activate or block the process of transcription.

Transcription actually begins when the enzyme RNA polymerase II binds to the promoter region of DNA to initiate the process of making a molecule of messenger mRNA. As indicated above, the sequence of bases in DNA—the order of A, T, C, and G—dictates the sequence of the mRNA which will be formed. Thus, an A in DNA can bind only to a U in mRNA. The DNA base G will bind only to the RNA base C, and so on. RNA polymerase connects these bases together in a process called elongation.

The second major stage of the process of making proteins based on the code of DNA is called translation. During translation, the mRNA—which was generated in the nucleus of a cell and now carries its transcript of the DNA code—moves to the cytoplasm, where it attaches temporarily to tiny structures called ribosomes. There, molecules of mRNA direct the assembly of small molecules called amino acids (of which 20 kinds exist) into proteins. Each amino acid is specified by a code of three bases. The helpers in this effort are molecules of transfer RNA (tRNA). Each tRNA molecule contains its own triplet code (to match the mRNA code), and each tRNA ferries a particular kind of amino acid to the mRNA-laden ribosomes.

Then, in the third step of protein synthesis, the amino acids are linked through chemical bonds to create a protein molecule. Proteins typically consist of hundreds of amino acids. Thus, the sequence of bases in DNA determines the sequence of mRNA, which then determines the linear sequence of amino acids in a protein. Depending on its sequence of amino acids, a protein may fold, twist, bend, pleat, coil, or otherwise contort itself until it assumes the three-dimensional shape that makes it functional.

In the body, proteins make up most of the structural elements of cells and tissues. They also function as enzymes, which regulate all of the body's chemical reactions.

Gene Expression and Factors in the Preimplantation Blastocyst

It is difficult to identify the genes and factors *in vivo* that affect the earliest events in mammalian development; maintain the undifferentiated, proliferating state of inner cell mass or epiblast cells; regulate implantation; and direct the differentiation of cells along specific developmental pathways, or cell lineages. The embryo itself is very small and, *in vivo*, is almost wholly inaccessible to study. Therefore, many

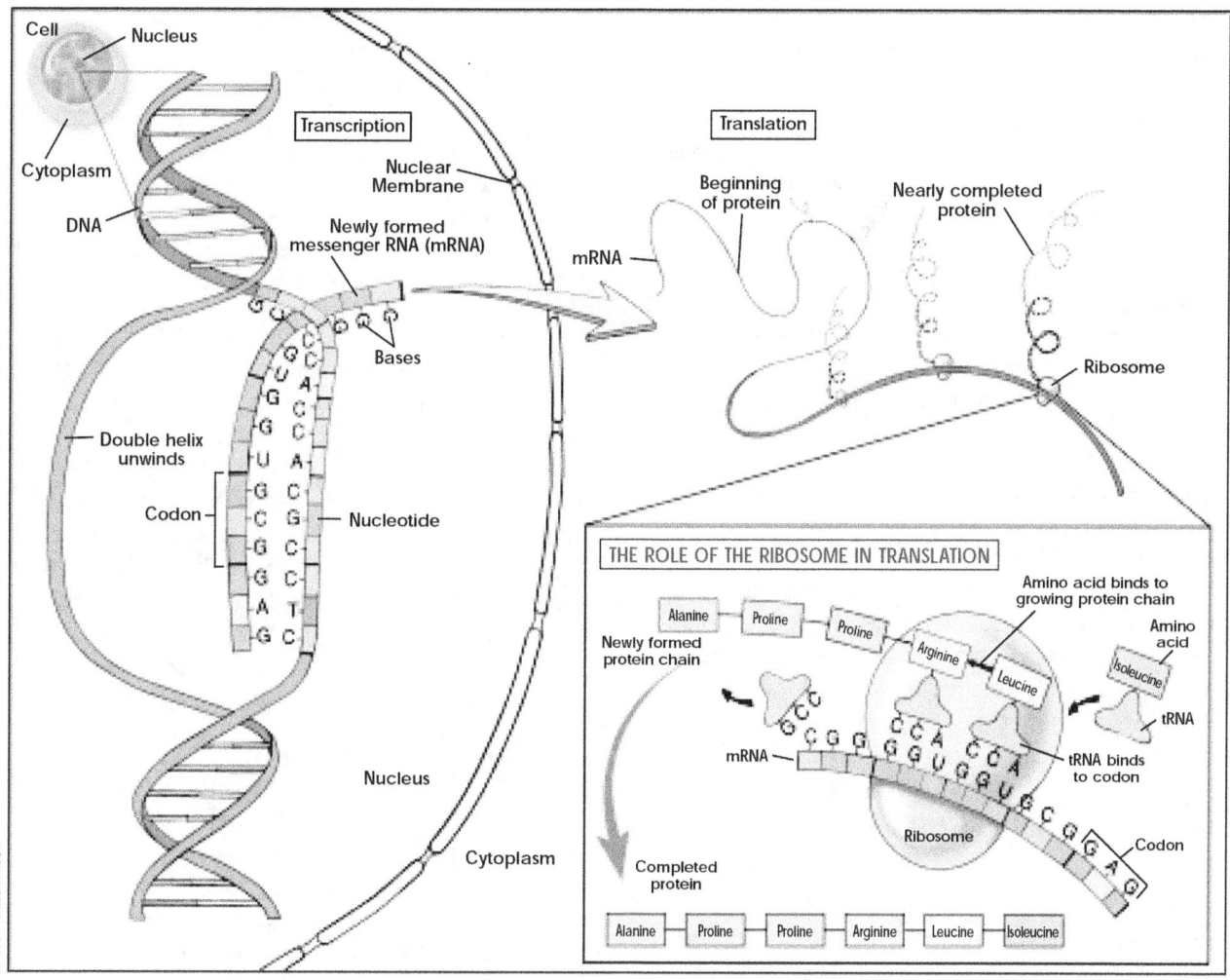

Figure A.6. Gene Transcription, Translation, and Protein Synthesis.

of the genetic and molecular influences that are now known to regulate early embryogenesis *in vivo* were identified by studying mouse embryonic stem cells *in vitro*.

For instance, Oct-4 is a transcription factor that has come to be recognized as a prototypical marker of undifferentiated, dividing cells. It is necessary for maintaining the undifferentiated state and proliferation of cells of the inner cell mass and the epiblast. Most of the studies of Oct-4 have been conducted in mouse embryos and ES cells. Oct-4 is expressed in the mouse oocyte, it disappears during the first cleavage of the zygote, and it reappears in the four-cell mouse embryo as the genome of the zygote begins to control embryonic development. Oct-4 persists in the inner cell mass of the blastocyst, but does not occur in differentiated trophectoderm cells, nor does it occur other differentiated cell types that arise after

gastrulation in the mouse. The gene for Oct-4, *Pou5f1*, is expressed in primordial germ cells, however [12, 32].

Oct-4 is a member of the class 5 POU (for Pit, Oct, and Unc) family of transcription factors, which bind promoter or enhancer sites in DNA. These proteins regulate gene transcription. The transcription factor Oct-4 can activate or repress gene expression; it binds to DNA at a distance from the start of transcription. Hence, depending on the target gene, Oct-4 may require the presence of co-activator proteins such as the E1A-like transcription factors and the Sox2 protein [37].

Another target of Oct-4 in mouse embryogenesis is the *Fgf4* gene. It encodes fibroblast growth factor-4 (FGF-4), a growth factor protein that is expressed together with Oct-4 in the inner cell mass and epiblast [32]. FGF-4 is a paracrine signal, meaning that it is released from one cell type and it acts on another. In this case, FGF-4 is released from proliferating inner cell mass cells and it affects the surrounding trophectoderm. FGF-4 may also act as an autocrine signal, meaning that it may affect the same inner cell mass cells that released it [13].

A series of recent experiments indicates that the level of Oct-4 expression—not simply its presence or absence in a cell—determines how mouse embryonic stem cells differentiate and whether they continue to proliferate [33] (see Appendix B. Mouse Embryonic Stem Cells).

Two proteins, leptin and STAT3, which are produced by maternal granulosa cells that surround the oocyte, are apparently secreted into the oocyte as it matures in its ovarian follicle. By the time the mouse or human zygote reaches the four-cell stage, leptin and STAT3 are concentrated in what may be the founder cell of the embryonic trophectoderm. Later, when the trophectoderm differentiates and separates from the inner cells mass of the blastocyst, leptin and STAT3 are expressed only in the trophectoderm, where they play a critical role during implantation [12].

Leukemia inhibitory factor (LIF), a cytokine, also plays an important role during implantation. The LIF gene is expressed in cultured mouse [31] and bovine blastocysts, as is the gene for its receptor. The mRNA for the receptor for LIF is expressed in human blastocysts [12, 47]. LIF, therefore, seems to be important for early mammalian blastocyst development, as well as implantation. It is also essential for the survival of the primordial germ cells, which will become eggs and sperm in the mature organism [22]. And if mouse embryonic stem (ES) cells are cultured from the inner cell mass of a blastocyst without the presence of "feeder" layers of cells, they require the addition of LIF to the culture medium in order to survive and proliferate [40]. Curiously, cultures of human ES cells do not respond to LIF [36, 48].

Regulation of Body Patterning in the Embryo

As the embryo forms, its overall body pattern is determined by the establishment of three clear axes—the anterior-posterior axis (head-tail), the dorsal-ventral (back-belly) axis, and left-right asymmetry. The establishment of these body axes at the correct time is fundamental to normal embryonic development. For instance, the central nervous system develops along the dorsal surface, with the largest concentration of neuronal tissue—the brain—at the anterior end of the embryo. The limbs develop symmetrically and bilaterally, whereas the heart—although it begins as a symmetrical structure—ultimately comes to point toward the left side of the trunk. Some internal structures are paired (the kidneys, lungs, adrenal glands, testes, and ovaries), whereas many are not (the heart, gut, pancreas, spleen, liver, and uterus) [19].

Information about the establishment of these body axes and their role in development is far from complete. For example, the anterior-posterior axis of the mouse blastocyst may be determined before it implants and is certainly established before gastrulation [15, 17]. An unanswered question, however, is whether this early embryonic axis helps determine the later development of the embryo. The early axis may play a role in primitive streak formation, and requires the expression of Wnt, which helps regulate the formation of one of embryo's chief signaling centers: the node [38].

As indicated above, an important group of cells that produces molecular signals that help determine the anterior-posterior axis of the mouse embryo is the anterior visceral endoderm (AVE). The AVE expresses different genes along its length. At E5.0 in the mouse, for example, the Hex gene—a member of the family of homeobox genes that help regulate body patterning of the mouse embryo—is expressed in the distal visceral endoderm. These cells migrate to become the AVE, which forms on the opposite side of the embryo from the primitive streak, thus establishing the anterior-posterior axis of the fetus [17].

Then, between E6.0 and E7.0 in the mouse, the anterior region of the AVE, where the heart will form, expresses Mrg1. The medial region expresses the transcription factor genes Otx2 and Lim1, as well as other genes. The region of the AVE that lies next to the part of the epiblast that will give rise to oral ectoderm and the forebrain expresses Hesx1, another homeobox gene. Collectively, the AVE and the genes it expresses help regulate the development of the anterior end of the embryo [3].

Other genes, notably Bmp4, also help shape the mouse embryo prior to gastrulation. BMP stands for bone morphogenetic protein, a family of proteins that help regulate the differentiation of mesenchymal cells, which are derived from mesoderm, including bone-forming osteoblasts, and adipocytes, which are fat cells. They also play a role in CNS development. *Bmp4*, which is expressed in the extraembryonic ectoderm next to the epiblast and also in the inner cell mass of the E3.5 and E4.5 mouse blastocyst, may activate genes in epiblast cells that then migrate to form the primitive streak. *Wnt3* apparently helps induce the formation of both the primitive streak and the node in mammals, although there is no evidence indicating that *Wnt3* expression is required for mesoderm induction. However, formation of the embryo's head region, obviously a key anterior structure, seems to require inhibition of the activities of *Wnt* and *Bmp4*—a potential role of the AVE [3, 18].

Therefore, coordinating the embryo's "decisions" about its body pattern is a hierarchy of genes. Overall, the *Hox* genes specify anterior-posterior polarity. Their normal function can be subverted by retinoic acid, which can activate *Hox* genes in inappropriate places. Less is known about the establishment of the dorsal-ventral axis. It may be determined in the blastocyst, or even in the oocyte [16]; it is clearly established when the notochord develops. Genes such as *Nodal* and *Lefty* help determine left-right asymmetry. Genes that regulate body patterning in embryonic development are well conserved throughout evolution among both vertebrates and invertebrates [19].

Regulation of Cell Differentiation in Early Embryogenesis

Myriad other genetic and molecular signals conspire to regulate cell differentiation in the embryo. Factors in a cell's environment bind to receptor molecules in its membrane and activate a series of intracellular responses that may result in gene activation or inactivation. The process by which a cell responds to an external signal is called signal transduction, and is itself the subject of many articles and books.

One of the earliest genes to be involved in cell differentiation in the preimplantation blastocyst are those that encode the GATA class of transcription factors. *GATA-6* is expressed in some inner cell mass cells of the E3.5 mouse blastocyst; *GATA-4* is expressed in the E5.5 parietal and visceral endoderm. *GATA-6* expression is required for the formation of the visceral endoderm; the role of *GATA-4* is less clear. Other genes such as *HNF-4*, which encodes a transcription factor, and *STAT3*, which encodes a protein important in a cytokine signaling pathway, are expressed later, during

the early differentiation of the visceral endoderm [18].

Other genes are expressed in the pregastrulation epiblast; examples are *Brachyury* and *Cripto*, which encode secreted growth factors. Still others, including *Nodal* and *Otx2*, are expressed in both the epiblast and the visceral endoderm [18].

A host of genes is expressed along the primitive streak. These include *HNF-3β* in the notochord, node, and floor plate (which will underlie the forebrain); *nodal, goosecoid, T, and Lim-1*, in the node; *Follistatin and T* for the remainder of the streak; and *FGF-4* just caudal to the node.

It is far easier to monitor the expression of particular genes than it is to identify their function(s) during development. One of the most useful kinds of experiments for determining the function of a gene involves its permanent inactivation—to create a knockout mouse, for example—followed by studies of impaired functions in the gene-deficient animal. Similar research strategies obviously cannot be used to determine the functions of specific genes in human embryogenesis. However, it is possible to identify human genes that are important for development by studying heritable abnormalities or congenital defects that have a genetic basis. Then, the function of the human genes—which almost certainly will have similar effects in mice—can be assessed in more detail by generating knockout mice that lack the gene.

THE CELL CYCLE

Many cells of the early embryo are in a constant state of dividing or of preparing to divide. The series of molecular events that regulate these processes is called the cell cycle (see Figure A.1. Cell Cycle).

The cell cycle includes four main phases: DNA synthesis (S phase), G2 (a gap phase during which the cell increases in size and prepares to divide), cell division (also called mitosis, M phase), and G1 (a gap phase of cell growth and replication of the centrioles). When a cell exits the cell cycle, to differentiate, for example, it is said to be in G0. Progression through the cell cycle is regulated by the activation of cyclin-dependent kinases (Cdks), enzymes that attach phosphate groups onto other proteins. Particular Cdks and their associated cyclins regulate the transition from one phase of the cell cycle to the next. For example, in mammalian cells, Cdk2 and cyclin E regulate the transition from G1 to S, whereas Cdk1 and cyclins A and B regulate the transition from S to G2. And recently, it has become clear that the cell cycle has several checkpoint mechanisms, during which the cell stops its progression through the cycle while it repairs damaged DNA [11].

The activity of the cell cycle varies, depending on the status of the cell and the cues—such as cytokine stimulation—the cell receives from its environment. Some cells "cycle" quickly, dividing in a matter of hours. Others cycle slowly, and some do not cycle at all. The epiblast cells of the postimplantation E5.5 to E6.0 mouse blastocyst, for example, have a mean cycle time of 11.5 hours. But a day later, at E6.5 to E7.0, epiblast cells have a mean cell cycle time of only 4.4 hours [23]. In contrast, the cycle time for cells in the cleavage-stage human embryo—a much earlier developmental stage—is approximately 36 hours [34]. And cells that are terminally differentiated—mature nerve cells in the brain, for example—have stopped dividing altogether. What factors regulate the cell cycle during development, or how the cell cycle alters gene expression or any other event in embryogenesis, remains largely unknown.

CELL DEATH IS A NORMAL PROCESS DURING EMBRYOGENESIS

It is a general characteristic of undifferentiated cells—including embryonic cells *in vivo* or *in vitro*— that when they stop dividing, they differentiate, become quiescent or senescent (stop their progress through the cell cycle and enter a period of temporary or permanent "rest"), or die. *In vivo* or *in vitro*, the process of cell death can occur by necrosis or apoptosis. The latter is a form of genetically controlled cell death that, in itself, is an important aspect of normal embryonic development *in vivo*. When the genetic program for apoptosis becomes activated, the cell commits a form of molecular suicide. Its DNA disintegrates in a characteristic manner, blebs (small pouches) form in the cell membrane, and the cell dies. The genetic controls for apoptosis differ, depending on the cell type, but all involve activating proteases called caspases, enzymes that destroy the protein components of cells.

As the body of an embryo develops, apoptosis helps shape it. For example, apoptosis helps control the spacing of nerve cells in the brain and spinal cord; it helps generate the space in the middle ear, and it causes the death of skin cells between fingers and toes—the typical "webbing" of fetal digits [19].

Many of the genes that regulate apoptosis were discovered in studies of the microscopic roundworm, *C. elegans*. The mammalian counterparts of these genes are very similar in terms of their DNA sequences, and are called homologues. For example, in *C. elegans,* the *ced-4* and *ced-3* genes are activated (in that order) prior to apoptosis. They, in turn, activate enzymes called caspases, which actually trigger apoptosis. But the regulatory pathway that leads to cell death is complex. Another apoptosis-control gene called *ced-9* can block activation of *ced-4* and *ced-3*, and thereby "rescue" a cell from apoptosis. The mammalian homologues of *ced-9* are members of the *BCL-2* gene family, which prevent apoptosis in mammalian cells—and in *C. elegans*, if they are introduced into cells from the worm [19].

Another mammalian apoptosis gene, *Apaf-1* works with caspase-9 to bring about cell death. It is interesting to note that the silencing of the *Apaf-1* gene—rather than a mutation in its DNA sequence—was recently linked to cancer metastasis [43]. In fact, several of the genes that normally regulate apoptosis inhibit the formation of tumors because they trigger the death of cells with damaged DNA that might otherwise replicate to produce a tumor. Because of their normal, protective function against the development of cancer, such genes are termed tumor-suppressor genes. Many tumor-suppressor genes, including *Apaf-1*, are associated with the so-called *p53* tumor-suppressor pathway. If even one of the apoptosis-regulating genes becomes mutated, the tumor-suppressor pathway can fail, a step toward the development of cancer.

SOME COMPARISONS BETWEEN EMBRYOGENESIS AND ONCOGENESIS

There are many molecular links between the regulation of normal embryogenesis and the induction of cancer, which is called oncogenesis. A comprehensive review of the similarities between the two exceeds the scope of this report. However, it is useful to point out that at least some of the genes, factors, and cell-cell interactions critical for normal embryonic development also play a role in—or are altered in—tumor development. The example cited above indicates that some of the genes that function during apoptosis in the embryo also protect the mature organism from developing tumors.

A different, and obvious, parallel between embryogenesis and oncogenesis can be observed in the spontaneous formation of tumors in the gonads of mammals, including humans. These unusual tumors, which include teratomas, embryonal carcinomas, and teratocarcinomas, develop from the germ cells in the testes or ovaries. The tumors have provoked a great deal of interest because they often contain highly differentiated cells and tissues such as teeth, hair, neural cells, and epithelial cells. The structures are disorganized, but often recognizable [2].

Although teratomas are benign, embryonal carcinomas and teratocarcinomas are highly malignant. The latter contain a kind of stem cell, called an embryonal carcinoma (EC) cell, which in mice and humans resembles embryonic stem (ES) cells. Human EC cells, unlike ES cells, typically have abnormal chromosomes. The chromosomes in mouse EC cells may appear to be normal, although they carry genetic defects. Nevertheless, mouse EC cells can contribute to normal embryonic development if they are introduced into a mouse blastocyst, which is then implanted in the uterus of a pseudopregnant female [2] (see Table A.1. Comparison of Mouse, Monkey, and Human ES, EG, and EC Cells).

Other genes recently identified as important in the development of human cancers are also active during embryonic development. For instance, the human breast cancer genes, BRCA1 and BRCA2, and their counterparts in mice are expressed in the three primary germ layers during embryogenesis, particularly in cell types undergoing the most rapid proliferation. The expression of these genes is dependent on the stage of the cell cycle, with peak expression during the G1/S transition and lowest expression in cells in the G1 or G0 phase. In mouse and nonhuman primate (cynomolgus monkey) embryos, the temporal and spatial patterns of Brca1 and Brca2 expression are virtually identical, despite the fact that the coding sequences for the genes and their promoters differ between the species. In humans, BRCA1 and BRCA2 probably function during the development of mammary epithelium, although little is known about their role in this process. Mutant forms of the genes appear to cause breast cancer

only if the mutations occur in the germ line. Somatic mutations of BRCA1 and BRCA2 are not linked to breast cancer [8].

DNA METHYLATION AND GENOMIC IMPRINTING AFFECT EMBRYONIC DEVELOPMENT

DNA methylation is the process of adding methyl groups to specific cytosine residues in the promoter regions of DNA. DNA methylation is a genome-wide phenomenon; it occurs in many genes depending on the stage of development and the differentiation status of a cell. When the methyl groups are bound at their designated sites in DNA, transcription factors cannot bind to the DNA and gene transcription is turned off. Also, DNA methylation causes a rearrangement of the structure of chromatin, the combination of DNA and protein that forms the chromosomes. DNA methylation patterns change during development, and their rearrangement in different tissues at different times is an important method for controlling gene expression [19].

Also important to embryonic development is the process of genomic imprinting, which causes certain to be genes turned on or off, depending on whether they are inherited from the mother or the father. Several mechanisms of genomic imprinting exist in mammals. A common method of imprinting is DNA methylation. Once methylated, or "marked," a gene may be activated or inactivated. Thus, the process of marking a gene as being inherited from either the father or the mother is genomic imprinting [19].

For most of the genes known to undergo imprinting, specific regulatory regions have been identified where methylation takes place. The methylation marks are acquired during gametogenesis, the process of sperm and egg formation, and they persist during the development of the pre- and post-implantation embryo [9, 44]. In contrast, the genes of nonimprinted embryos acquire their methylation patterns after blastocyst implantation, as do ES cells in vitro [50].

The genomes of germ cells and the zygote are largely demethylated, although the sites associated with parental-specific imprints remain methylated. In the preimplantation blastocyst, the nonimprinted genes of undifferentiated cells remain demethylated, which

Table A.1. Comparison of Mouse, Monkey, and Human Pluripotent Stem Cells					
Marker Name	Mouse EC/ ES/EG cells	Monkey ES cells	Human ES cells	Human EG cells	Human EC cells
SSEA-1	+	–	–	+	–
SSEA-3	–	+	+	+	+
SEA-4	–	+	+	+	+
TRA-1-60	–	+	+	+	+
TRA-1-81	–	+	+	+	+
Alkaline phosphatase	+	+	+	+	+
Oct-4	+	+	+	Unknown	+
Telomerase activity	+ ES, EC	Unknown	+	Unknown	+
Feeder-cell dependent	ES, EG, some EC	Yes	Yes	Yes	Some; relatively low clonal efficiency
Factors which aid in stem cell self-renewal	LIF and other factors that act through gp130 receptor and can substitute for feeder layer	Co-culture with feeder cells; other promoting factors have not been identified	Feeder cells + serum; feeder layer + serum-free medium + bFGF	LIF, bFGF, forskolin	Unknown; low proliferative capacity
Growth characteristics *in vitro*	Form tight, rounded, multi-layer clumps; can form EBs	Form flat, loose aggregates; can form EBs	Form flat, loose aggregates; can form EBs	Form rounded, multi-layer clumps; can form EBs	Form flat, loose aggregates; can form EBs
Teratoma formation *in vivo*	+	+	+	–	+
Chimera formation	+	Unknown	+	–	+

> **KEY**
> ES cell = Embryonic stem cell
> EG cell = Embryonic germ cell
> EC cell = Embryonal carcinoma cell
> SSEA = Stage-specific embryonic antigen
> TRA = Tumor rejection antigen-1
> LIF = Leukemia inhibitory factor
> bFGF = Basic fibroblast growth factor
> EB = Embryoid bodies

means that most of their genes are capable of being expressed. But before gastrulation, as the three germ layers prepare to differentiate, the DNA of the embryo's somatic cells becomes remethylated and genes are selectively turned on or off. The only cells that escape this phenomenon are the primordial germ cells (PGCs). They gradually remove their genomic imprinting marks, which exist in the form of parentally specified DNA methylation patterns. This phenomenon of erasing the marks for genomic imprinting occurs as the PGCs migrate to the gonadal ridges, which in the mouse occurs on E13.5 [23]. Then, as the germ cells mature, their genomes acquire new imprints due to the activity of a specific DNA methyltransferase, which adds methyl groups to DNA [50].

REFERENCES

1. Alberts, B., Bray, D., Lewis, J., Raff, M., Roberts, K., and Watson, J.D. (1994). Molecular biology of the cell, (New York: Garland Publishing, Inc.).

2. Andrews, P.W., Przyborski, S.A., and Thomson, J. (2001). Embryonal carcinoma cells as embryonic stem cells. Marshak, D.R., Gardner, D.K., and Gottlieb, D. eds. Cold Spring Harbor Laboratory Press, 231-266.

3. Beddington, R.S. and Robertson, E.J. (1999). Axis development and early asymmetry in mammals. Cell. 96, 195-209.

4. Bongso, A., personal communication.

5. Brook, F.A. and Gardner, R.L. (1997). The origin and efficient derivation of embryonic stem cells in the mouse. Proc. Natl. Acad. Sci. U. S. A. 94, 5709-5712.

6. Burdsal, C.A., Flannery, M.L., and Pedersen, R.A. (1998). FGF-2 alters the fate of mouse epiblast from ectoderm to mesoderm in vitro. Dev. Biol. 198, 231-244.

7. Carayannopoulos, M.O., Chi, M.M., Cui, Y., Pingsterhaus, J.M., McKnight, R.A., Mueckler, M., Devaskar, S.U., and Moley, K.H. (2000). GLUT8 is a glucose transporter responsible for insulin-stimulated glucose uptake in the blastocyst. Proc. Natl. Acad. Sci. U. S. A. 97, 7313-7318.

8. Chodosh, L.A. (1998). Expression of BRCA1 and BRCA2 in normal and neoplastic cells. J. Mammary Gland Biol. Neoplasia. 3, 389-402.

9. Constância, M., Pickard, B., Kelsey, G., and Reik, W. (1998). Imprinting mechanisms. Genome Res. 8, 881-900.

10. Cronier, L., Bastide, B., Defamie, N., Niger, C., Pointis, G., Gasc, J.M., and Malassine, A. (2001). Involvement of gap junctional communication and connexin expression in trophoblast differentiation of the human placenta. Histol. Histopathol. 16, 285-295.

11. D'Urso, G. and Datta, S. (2001). Cell cycle control, checkpoints, and stem cell biology. Marshak, D.R., Gardner, D.K., and Gottlieb, D. eds. Cold Spring Harbor Laboratory Press, 61-94.

12. Edwards, R.G. (2000). The role of embryonic polarities in preimplantation growth and implantation of mammalian embryos. Hum. Reprod. 15 Suppl 6, 1-8.

13. Feldman, B., Poueymirou, W., Papaioannou, V.E., DeChiara, T.M., and Goldfarb, M. (1995). Requirement of FGF-4 for postimplantation mouse development. Science. 267, 246-249.

14. Fong, C.Y., Bongso, A., Ng, S.C., Kumar, J., Trounson, A., and Ratnam, S. (1998). Blastocyst transfer after enzymatic treatment of the zona pellucida: improving in-vitro fertilization and understanding implantation. Hum. Reprod. 13, 2926-2932.

15. Gardner, R.L. (1997). The early blastocyst is bilaterally symmetrical and its axis of symmetry is aligned with the animal-vegetal axis of the zygote in the mouse. Development. 124, 289-301.

16. Gardner, D.K. (1998). Changes in requirements and utilization of nutrients during mammalian preimplantation embryo development and their significance in embryo culture. Theriogenology. 49, 83-102.

17. Gardner, R.L. (1999). Polarity in early mammalian development. Curr. Opin. Genet. Dev. 9, 417-421.

18. Gardner, R.L. (2001). The initial phase of embryonic patterning in mammals. Int. Rev. Cytol. 203, 233-290.

19. Gilbert, S.F. (2000). Developmental biology. (Sunderland, MA: Sinauer Associates).

20. Gossler, A. (1992). Early embryonic development of animals, Hennig, W., Nover, L., and Scheer, U. eds. (Berlin, New York: Springer-Verlag).

21. Guillemot, F., Nagy, A., Auerbach, A., Rossant, J., and Joyner, A.L. (1994). Essential role of Mash-2 in extra-embryonic development. Nature. 371, 333-336.

22. Hara, T., Tamura, K., de Miguel, M.P., Mukouyama, Y., Kim, H., Kogo, H., Donovan, P.J., and Miyajima, A. (1998). Distinct roles of oncostatin M and leukemia inhibitory factor in the development of primordial germ cells and sertoli cells in mice. Dev. Biol. 201, 144-153.

23. Hogan, B., Beddington, R., Constantini, F., and Lacy, E. (1994). Manipulating the mouse embryo a laboratory manual, (Cold Spring Harbor, New York: Cold Spring Harbor Laboratory Press).

24. Hogan, B.L. (1999). Morphogenesis. Cell. 96, 225-233.

25. Hogan, B. (2001). Primordial germ cells as stem cells. Marshak, D.R., Gardner, D.K., and Gottlieb, D. eds. Cold Spring Harbor Laboratory Press, 189-204.

26. Janatpour, M.J., Utset, M.F., Cross, J.C., Rossant, J., Dong, J., Israel, M.A., and Fisher, S.J. (1999). A repertoire of differentially expressed transcription factors that offers insight into mechanisms of human cytotrophoblast differentiation. Dev. Genet. 25, 146-157.

27. Johnson, M.H., Maro, B., and Takeichi, M. (1986). The role of cell adhesion in the synchronization and orientation of polarization in 8-cell mouse blastomeres. J. Embryol. Exp. Morphol. 93, 239-255.

28. Jones, J.M. and Thomson, J.A. (2000). Human embryonic stem cell technology. Semin. Reprod. Med. 18, 219-223.

29. Kunath, T., Strumpf, D., Rossant, J., and Tanaka, S. (2001). Trophoblast stem cells. Marshak, D.R., Gardner, D.K., and Gottlieb, D. eds. Cold Spring Harbor Laboratory Press, 267-288.

30. Marshak, D.R., Gottlieb, D., Kiger, A.A., Fuller, M.T., Kunath, T., Hogan, B., Gardner, R.L., Smith, A., Klar, A.J.S., Henrique, D., D'Urso, G., Datta, S., Holliday, R., Astle, C.M., Chen, J., Harrison, D.E., Xie, T., Spradling, A., Andrews, P.W., Przyborski, S.A., Thomson, J.A., Kunath, T., Strumpf, D., Rossant, J., Tanaka, S., Orkin, S.H., Melchers, F., Rolink, A., Keller, G., Pittenger, M.F., Marshak, D.R., Flake, A.W., Panicker, M.M., Rao, M., Watt, F.M., Grompe, M., Finegold, M.J., Kritzik, M.R., Sarvetnick, N., and Winton, D.J. (2001e). Stem cell biology, Marshak, D.R., Gardner, R.L., and Gottlieb, D. eds. (Cold Spring Harbor, New York: Cold Spring Harbor Laboratory Press).

31. Nichols, J., Davidson, D., Taga, T., Yoshida, K., Chambers, I., and Smith, A. (1996). Complementary tissue-specific expression of LIF and LIF-receptor mRNAs in early mouse embryogenesis. Mech. Dev. *57*, 123-131.

32. Nichols, J., Zevnik, B., Anastassiadis, K., Niwa, H., Klewe-Nebenius, D., Chambers, I., Scholer, H., and Smith, A. (1998). Formation of pluripotent stem cells in the mammalian embryo depends on the POU transcription factor Oct4. Cell. *95*, 379-391.

33. Niwa, H., Miyazaki, J., and Smith, A.G. (2000). Quantitative expression of Oct-3/4 defines differentiation, dedifferentiation or self-renewal of ES cells. Nat. Genet. *24*, 372-376.

34. Odorico, J.S., Kaufman, D.S., and Thomson, J.A. (2001). Multilineage Differentiation from Human Embryonic Stem Cell Lines. Stem Cells. *19*, 193-204.

35. Pelton, T.A., Bettess, M.D., Lake, J., Rathjen, J., and Rathjen, P.D. (1998). Developmental complexity of early mammalian pluripotent cell populations *in vivo* and *in vitro*. Reprod. Fertil. Dev. *10*, 535-549.

36. Pera, M.F., Reubinoff, B., and Trounson, A. (2000). Human embryonic stem cells. J. Cell Sci. *113 (Pt 1)*, 5-10.

37. Pesce, M., Anastassiadis, K., and Scholer, H.R. (1999). Oct-4: lessons of totipotency from embryonic stem cells. Cells Tissues Organs. *165*, 144-152.

38. Rossant, J., personal communication.

39. Shinohara, T., Orwig, K.E., Avarbock, M.R., and Brinster, R.L. (2000). Spermatogonial stem cell enrichment by multi-parameter selection of mouse testis cells. Proc. Natl. Acad. Sci. U. S. A. *97*, 8346-8351.

40. Smith, A.G., Heath, J.K., Donaldson, D.D., Wong, G.G., Moreau, J., Stahl, M., and Rogers, D. (1988). Inhibition of pluripotential embryonic stem cell differentiation by purified polypeptides. Nature. *336*, 688-690.

41. Smith, A. (2001). Embryonic stem cells. Marshak, D.R., Gardner, D.K., and Gottlieb, D. eds. Cold Spring Harbor Laboratory Press, 205-230.

42. Smith, A.G. (2001). Origins and properties of mouse embryonic stem cells. Annu. Rev. Cell. Dev. Biol. 1-22.

43. Soengas, M.S., Capodieci, P., Polsky, D., Mora, J., Esteller, M., Opitz-Araya, X., McCombie, R., Herman, J.G., Gerald, W.L., Lazebnik, Y.A., Cordon-Cardo, C., and Lowe, S.W. (2001). Inactivation of the apoptosis effector Apaf-1 in malignant melanoma. Nature. *409*, 207-211.

44. Surani, M.A. (1998). Imprinting and the initiation of gene silencing in the germ line. Cell. *93*, 309-312.

45. Tanaka, M., Gertsenstein, M., Rossant, J., and Nagy, A. (1997). Mash2 acts cell autonomously in mouse spongiotrophoblast development. Dev. Biol. *190*, 55-65.

46. Tanaka, S., Kunath, T., Hadjantonakis, A.K., Nagy, A., and Rossant, J. (1998). Promotion of trophoblast stem cell proliferation by FGF4. Science. *282*, 2072-2075.

47. Teruel, M., Smith, R., and Catalano, R. (2000). Growth factors and embryo development. Biocell. *24*, 107-122.

48. Thomson, J.A., Itskovitz-Eldor, J., Shapiro, S.S., Waknitz, M.A., Swiergiel, J.J., Marshall, V.S., and Jones, J.M. (1998). Embryonic stem cell lines derived from human blastocysts. Science. *282*, 1145-1147.

49. Trounson, A.O., Gardner, D.K., Baker, G., Barnes, F.L., Bongso, A., Bourne, H., Calderon, I., Cohen, J., Dawson, K., Eldar-Geve, T., Gardner, D.K., Graves, G., Healy, D., Lane, M., Leese, H.J., Leeton, J., Levron, J., Liu, D.Y., MacLachlan, V., Munné, S., Oranratnachai, A., Rogers, P., Rombauts, L., Sakkas, D., Sathananthan, A.H., Schimmel, T., Shaw, J., Trounson, A.O., Van Steirteghem, A., Willadsen, S., and Wood, C. (2000). Handbook of *in vitro* fertilization, (Boca Raton, London, New York, Washington, D.C.: CRC Press).

50. Tucker, K.L., Beard, C., Dausmann, J., Jackson-Grusby, L., Laird, P.W., Lei, H., Li, E., and Jaenisch, R. (1996). Germ-line passage is required for establishment of methylation and expression patterns of imprinted but not of nonimprinted genes. Genes Dev. *10*, 1008-1020.

APPENDIX B:

MOUSE EMBRYONIC STEM CELLS

MOUSE EMBRYONIC STEM CELL CULTURES

The techniques for culturing mouse embryonic stem (ES) cells from the inner cell mass of the preimplantation blastocyst were first reported 20 years ago [6, 11], and versions of these standard procedures are used today in laboratories throughout the world. Additionally, studies of embryonal carcinoma (EC) cells from mice and humans [2, 30] have helped establish parameters for growing and assessing ES cells. It is striking that, to date, only three species of mammals have yielded long-term cultures of self-renewing ES cells: mice, monkeys, and humans [21, 34, 35, 36] (see Figure B.1. Origins of Mouse Pluripotent Stem Cells).

In mice, the efficiency of generating ES cells is influenced by the genetic strain of laboratory mice and individual factors that affect pregnant females. Only a few strains of laboratory mice—notably 129, C57BL/6, and a hybrid strain—yield cultures of ES cells. Even then, ES cells derived from C57BL/6 blastocysts do not behave as reliably as do ES cells from the 129 strain of mice. The former are more difficult to propagate *in vitro*, generate chimeras less efficiently than do ES cells from the 129 strain of mice, and infrequently contribute to the germ line [4].

Another influence on the efficiency with which ES cells can be cultured from mouse blastocysts is the pregnancy status of the female. Pregnant mice that are in diapause tend to yield ES cells with greater success. Diapause occurs in female mice that have produced one litter and are still nursing when they become pregnant again. Diapause is a naturally occurring delay in the process of blastocyst implantation, which causes an arrest in embryonic development and a small increase in the number of epiblast cells [28]. These findings have led to the notion that genetic factors that are peculiar to specific strains of inbred mice, and other *in vivo* influences such as diapause,

determine, to a great extent, whether mouse ES cells can be derived from a given blastocyst.

Generating cultures of mouse or human ES cells that remain in a proliferating, undifferentiated state is a multistep process that typically includes the following. First, the inner cell mass of a preimplantation blastocyst is removed from the trophectoderm that surrounds it. (For cultures of human ES cells, blastocysts are generated by *in vitro* fertilization and donated for research.) The small plastic culture dishes used to grow the cells contain growth medium supplemented with fetal calf serum, and are sometimes coated with a "feeder" layer of nondividing cells. The feeder cells are often mouse embryonic fibroblast (MEF) cells that have been chemically inactivated so they will not divide. Mouse ES cells can be grown *in vitro* without feeder layers if the cytokine leukemia inhibitory factor (LIF) is added to the culture medium (see below). Human ES cells, however do not respond to LIF.

Second, after several days to a week, proliferating colonies of cells are removed and dispersed into new culture dishes, each of which also contains an MEF feeder layer. Under these *in vitro* conditions, the ES cells aggregate to form colonies. Some colonies consist of dividing, nondifferentiated cells; in other colonies, cells may be differentiating. It is difficult to maintain human ES cells in dispersed cultures where cells do not aggregate, although mouse ES cells can be cultured this way. Depending on the culture conditions, it may also be difficult to prevent the spontaneous differentiation of mouse or human ES cells.

In the third major step required to generate ES cell lines, the individual, nondifferentiating colonies are dissociated and replated into new dishes, a step called passage. This replating process establishes a "line" of ES cells. The line of cells is "clonal" if a single ES cell generates it. Following some version of this fundamental procedure, human and mouse ES cells can be grown and passaged for two or more years,

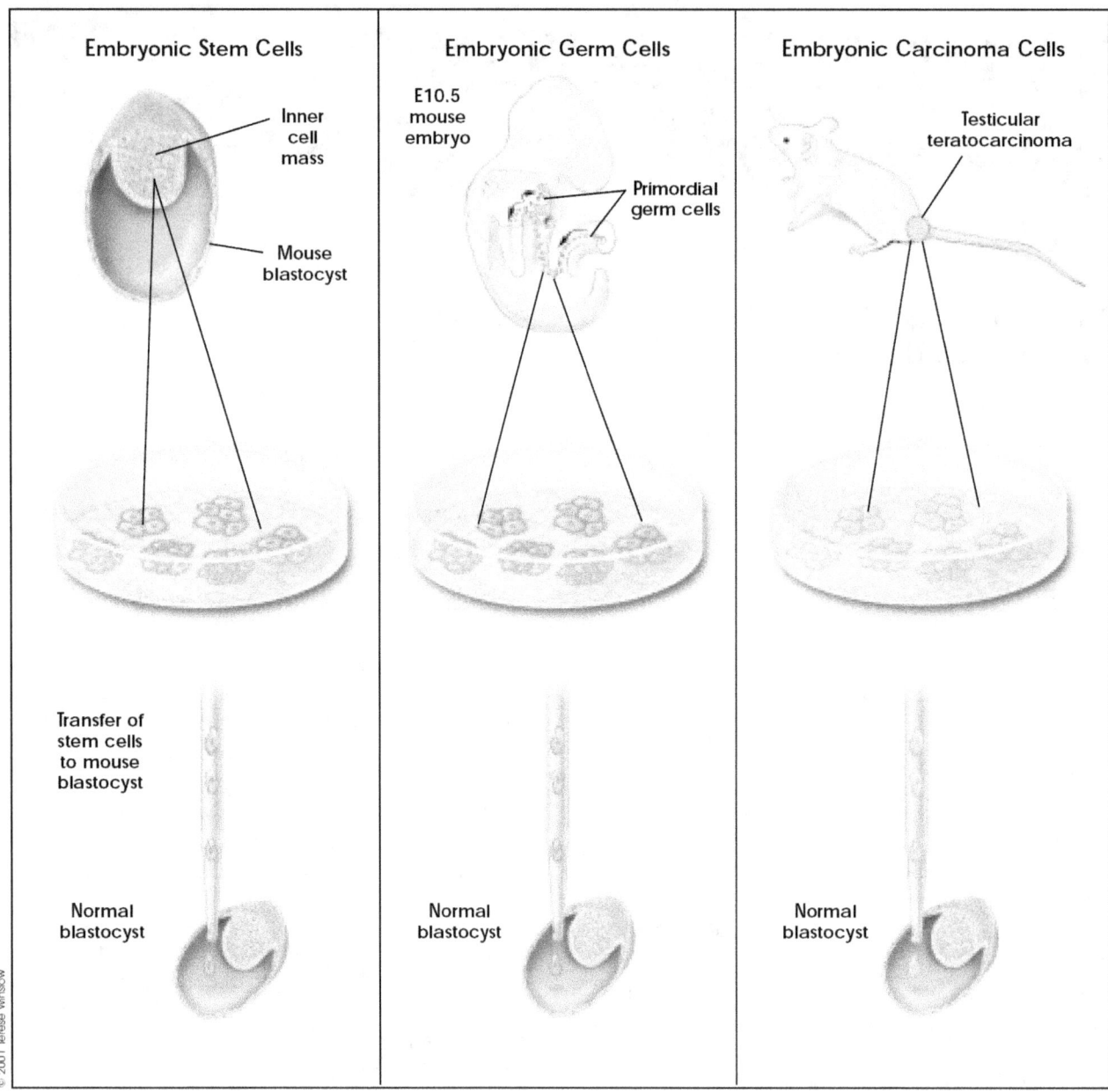

Figure B.1. Origins of Mouse Pluripotent Stem Cells.

through hundreds of population doublings, and still maintain a normal complement of chromosomes, called a karyotype [31, 35].

MAINTAINING MOUSE EMBRYONIC STEM CELLS IN THEIR UNDIFFERENTIATED STATE

Leukemia Inhibitory Factor and STAT3 Activation

Mouse ES cells can be maintained in a proliferative, undifferentiated state *in vitro* by growing them on feeder layers of MEF cells. An alternative to culture on feeder layers is the addition of leukemia inhibitory factor (LIF) to the growth medium [31, 39]. LIF is produced by feeder cells and, in their absence, allows mouse ES cells *in vitro* to continue proliferating without differentiating [20]. LIF exerts its effects by binding to a two-part receptor complex that consists of the LIF receptor and the gp130 receptor. The binding of LIF triggers the activation of the latent transcription factor STAT3, a necessary event *in vitro* for the continued proliferation of mouse ES cells [5, 12, 14]. Recent evidence indicates that two transcription factors, STAT3 and Oct-4, may interact and perhaps affect the function of a common set of target genes [15].

In vivo, signaling through the gp130 receptor is not necessary for normal, early embryonic development but is required to maintain the epiblast during diapause. After gastrulation, LIF signaling and STAT3 activation promote the differentiation of specific cell lineages such as the myeloid cells of the hemato-poietic system or the astrocyte precursor cells in the central nervous system [9].

The self-renewal of mouse ES cells also appears to be influenced by SHP-2 and ERK activity. SHP-2 is a tyrosine phosphatase, an enzyme that removes phosphate groups to the tyrosine residues of various proteins. SHP-2 interacts with the intracellular (amino terminus) domain of the gp130 receptor. ERK (which stands for extracellular regulated kinase) is one of several kinds of enzymes that becomes activated when the gp130 receptor and other cell-surface receptors are stimulated. Both ERK and SHP-2 are components of a signal-transduction pathway that counteracts the proliferative effects of STAT3 activation. Therefore, if ERK and SHP-2 are active, they inhibit ES cell self-renewal [5] (see Figure B.2. The LIF-STAT3 Signaling Pathway Promotes Embryonic Stem Cell Self-Renewal).

It is possible that some of the components of signaling pathways in cultured mouse ES cells are unique to these cells. For example, mouse ES cells *in vitro* express high amounts of a modified version of an adapter protein, Gab1. The unusual form of Gab1 that occurs in ES cells may suppress interactions of specific receptors to the Ras-ERK signaling pathway [31]. Further, the expression of this altered form of Gab1 may be promoted by the transcription factor Oct-4. In mouse ES cells, Oct-4 expression and increased synthesis of Gab1 may help suppress induction of differentiation [30].

Thus, the emerging picture is that the effects of various signaling pathways must be balanced in a particular way for ES cells to remain in a self-renewing state. If the balance shifts, ES cells begin to differentiate [29, 30].

Expression of Oct-4 in Undifferentiated, Pluripotent Cells

One of the hallmarks of an undifferentiated, pluripotent cell is the expression of the *Pou5f1* gene, which encodes the transcription factor Oct-4 (also

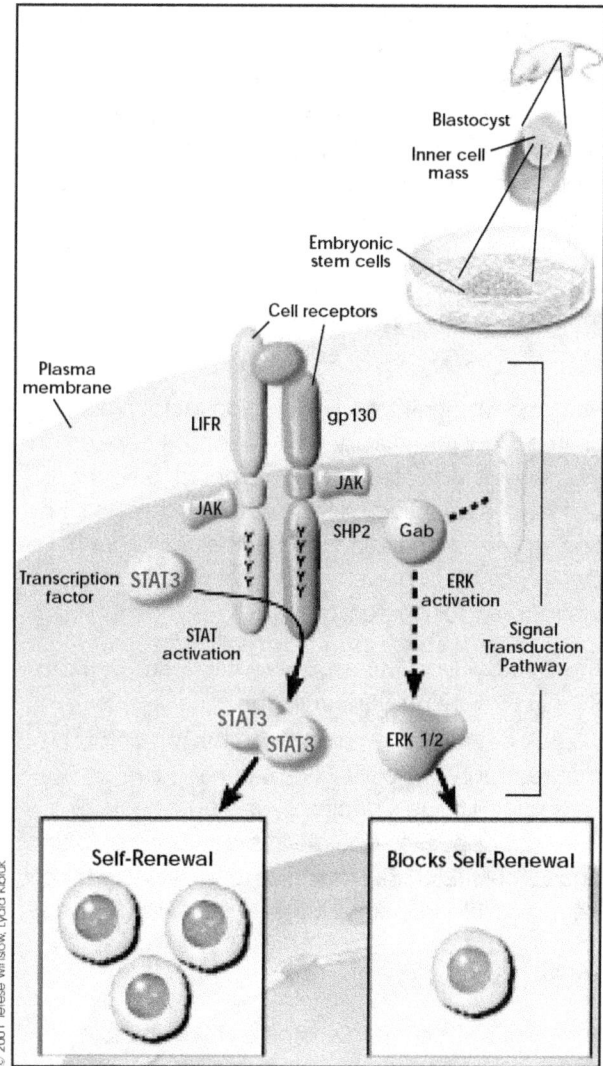

Figure B.2. The LIF-STAT3 Signaling Pathway Promotes Embryonic Stem Cell Self-Renewal.

called Oct-3 or Oct-3/4). Oct-4 is present in the mouse zygote, and is required throughout blastocyst development to establish [13] and maintain [15] the pluripotency of the inner cell mass and the epiblast. Oct-4 is also expressed in the primordial germ cells of mice and in mature germ cells [19, 23, 26].

Mouse ES cells *in vitro* can replicate indefinitely and produce 10^9 to 10^{10} (1 to 10 billion) cells without differentiating. *In vitro*, undifferentiated, proliferating mouse [18] and human [21] ES cells express Oct-4. Studies of Oct-4 expression and function in human cells are incomplete, however, and most of the information about Oct-4 comes from the study of mouse ES cells *in vitro*.

As is the case with inner cell mass and epiblast cells *in vivo*, Oct-4 expression *in vitro* is required to maintain the pluripotent, undifferentiated state of ES cells. If Oct-4 expression is inhibited in cultured mouse ES cells, the cells generate trophectoderm. If Oct-4 expression is artificially increased, mouse ES cells differentiate into primitive endoderm and mesoderm. Therefore, the level of Oct-4 expression dictates a significant aspect of the developmental program of mouse ES cells, making the protein a candidate "master regulator" of ES cell pluripotency [15].

How and why the Oct-4 transcription factor plays such an important role in early embryogenesis depend on the genes it regulates. Seven to eight target genes for Oct-4 have been identified to date; it activates some and represses others. In fact, the overall impact of Oct-4 may be to prevent the expression of genes that are required for differentiation [19].

The Cell Cycle of Mouse Embryonic Stem Cells: Its Role in Preventing Differentiation

Like the cells of the epiblast in the preimplantation mouse embryo, mouse ES cells *in vitro* have an unusual cell cycle. Specifically, the G1 checkpoint does not appear to operate in proliferating epiblast and ES cells [25, 38]. This may explain why it has not been possible to induce quiescence—withdrawal from the cell cycle to a G1 or G0 state—in undifferentiated ES cells [29].

However, if ES cells begin to differentiate by forming embryoid bodies, cyclin D expression increases, the G1 phase of the cell cycle becomes longer, and the rate of cell division slows [25]. This can occur if LIF or feeder layers are withdrawn from mouse ES cell cultures. Then, cell division continues for only a few days as the process of differentiation begins [29]. Perhaps constant cell proliferation somehow inhibits cell differentiation, and once the signals for cell division are removed, differentiation can occur [37].

Markers of Undifferentiated Embryonic Stem Cells

ES and EC cells, as well as cells of the inner cell mass of mouse blastocysts, express a panel of surface markers that are used to characterize undifferentiated, pluripotent embryonic cells. (see Table B.1. Comparison of Mouse, Monkey, and Human Pluripotent Stem Cells). The markers also distinguish mouse ES and EC cells from human ES and EC cells. For example mouse ES and EC cells express the stage-specific embryonic antigen SSEA-1, whereas

human ES and EC cells do not. But human ES and EC cells express SSEA-3 and SSEA-4, whereas mouse ES and EC cells do not [21, 35].

Human EG cells, which are derived from primordial germ cells, express all three markers: SSEA-1, SSEA-3, and SSEA-4. The biological significance of the expression patterns of these surface antigens is unclear, but SSEA-1 expression may be related to the growth characteristic of the cells *in vitro*. Undifferentiated human ES and EC cells tend to grow in flat, relatively loose colonies. In contrast, mouse ES and EC colonies tend to be multilayered and compact [27]. Alternatively, the surface expression of various SSEAs may reflect a difference in the developmental stages of the cells [17].

Other markers used to identify ES cells are the surface antigens TRA1-60, TRA1-81, and the enzyme alkaline phosphatase. All occur in human ES [3, 27, 35], as they do in their mouse counterparts.

Genomic Imprinting in Embryonic Stem Cells

It is known that if genomic imprinting patterns are disturbed before blastocyst implantation *in vivo*, fetal abnormalities may result. In genomic imprinting, DNA methylation marks certain genes, depending on whether they are inherited from the mother or the father. The marked genes are turned on or off in a non-random pattern that is determined by parental origin. Imprinting marks are erased in the primordial germ cells and then reestablished during the formation of eggs and sperm.

However, when embryonic development occurs *in vitro* or when ES cells are grown in tissue culture, normal patterns of genomic imprinting may be disturbed. For example, mouse embryos that were grown *in vitro* in the presence of fetal calf serum—a very different environment than the oviduct—and then allowed to develop *in vivo*, showed abnormal genomic imprinting patterns and abnormal development. Apparently, the presence of fetal calf serum, a common ingredient in mouse and human ES cultures, decreases the expression of certain imprinted genes [8].

How or whether the use of fetal calf serum for culturing mouse or human ES cells affects genomic imprinting and the behavior of ES cells *in vitro* is not known. But for mouse ES cells, the parental imprinting pattern apparently persists *in vitro* [16, 22]. The imprinting pattern of human ES cells *in vitro* has not yet been determined.

Table B.1. Comparison of Mouse, Monkey, and Human Pluripotent Stem Cells

Marker Name	Mouse EC/ ES/EG cells	Monkey ES cells	Human ES cells	Human EG cells	Human EC cells
SSEA-1	+	–	–	+	–
SSEA-3	–	+	+	+	+
SEA-4	–	+	+	+	+
TRA-1-60	–	+	+	+	+
TRA-1-81	–	+	+	+	+
Alkaline phosphatase	+	+	+	+	+
Oct-4	+	+	+	Unknown	+
Telomerase activity	+ ES, EC	Unknown	+	Unknown	+
Feeder-cell dependent	ES, EG, some EC	Yes	Yes	Yes	Some; relatively low clonal efficiency
Factors which aid in stem cell self-renewal	LIF and other factors that act through gp130 receptor and can substitute for feeder layer	Co-culture with feeder cells; other promoting factors have not been identified	Feeder cells + serum; feeder layer + serum-free medium + bFGF	LIF, bFGF, forskolin	Unknown; low proliferative capacity
Growth characteristics *in vitro*	Form tight, rounded, multi-layer clumps; can form EBs	Form flat, loose aggregates; can form EBs	Form flat, loose aggregates; can form EBs	Form rounded, multi-layer clumps; can form EBs	Form flat, loose aggregates; can form EBs
Teratoma formation *in vivo*	+	+	+	–	+
Chimera formation	+	Unknown	+	–	+

KEY

ES cell	=	Embryonic stem cell	TRA	=	Tumor rejection antigen-1
EG cell	=	Embryonic germ cell	LIF	=	Leukemia inhibitory factor
EC cell	=	Embryonal carcinoma cell	bFGF	=	Basic fibroblast growth factor
SSEA	=	Stage-specific embryonic antigen	EB	=	Embryoid bodies

Targeted Differentiation of Mouse Embryonic Stem Cells.

Outlined here are three different ways to direct mouse ES cell differentiation *in vitro*. In the first example, mouse ES cells are directed to generate primitive blood vessels. In the second, mouse ES cells are directed to become neurons that release the transmitters dopamine and serotonin. And in the third— a series of experiments conducted by the same lab group that generated dopamine neurons—very similar conditions are used to direct the differentiation of mouse ES cells to yield pancreatic islet cells that secrete insulin.

Making Vascular Progenitors from Mouse Embryonic Stem Cells

In the mouse embryo, blood cells and blood vessels are formed at roughly the same time, when blood islands first appear in the wall of the yolk sac. A prevailing idea is that blood cells and blood vessels arise from a common precursor cell derived from mesoderm, the hemangioblast. After hemangioblasts differentiate from the mesoderm, they aggregate to form blood islands. The inner cells of the blood islands become hematopoietic stem cells, or blood-forming cells. The outer cells of the blood islands become angioblasts, which give rise to the blood vessels. A recent study showed that mouse ES cells *in vitro* could be induced to follow this *in vivo* developmental pathway.

In vivo, blood vessel formation occurs in two ways: by vasculogenesis and angiogenesis. Vasculogenesis helps establish the blood islands and the capillary network that connects them. During angiogenesis, new blood vessels form by remodeling or adding to existing vessels. Both vasculogenesis and angiogenesis are regulated by the actions of a series of paracrine growth factors, which include fibroblast growth factor–2 (FGF-2), vascular endothelial growth factor (VEGF), and later (in the adult) platelet-derived growth factor (PDGF) and transforming growth factor beta (TGFß). Each of these growth factors binds to specific receptors. VEGF, for instance, binds to two different receptors: VEGF-R1, also known as Flt1, and VEGF-R2, also known as Flk1 [7].

To make vascular progenitors from mouse ES cells, Shin-Ichi Nishikawa of Kyoto University Graduate School of Medicine in Japan and his colleagues tried to mimic this *in vivo* pathway for blood vessel formation [40]. They grew undifferentiated ES cells on collagen-coated dishes in medium containing fetal calf serum but no leukemia inhibitory factor (LIF). This induced the generation of cells that express Flk1, a receptor for VEGF. Several days later, the cells began to differentiate. Nearly all the mouse ES cells expressed α-smooth muscle actin (SMA), a marker for mural cells. (Mural cells, which include pericytes and smooth muscle cells, normally interact *in vivo* with endothelial cells to make blood vessels.) When VEGF was added to the culture medium, sheets of endothelial cells formed that expressed platelet-endothelial cell adhesion molecule (PECAM1) and other endothelial cell markers. At this point, the culture contained two differentiating cell types, endothelial cells and mural cells.

Therefore, it appeared that the mouse ES cells had differentiated into Flk1+ precursor cells, which then gave rise to both mural cells and endothelial cells

in vitro. To test that hypothesis, single Flk1+ cells were cultured. The individual ES cells generated three kinds of colonies: pure mural cells (SMA+), pure endothelial cells (PECAM1+), and mixed mural and endothelial cells. That result indicated that ES cells can give rise to Flk1+ cells that are precursors for both mural and endothelial cells.

The next test was to see whether the mural cells and endothelial cells generated from Flk1+ precursors could assemble into primitive blood vessels *in vitro*. They did. By growing hundreds of Flk1+ cells in collagen gel suspensions with fetal calf serum and VEGF, tube-like structures formed within three to five days. This change in the culture conditions allowed the ES cells to grow in suspension and interact with each other. As a result, the cells spontaneously organized themselves into tube-like structures that resemble blood vessels *in vivo*. The tubes were composed of endothelial (PECAM1+) cells and mural (SMA+) cells. Occasionally, they formed branching structures, which is typical of the organization of blood vessels *in vivo*. Also, blood cells (bearing the markers CD45 and Ter119) formed inside the tubes, which also mimicked the organization of blood islands in the early embryo *in vivo*.

The final test was to see whether the Flk1+ cells generated from mouse ES cells *in vitro* would differentiate into endothelial cells and mural cells *in vivo*. Again, they did. Flk1+ cells were engineered to express LacZ (which allows the cells to be tracked visually) and injected into the developing hearts of stage 16-17 chick embryos. The donor mouse cells populated blood vessels in the chicks' head, yolk sac, heart, and regions between the somites, forming endothelial cells and mural cells in those regions.

Thus, undifferentiated mouse ES cells can be directed to differentiate into Flk1+ precursors that give rise to endothelial cells and mural cells *in vitro* and *in vivo*. Further, the differentiated cells can form tube-like vascular structures *in vitro*. The experiments not only demonstrate the power of directed differentiation of ES cells into individual cell types, they also show that ES cells can generate multiple cell types that then spontaneously organize themselves into tissues that resemble those *in vivo*. In addition, the experiments by Nishikawa and his co-workers [40] reveal that Flk1+ cells are important for generating blood vessels *in vivo*.

Making Dopamine Neurons from Mouse Embryonic Stem Cells

A second example of the directed differentiation of mouse ES cells *in vitro* yielded the formation of particular kinds of neurons that normally occur in the mammalian midbrain and hindbrain. For a long time, the goal of efficiently inducing the formation of these neurons—which release the neurotransmitters dopamine and serotonin, respectively— was highly desired, but elusive. In Parkinson's Disease, a key population of midbrain neurons that releases dopamine dies. So finding a way to grow large quantities of nerve cells *in vitro* that might be able to replace lost dopamine neurons *in vivo* is a clinical priority (see Chapter 8. Rebuilding the Nervous System with Stem Cells).

Last year, Ron McKay and his colleagues reported an efficient technique for inducing mouse ES cells *in vitro* to differentiate into dopamine neurons of the midbrain and serotonin neurons, which normally populate the hindbrain. Like Nishikawa and his colleagues [40], McKay and his collaborators [10] triggered the differentiation of mouse ES cells *in vitro* at various stages by changing the growth conditions to mimic, in part, those that occur during embryogenesis *in vivo*. The resulting differentiated nerve cells look and function like their *in vivo* counterparts.

During embryogenesis, central nervous system (CNS) development is a long, complex process that depends on a highly coordinated series of cellular and molecular events. Different signals direct the formation of the neurectoderm from the epiblast, a process that ultimately results in the formation of the CNS, the brain and spinal cord. Later, other signals regulate the development of different parts of the brain. For example, early in the formation of the brain, the homeobox genes *OTX1* and *OTX2* are expressed [28]. Cells of the epiblast express *OTX2* before the onset of gastrulation. Then, during gastrulation, *OTX2* is expressed in the anterior neurectoderm, where it is necessary for the formation of the midbrain and forebrain. Meanwhile, *OTX1* expression occurs in the region of the neurectoderm that gives rise to the dorsal forebrain. Interactions between *OTX1* and *OTX2* are thought to help shape the midbrain and hindbrain [1].

Once these major brain structures form, various genes control the development of individual nerve cell types. For example, the genes *Pax2, Pax5, Wnt1,*

En1, and *Nurr1* help control the differentiation of neurons that release the transmitters dopamine and serotonin [24, 33]. Furthermore, when the proteins sonic hedgehog (SHH) and fibroblast growth factor-8 (FGF-8) are added to explant cultures (small chunks of tissue maintained *in vitro*) of neural plate, the development of midbrain neurons is enhanced [41].

Taking into account these and other findings, McKay and his coworkers devised an *in vitro* system for controlling the differentiation of mouse ES cells into midbrain neurons that release dopamine and hindbrain neurons that release serotonin [11]. The culture conditions they used differ from those devised by Nishikawa and his colleagues (described above), but the starting material—undifferentiated, proliferating mouse ES cells—was the same in both experiments. McKay and his colleagues cultured mouse ES cells in five distinct stages, each of which they identified by the changes in culture conditions and the behavior of the cells (see Figure B.3. Directed Differentiation of Mouse Embryonic Stem Cells Into Neurons or Pancreatic Islet-Like Clusters).

In stage 1, undifferentiated mouse ES cells were dissociated into single cells and plated at low density. They proliferated in plastic culture dishes coated with gelatin. The growth media contained LIF and fetal calf serum and was supplemented with amino acids, conditions that promoted the proliferation of undifferentiated ES cells. In stage 2, the cells were induced to form embryoid bodies by dissociating them and replating at a higher density on a nonadherent surface. These conditions allowed the cells to aggregate and begin the process of differentiation. After four days, the cells were replated on an adherent substrate in the original (stage 1) growth medium. Twenty-four hours later, the growth medium was replaced with serum-free insulin/transferrin/selenium/fibronectin (ITSFn) medium. This switch to a serum-free medium (one lacking fetal calf serum) caused many cells to die but allowed the survival of cells that express nestin. This intermediate filament protein is used as a marker to identify CNS stem cells *in vivo* and *in vitro*, although it is also expressed by other cell types. Stage 1 neurons expressed high levels of *OXT2*, which decreased in stages 2 and 3. *OXT1* was not expressed until the cells reached stage 3.

Guiding the mouse ES cells through stages 4 and 5 of *in vitro* development yielded fully differentiated dopaminergic and serotoninergic neurons. After 6 to

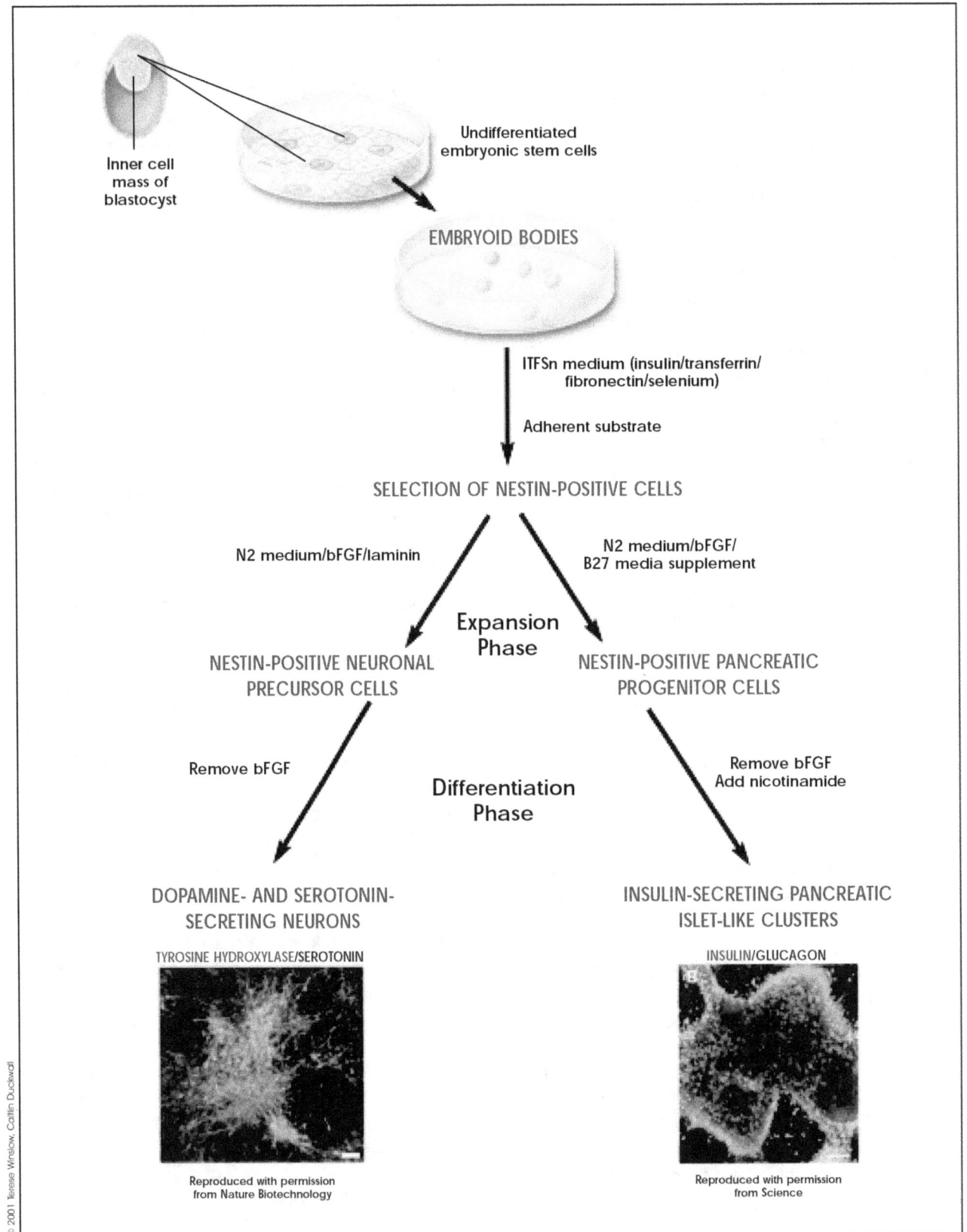

Figure B.3. Directed Differentiation of Mouse Embryonic Stem Cells Into Neurons or Pancreatic Islet-Like Clusters.

10 days in the medium that selects for cells that express nestin, the cells were dissociated and induced to divide in another medium, N2, supplemented with laminin and basic FGF, a growth factor that induces proliferation. Other critical additives to yield stage 4 cells were SHH and FGF-8. Cells at stages 3 and 4 express genes that, in vivo, trigger the development of dopaminergic and serotinergic neurons—namely, Pax2, Pax5, Wnt1, En1, and Nurr1. Stage 5, the final stage of differentiation, was achieved by removing basic FGF from the growth medium (which made the cells stop dividing) and growing the cells for 6 to 15 days in N2 medium supplemented with laminin and ascorbic acid, a combination of additives that induces the differentiation of serotonin neurons.

This complex, multistage differentiation process yielded a higher percentage (30 percent) of neurons that express tyrosine hydroxylase (TH, the rate-limiting enzyme in the synthesis of dopamine) than any other reported in vivo or in vitro technique. The cells were confirmed to be true dopamine neurons by several functional assays. The neurons secreted dopamine into the culture medium, showed the electrical activity typical of neurons, and responded to the addition of a high concentration of potassium ions (via the addition of potassium chloride) by releasing more dopamine, much as they would in vivo. A separate population of neurons in the mouse ES cell cultures stained positive for serotonin. The differentiation of serotoninergic neurons could be induced by adding only SHH to the culture medium; addition of FGF-8 was not required. Thus, mouse ES cells in vitro can be directed to differentiate at a high efficiency into neurons that release either dopamine or serotonin.

Making Pancreatic Islet Cells from Mouse Embryonic Stem Cells

The experimental strategy is similar to that described above [10] and is based on a five-stage, in vitro system. As before (to differentiate neurons that produce dopamine), undifferentiated mouse ES cells are induced to proliferate in LIF-supplemented medium (stage 1). Then, the cells are induced to form embryoid bodies (EBs) in serum-free ITSFn medium without LIF (stage 2). ES stage 1 cells expressed Oct-4, a transcription factor that characterizes undifferentiated, proliferating, pluripotent cells. Again, cells that express nestin survive in serum-free medium, whereas other cell types do not, thus creating an environment that

"selects" for nestin-positive cells (stage 3). As before, cells that express nestin are expanded by adding the mitogen basic FGF to the serum-free medium (stage 4). When basic FGF is withdrawn, the cells stop dividing and begin their final stages of differentiation. It is at this point that the techniques for generating neurons that release dopamine and pancreatic islet cells that release insulin diverge.

To generate neurons that release dopamine, ES-derived cells were cultured in medium that contained SHH and FGF-8 and later, an N2 medium supplemented with laminin and ascorbic acid [10]. To generate pancreatic islet cells, however, B27 culture medium was used for stage 4, and nicotinamide was added to stage 5 cultures. Another change in the pancreatic islet culture system was to co-culture individual stage 4 or 5 ES cells, which were tagged with the marker green fluorescent protein (GFP), with nontagged ES cells. This meant that an individual, tagged ES cell could be followed so its developmental fate could be traced, a technique that made possible the clonal analysis of the labeled ES cell and its progeny. Tagged, GFP-expressing ES cells gave rise to both pancreatic islet cells and neurons, indicating that the same cell acted as the precursor for both differentiated cell types (see Figure B.3. Directed Differentiation of Mouse Embryonic Stem Cells Into Neurons or Pancreatic Islet-Like Clusters).

The tests that identified the differentiated cells types as pancreatic islet cells and neurons included assays of various markers. The ES cells at stages 1 and 5 expressed GATA-4 and HNFb, markers for embryonic endoderm and extra-embryonic endoderm. This indicates that endodermal markers are present in undifferentiated ES cells. But stage 5 cells express additional markers that are characteristic of endocrine pancreatic islet cells: mouse insulin I and II, islet amyloid polypeptide, and the glucose transporter GLUT-2. Other cells stained positive for glucagon, a hormone produced by the alpha cells of the pancreas, and somatostatin, a peptide hormone produced by pancreatic endocrine cells in vivo. Nerve cells that surrounded the clusters of islet cells—a spontaneously forming, in vitro arrangement of cell types that mimicked their arrangement in vivo—stained positive for neuron-specific tubulin. No cells stained positive for both pancreatic islet markers and neuronal markers, indicating that the two cell types had differentiated completely from a common precursor cell.

Other tests demonstrated the functional properties of the pancreatic islet cells differentiated from mouse ES cells. Adding glucose to the culture medium triggered the release of insulin in a dose-dependent manner. Agonists and antagonists of insulin release *in vivo* stimulated or blocked insulin release *in vitro*, indicating that the pharmacological responses of the ES-derived islet cells *in vitro* mirrored *in vivo* responses. Finally, when cell clusters of the cultured pancreatic islets were grafted under the skin of diabetic mice (whose diabetes was induced by treatment with streptozocin), the grafts survived and became infiltrated with blood vessels. The ES-derived pancreatic islets released only one-fiftieth the amount of insulin they released as islet cells *in vivo*, however, the diabetic mice experienced no correction of their hyperglycemia (see Chapter 7. Stem Cells and Diabetes; and Figure 7.2. Development of Insulin Secreting Pancreatic-Like Cells from Mouse Embryonic Stem Cells).

Taken together, the three studies show that the differentiation of lines of mouse ES cells can be directed *in vitro* to yield vascular structures [40], neurons that release dopamine and serotonin [10], and endocrine pancreatic islet cells. In all three cases, proliferating, undifferentiated mouse ES cells provided the starting material and functional, differentiated cells were the result. Also, in all three experiments, the onset of mouse ES cell differentiation was triggered by withdrawing the cytokine LIF, which promotes the division of undifferentiated mouse ES cells, but — inexplicably — does *not* have the same effect on human ES cells. In addition, the ES cells in all three examples cited were induced to aggregate, a change in their three-dimensional environment that presumably allowed some of the cell-cell interactions to occur *in vitro* that would occur *in vivo* during normal embryonic development.

Collectively, these three studies provide some of the best examples of directed differentiation of mouse ES cells *in vitro*. Two of them showed that a single precursor cell can give rise to multiple, differentiated cell types[10, 40], and all of three studies demonstrated that the resulting differentiated cells function as their *in vivo* counterparts do.

These two criteria – demonstrating that a single cell can give rise to multiple cells types (clonal analysis), and that the functional properties of the differentiated cells – form the basis of an acid test for all claims of directed differentiation of either ES cells or of adult stem cells. Unfortunately, very few experiments meet these criteria, which too often makes it impossible to assess whether a differentiated cell type resulted from the experimental manipulation that was reported.

REFERENCES

1. Acampora, D. and Simeone, A. (1999). The TINS Lecture. Understanding the roles of Otx1 and Otx2 in the control of brain morphogenesis. Trends. Neurosci. 22, 116-122.

2. Andrews, P.W., Casper, J., Damjanov, I., Duggan-Keen, M., Giwercman, A., Hata, J., von Keitz, A., Looijenga, L.H., Millan, J.L., Oosterhuis, J.W., Pera, M., Sawada, M., Schmoll, H.J., Skakkebaek, N.E., van Putten, W., and Stern, P. (1996). Comparative analysis of cell surface antigens expressed by cell lines derived from human germ cell tumours. Int. J. Cancer. 66, 806-816.

3. Andrews, P.W., Damjanov, I., Simon, D., Banting, G.S., Carlin, C., Dracopoli, N.C., and Fogh, J. (1984). Pluripotent embryonal carcinoma clones derived from the human teratocarcinoma cell line Tera-2. Differentiation *in vivo* and *in vitro*. Lab. Invest. 50, 147-162.

4. Brook, F.A. and Gardner, R.L. (1997). The origin and efficient derivation of embryonic stem cells in the mouse. Proc. Natl. Acad. Sci. U. S. A. 94, 5709-5712.

5. Burdon, T., Chambers, I., Stracey, C., Niwa, H., and Smith, A. (1999). Signaling mechanisms regulating self-renewal and differentiation of pluripotent embryonic stem cells. Cells Tissues Organs. 165, 131-143.

6. Evans, M.J. and Kaufman, M.H. (1981). Establishment in culture of pluripotential cells from mouse embryos. Nature. 292, 154-156.

7. Gilbert, S.F. (2000). Developmental biology. (Sunderland, MA: Sinauer Associates).

8. Khosla, S., Dean, W., Brown, D., Reik, W., and Feil, R. (2001). Culture of preimplantation mouse embryos affects fetal development and the expression of imprinted genes. Biol. Reprod. 64, 918-926.

9. Kishimoto, T., Taga, T., and Akira, S. (1994). Cytokine signal transduction. Cell. 76, 253-262.

10. Lee, S.H., Lumelsky, N., Studer, L., Auerbach, J.M., and McKay, R.D. (2000). Efficient generation of midbrain and hindbrain neurons from mouse embryonic stem cells. Nat. Biotechnol. 18, 675-679.

11. Martin, G.R. (1981). Isolation of a pluripotent cell line from early mouse embryos cultured in medium conditioned by teratocarcinoma stem cells. Proc. Natl. Acad. Sci. U. S. A. 78, 7634-7638.

12. Matsuda, T., Nakamura, T., Nakao, K., Arai, T., Katsuki, M., Heike, T., and Yokota, T. (1999). STAT3 activation is sufficient to maintain an undifferentiated state of mouse embryonic stem cells. EMBO J. 18, 4261-4269.

13. Nichols, J., Zevnik, B., Anastassiadis, K., Niwa, H., Klewe-Nebenius, D., Chambers, I., Scholer, H., and Smith, A. (1998). Formation of pluripotent stem cells in the mammalian embryo depends on the POU transcription factor Oct4. Cell. 95, 379-391.

14. Niwa, H., Burdon, T., Chambers, I., and Smith, A. (1998). Self-renewal of pluripotent embryonic stem cells is mediated via activation of STAT3. Genes Dev. 12, 2048-2060.

15. Niwa, H., Miyazaki, J., and Smith, A.G. (2000). Quantitative expression of Oct-3/4 defines differentiation, dedifferentiation or self-renewal of ES cells. Nat. Genet. 24, 372-376.

16. O'Shea, K.S. (1999). Embryonic stem cell models of development. Anat. Rec. 257, 32-41.

17. Pera, M., personal communication.

18. Pesce, M., Gross, M.K., and Scholer, H.R. (1998). In line with our ancestors: Oct-4 and the mammalian germ. Bioessays. 20, 722-732.

19. Pesce, M., Wang, X., Wolgemuth, D.J., and Scholer, H. (1998). Differential expression of the Oct-4 transcription factor during mouse germ cell differentiation. Mech. Dev. 71, 89-98.

20. Rathjen, P.D., Toth, S., Willis, A., Heath, J.K., and Smith, A.G. (1990). Differentiation inhibiting activity is produced in matrix-associated and diffusible forms that are generated by alternate promoter usage. Cell. 62, 1105-1114.

21. Reubinoff, B.E., Pera, M.F., Fong, C.Y., Trounson, A., and Bongso, A. (2000). Embryonic stem cell lines from human blastocysts: somatic differentiation in vitro. Nat. Biotechnol. 18, 399-404.

22. Rohwedel, j., Sehlmeyer, U., Shan, J., Meister, A., and Wobus, A.M. (1996). Primordial germ cell-derived mouse embryonic germ (EG) cells in vitro resemble undifferentiated stem cells with respect to differentiation capacity and cell cycle distribution. Cell. Biol. Int. 20, 279-587.

23. Rosner, J.L. (1990). Reflections of science as a product. Nature. 345, 108.

24. Rowitch, D.H. and McMahon, A.P. (1995). Pax-2 expression in the murine neural plate precedes and encompasses the expression domains of Wnt-1 and En-1. Mech. Dev. 52, 3-8.

25. Savatier, P., Lapillonne, H., van Grunsven, L.A., Rudkin, B.B., and Samarut, J. (1996). Withdrawal of differentiation inhibitory activity/leukemia inhibitory factor up-regulates D-type cyclins and cyclin-dependent kinase inhibitors in mouse embryonic stem cells. Oncogene. 12, 309-322.

26. Schöler, H.R., Ruppert, S., Suzuki, N., Chowdhury, K., and Gruss, P. (1990). New type of POU domain in germ line-specific protein Oct-4. Nature. 344, 435-439.

27. Shamblott, M.J., Axelman, J., Wang, S., Bugg, E.M., Littlefield, J.W., Donovan, P.J., Blumenthal, P.D., Huggins, G.R., and Gearhart, J.D. (1998). Derivation of pluripotent stem cells from cultured human primordial germ cells. Proc. Natl. Acad. Sci. U. S. A. 95, 13726-13731.

28. Simeone, A. (1998). Otx1 and Otx2 in the development and evolution of the mammalian brain. EMBO J. 17, 6790-6798.

29. Smith, A.G. (2001). Embryonic stem cells. Marshak, D.R., Gardner, D.K., and Gottlieb, D. eds. (Cold Spring Harbor, New York: Cold Spring Harbor Laboratory Press). 205-230.

30. Smith, A., personal communication.

31. Smith, A.G. (2001). Origins and properties of mouse embryonic stem cells. Annu. Rev. Cell. Dev. Biol.

32. Stevens, L.C. (1970). The development of transplantable teratocarcinomas from intratesticular grafts of pre-and postimplantation mouse embryos. Dev. Biol. 21, 364-382.

33. Stoykova, A. and Gruss, P. (1994). Roles of Pax-genes in developing and adult brain as suggested by expression patterns. J. Neurosci. 14, 1395-1412.

34. Thomson, J.A., Kalishman, J., Golos, T.G., Durning, M., Harris, C.P., Becker, R.A., and Hearn, J.P. (1995). Isolation of a primate embryonic stem cell line. Proc. Natl. Acad. Sci. U. S. A. 92, 7844-7848.

35. Thomson, J.A., Itskovitz-Eldor, J., Shapiro, S.S., Waknitz, M.A., Swiergiel, J.J., Marshall, V.S., and Jones, J.M. (1998). Embryonic stem cell lines derived from human blastocysts. Science. 282, 1145-1147.

36. Thomson, J.A. and Marshall, V.S. (1998). Primate embryonic stem cells. Curr. Top. Dev. Biol. 38, 133-165.

37. Weissman, I.L. (2000). Stem cells: units of development, units of regeneration, and units in evolution. Cell. 100, 157-168.

38. Wianny, F., Real, F.X., Mummery, C.L., van Rooijen, M., Lahti, J., Samarut, J., and Savatier, P. (1998). G1-phase regulators, Cyclin D1, Cyclin D2, and Cyclin D3: up-regulation at gastrulation and dynamic expression during neurolation. Dev. Dyn. 212, 49-62.

39. Williams, R.L., Hilton, D.J., Pease, S., Willson, T.A., Stewart, C.L., Gearing, D.P., Wagner, E.F., Metcalf, D., Nicola, N.A., and Gough, N.M. (1988). Myeloid leukaemia inhibitory factor maintains the developmental potential of embryonic stem cells. Nature. 336, 684-687.

40. Yamashita, J., Itoh, H., Hirashima, M., Ogawa, M., Nishikawa, S., Yurugi, T., Naito, M., Nakao, K., and Nishikawa, S. (2000). Flk1-positive cells derived from embryonic stem cells serve as vascular progenitors. Nature. 408, 92-96.

41. Ye, W., Shimamura, K., Rubenstein, J.L., Hynes, M.A., and Rosenthal, A. (1998). FGF and Shh signals control dopaminergic and serotonergic cell fate in the anterior neural plate. Cell. 93, 755-766.

This page intentionally left blank

HUMAN EMBRYONIC STEM CELLS AND HUMAN EMBRYONIC GERM CELLS

METHODS FOR GROWING HUMAN EMBRYONIC STEM CELLS IN VITRO

To grow cultures of human ES cells, Thomson and his collaborators used 36 fresh or frozen embryos generated in IVF laboratories from couples undergoing treatment for infertility. From the 14 embryos that developed to the blastocyst stage, they established 5 human ES cell lines—H1, H7, H9, H13 and H14 [35]. Four of the 5 lines were derived from frozen embryos provided to Thomson's laboratory by Josef Itskovitz-Eldor, of the Rambam Medical Center in Haifa, Israel. The ES cell line from the fifth, fresh embryo was derived from an embryo donated in Wisconsin.

To generate human ES cell cultures, cells from the inner cell mass of a human blastocyst were cultured in a multi-step process. The pluripotent cells of the inner cell mass were separated from the surrounding trophectoderm by immunosurgery, the antibody-mediated dissolution of the trophectoderm. The inner cell masses were plated in culture dishes containing growth medium supplemented with fetal bovine serum on feeder layers of mouse embryonic fibroblasts that had been gamma-irradiated to prevent their replication. After 9 to 15 days, when inner cell masses had divided and formed clumps of cells, cells from the periphery of the clumps were chemically or mechanically dissociated and replated in the same culture conditions. Colonies of apparently homogeneous cells were selectively removed, mechanically dissociated, and replated. These were expanded and passaged, thus creating a cell line. None of the initial 5 human ES cell lines generated in this manner was derived clonally (cloned from a single cell and are, therefore, genetically identical) [35] (see Figure C.1. Techniques for Generating Embryonic Stem Cell Cultures).

The five original human ES cell lines continued to divide without differentiating for 5 to 6 months [35]. Since then, the H9 line has divided for nearly two years *in vitro*, for more than 300 population doublings and has yielded two subclones, H9.1 and H9.2 [1][1]. All the ES cell lines express high levels of telomerase [1, 36], the enzyme that helps maintain telomeres which protect the ends of chromosomes. Telomerase activity and long telomeres are characteristic of proliferating cells in embryonic tissues and of germ cells. Human somatic cells, however, do not show telomerase activity and their telomeres are considerably shorter. Unlike ES cells, differentiated somatic cells also stop dividing in culture—a phenomenon called replicative senescence (see Figure C.2. Telomeres and Telomerase).

Three of the human ES cell lines generated by Thomson were XY (male) and two were XX (female); all maintained a normal karyotype. Like monkey ES cells [34], human ES cells express a panel of surface makers that include the stage-specific embryonic antigens SSEA-3 and SSEA-4, as well as TRA-1-60, TRA-1-81, and alkaline phosphatase [14, 25, 26, 35]. Mouse ES cells do not express SSEA-3 or SSEA-4; they express SSEA-1, which human and monkey ES cells do not. Human ES cells also express the transcription factor Oct-4 [26], as mouse ES cells do.

A somewhat different technique for deriving and culturing human ES cells has now been reported by

---

[1] The H9.1 and H9.2 clonal cell lines were produced by first plating 105 of the parent H9 cells per well in tissue-culture plates. The culture medium contained KnockOut Dulbecco's modified minimal essential medium (a serum-free substitute for the 20% fetal bovine serum used in the 1998 experiments), and basic FGF, which is necessary to maintain cell proliferation and prevent differentiation. To generate clonal cell lines from individual H9 ES cells, 384 single cells were removed from these cultures and transferred individually to the wells of larger plates that contained non-dividing mouse embryonic fibroblasts (MEF) as feeder layers. The single ES cells proliferated and, every 7 days, were dissociated and replated, a process that generate two clonal cell lines, H9.1 and H9.2.

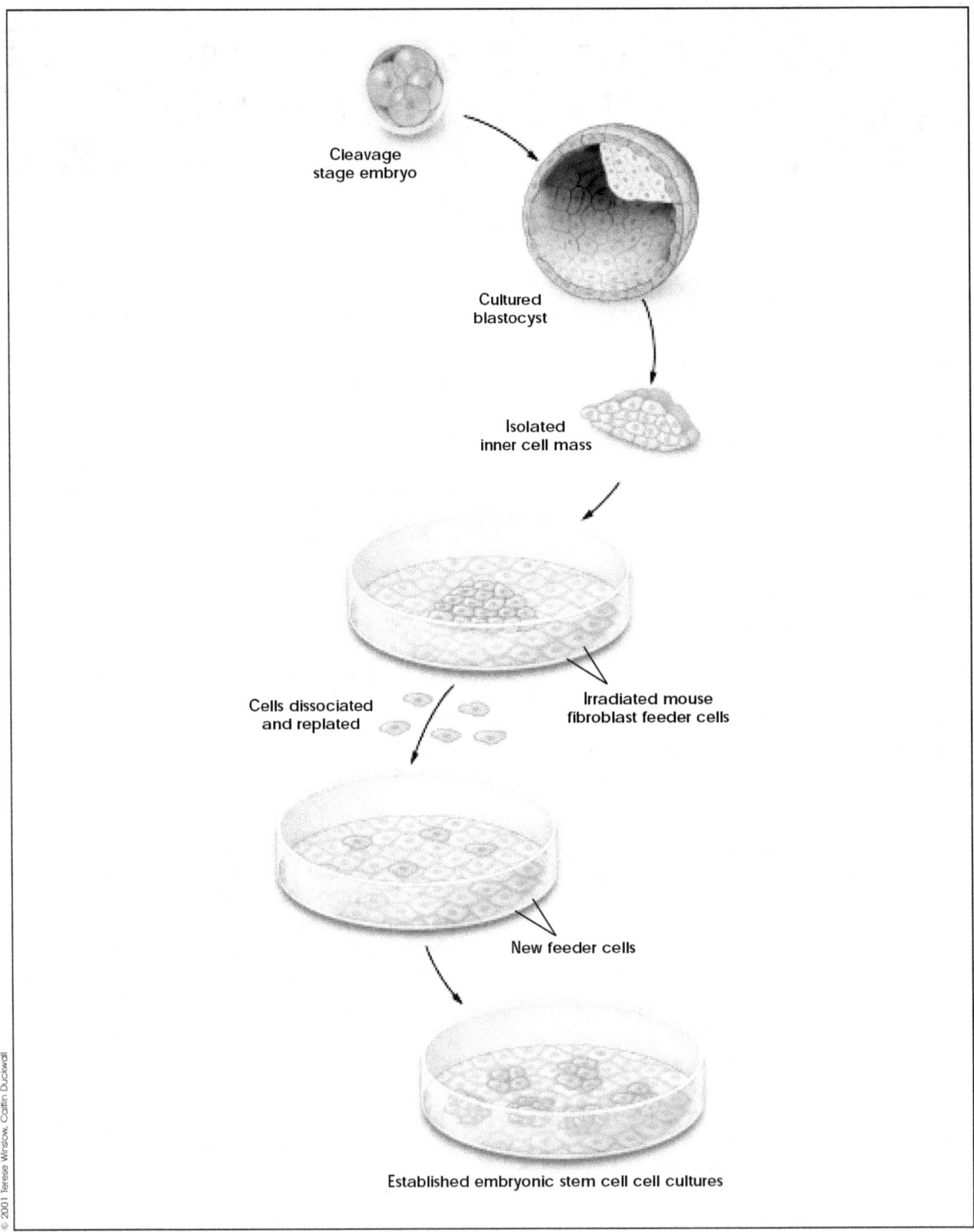

Figure C.1. Techniques for Generating Embryonic Stem Cell Cultures.

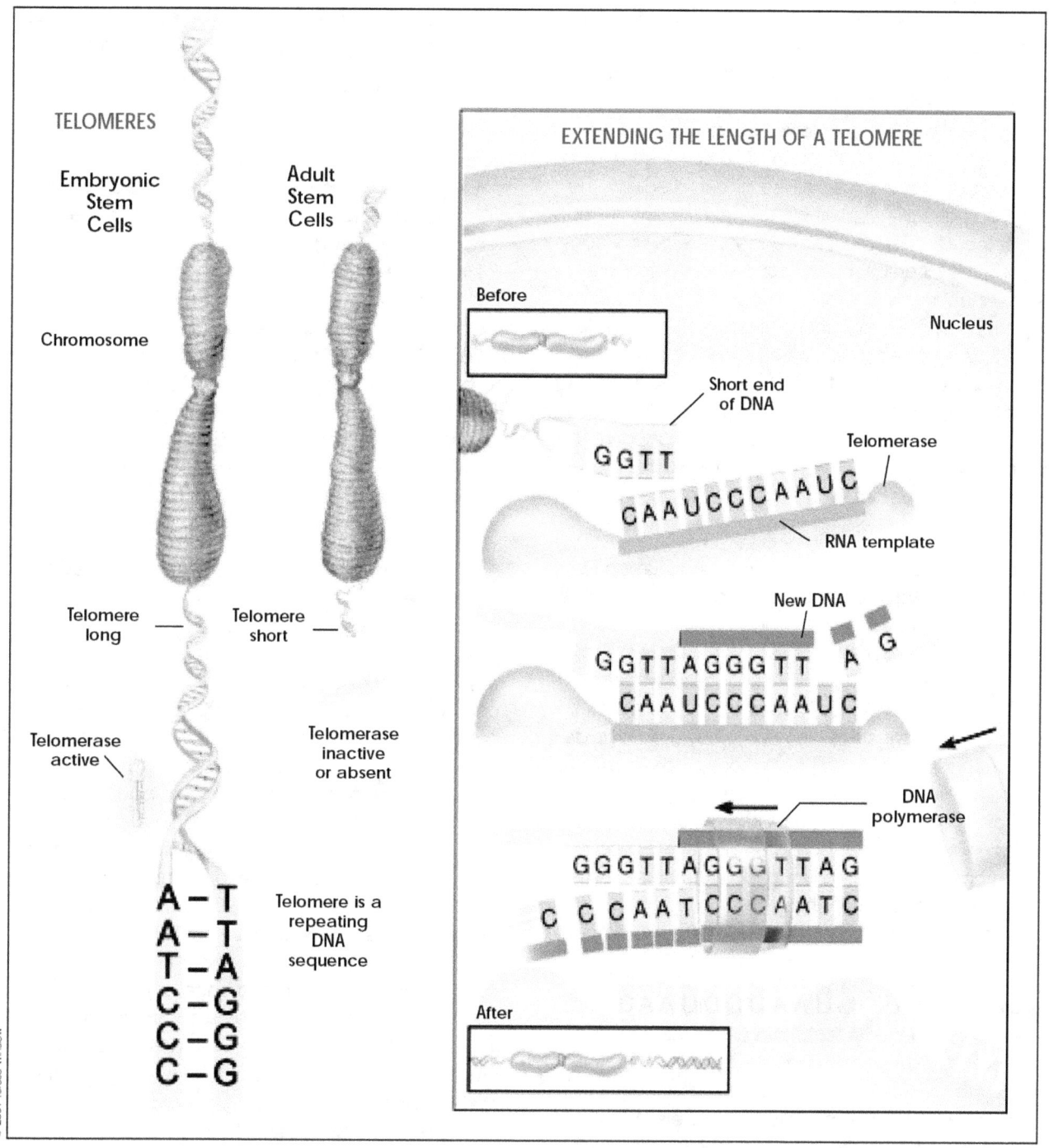

Figure C.2. Telomeres and Telomerase.
A telomere is a repeating sequence of double-stranded DNA located at the ends of chromosomes. Greater telomere length is associated with immortalized cell lines such as embryonic stem cells and cancer cells. As cells divide and differentiate throughout the lifespan of an organism or cell line, the telomeres become progressively shortened and lose the ability to maintain their length. Telomerase is an enzyme that lengthens telomeres by adding on repeating sequences of DNA. Telomerase binds to the ends of the telomere via an RNA template that is used for the attachment of a new strand of DNA. Telomerase adds several repeated DNA sequences then releases and a second enzyme, DNA Polymerase, attaches the opposite or complementary strand of DNA completing the double stranded extension of the chromosome ends. High levels of telomerase activity are detected in embryonic stem cells and cancer cells, whereas little or no telomerase activity is present in most mature, differentiated cell types. The functions of telomeres and telomerase appear to be important in cell division, normal development, and aging.

investigators in Singapore and Australia. The human blastocysts are cultured in Singapore, where mono-layer cultures of human ES cells growing on feeder layers are prepared. The primary cultures are shipped to Australia, where the colonies of growing cells are dissociated mechanically and replated. LIF and fetal bovine serum are added to the growth medium. The cells do not grow well without serum, although it is not clear that LIF has any effect. Under these *in vitro* conditions, the ES cells tend to clump and differentiate spontaneously as they are passaged. *In vivo*, after injection into the testes of immunocompromised mice, the ES cells differentiate into bone, cartilage, squa-mous and cuboidal epithelium, neural cells, glandular epithelium, and striated muscle [25, 26]. Six human ES cell lines have been generated from 12 blastocysts, a high yield by any standard. The original two cell lines were generated from fresh embryos; the other four cells lines were generated from frozen embryos [23].

Recent reports have identified additional human ES cell lines that have been developed. New derivations have been conducted from the blastocyst of frozen embryos at two centers in India (National Centre for Biological Sciences, University of Agriculture Sciences, Bangalore; Harkishondas Hospital in collaboration with Reliance Biotechnology, Bombay). They used deriva-tion techniques that differ from those of the Thomson laboratory including the use of laser ablation for the removal of the inner cell mass [22, 24, 33, 36]. An additional preparation of human ES cell lines has been conducted in San Francisco [10]. There are no publications to date on these cell lines and the extent of the research being conducted is not known.

By several criteria, all of the human ES cell lines gen-erated to date are pluripotent. When injected under the skin or into the testes of immunocompromised mice—an *in vivo* method of determining pluripotency —the human ES cells form teratomas that contain derivatives of all three primary germ layers. When allowed to differentiate *in vitro* (by culturing the cells in the absence of MEF feeder layers), the human ES cells differentiate spontaneously. Subsequent studies indicate that *in vitro* differentiation of these human ES cell lines is extensive; the cells can generate many cell types that are derived from all three primary germ layers [1, 14, 25, 26]. However, the extent to which these human ES cell lines will differentiate *in vitro* does not match their more extensive differen-tiation capability *in vivo* (in teratomas) [19].

METHODS FOR THE DERIVATION AND CULTURE OF HUMAN EMBRYONIC GERM CELLS

To derive cultures of human embryonic germ (EG)-like cells, Gearhart and his colleagues grew cells from 38 initial cultures of primordial germ cells (PGC), which were obtained from the gonadal ridge and mesen-tery of 5 to 9-week gestation fetal tissue. (PGCs give rise to the germ cells, eggs and sperm, in the adult.) The PGCs were mechanically and chemically disso-ciated, then plated on a feeder layer of non-dividing, mouse STO fibroblasts in growth medium supple-mented with fetal bovine serum [31]. Unlike the growth conditions initially reported for human ES cells [35], the medium for human PGCs cells also con-tained the cytokine, leukemia inhibitory factor (LIF), a mitogen (basic fibroblast growth factor, bFGF), and forskolin.

After one to three weeks *in vitro*, the human PGCs had formed dense, multilayered colonies of cells that resembled mouse ES or EG cells. Cells in these colonies expressed SSEA-1, SSEA-3, SSEA-4, TRA1-60, TRA-1-81, and alkaline phosphatase. A small, variable percentage (1 to 20 %) of the PGC-derived cell colonies spontaneously formed embryoid bodies. The growth medium for embryoid body cultures lacked LIF, bFGF, and forskolin. The embryoid bodies were collected from the cultures and either examined for the cell types they contained, or replated into single wells of a tissue culture plate for 14 days. The range of cell types in the human PGC-derived embryoid bodies included derivatives of all three embryonic germ layers—endoderm, mesoderm, and ecto-derm—based on the appearance of the cells and the surface markers they expressed. This result was interpreted to mean that the PGC-derived cells were pluripotent, however, it was not possible to demon-strate pluripotency *in vivo* by generating the forma-tion of teratomas in mice [31].

In their next series of experiments, Gearhart and his collaborators devised methods for growing stem cells derived from human EG cells. The process requires the generation of embryoid bodies, which form spon-taneously from EG cells that remain attached to the substrate. The embryoid bodies then float freely in the culture medium. Each embryoid body consists of an unpredictable mix of partially differentiated cell types, but allowing the embryoid bodies to form is the most consistent way of allowing EG-derived cells to differentiate [11]. The process involves several stages of cell derivation in a different kinds of growth media. Cells from low-serum cultures were passaged, chemically dissociated, and resuspended in a culture media that contains 50% fetal bovine serum, and frozen in this state. To measure proliferation, cultures are derived from the frozen embryoid bodies and grown in the same media used to grow the dissociated cells. Clonal cell lines are then derived from the embryoid body-derived cultures [32].

The embryoid body-derived cells resulting from this process have high proliferative capacity and gene expression patterns that are representative of multiple cell lineages. This suggests that the embryoid body-derived cells are progenitor or precursor cells for a variety of differentiated cell types [11].

Recently, Neil Hanley and David Wilson from the University of Southampton, United Kingdom, have derived EG cells from the primordial germ cells of the fetal gonadal ridge. Using material at 8 -10 weeks gestation, cells were derived slightly differently form the methods of Shamblott et al using a combination of irradiated fibroblast feeder layers and gelatin coated tissue culture dishes [12]. This method and the further characterization of the alkaline phosphatase/ SSEA1-positive EG cells currently remains unpublished.

DIRECTED DIFFERENTIATION OF HUMAN EMBRYONIC STEM CELLS AND EMBRYONIC GERM CELLS IN VITRO

As with cultures of mouse ES cells, human ES cells begin to differentiate if they are removed from feeder layers and grown in suspension culture on a non-adherent surface. The human ES cells form embryoid bodies which, in the early stages, may be simple or cystic and filled with fluid. Although human embryoid bodies vary in their cellular content, many include cells that look like neurons and heart muscle cells [14, 25, 26].

After the human embryoid bodies form, they can be dissociated and replated in monolayer cultures which are then exposed to specific growth factors that influence further cell differentiation. Some growth factors induce cell types that would normally be derived from ectoderm in the embryo; these include retinoic acid, epidermal growth factor (EGF), bone morphogenic protein 4 (BMP4), and basic fibroblast growth factor (bFGF). Other growth factors, such as activin-A and transforming growth factor–beta 1 (TGF-ß1) trigger the differentiation of mesodermally-derived cells. Two other factors, hepatocyte growth factor (HGF) and nerve growth factor (NGF), promote differentiation into all three germ layers, including endoderm. When these eight growth factors were added individually to cell cultures derived from embryoid bodies (generated from the H9 line from Thomson's laboratory), the cells differentiated into 11 cell types that represented all three germ layers. The identify of the differentiated human embryoid body-derived cells was determined by their morphology, growth characteristics and expression of messenger RNA (mRNA) for specific markers [30] (see Figure A.6 Gene Transcription, Translation, and Protein Synthesis).

Human embryoid body-derived cells will differentiate spontaneously into many kinds of cells, without the addition of growth factors. However, the addition of one of a number of growth factors resulted in cultures that were more likely to be populated by only one or two types of differentiated cells, as measured by mRNA transcripts expressed by the cells. Human embryoid body-derived cultures treated with bFGF differentiated largely into epidermal epithelial cells that express keratin, a protein in skin. Cells in activin-A–treated cultures formed muscle cell-like syncytium —fused, multinucleated populations of similar cells— that express the enzyme muscle-specific enolase. And cultures treated with retinoic acid differentiated into cells that resemble neurons and express neurofilament H. However, the same growth factor typically induced the expression of multiple markers; none of the resulting cell populations was homogeneous [30].

Spontaneous differentiation of human ES cells into hematopoietic cells, which form all the lineages of blood cells, is rare in vitro. However, by co-culturing human ES cells with mouse bone marrow stromal cells (irradiated to prevent their replication) in growth medium that contains fetal bovine serum, but no added growth factors, the cells differentiate to form what appear to be hematopoietic precursor cells. The partly differentiated cells express CD34, a marker for blood cell precursors. If these partly differentiated human ES cells are replated under conditions that allow them to form colonies of hematopoietic cells, they differentiate into erythroid cells, macrophages, granulocytes, and megakaryocytes [19] (see Chapter 5. Hematopoietic Stem Cells).

As indicated, human ES cells maintained *in vitro* have tendency to differentiate spontaneously, a characteristic that may not always be desirable. Thus, it may be necessary to devise methods that allow undifferentiated ES cells be selected from a culture that contains a mixture of differentiated, partially differentiated, and undifferentiated cells types. The undifferentiated ES cells could then be used for the purposes of directed differentiation, or they could be removed from cultures in which the differentiated cell types are the desired product. In either case, a suggested method for identifying undifferentiated ES cells is to introduce a marker gene—such as that encoding green fluorescence protein (GFP)—whose expression is driven by a gene that is specifically expressed in proliferating, undifferentiated cells, such as *Rex1*. Then, undifferentiated cells that express GFP can be selectively removed from human ES cultures by using a fluorescence activated cells sorter (FACS) [9] (see Appendix E.i. Markers: How Do Researchers Use Them to Identify Stem Cells?).

Joseph Itskovitz-Eldor and his colleagues are trying to direct the differentiation of human ES cells into cardiac myocytes. They use several of the human ES lines generated in James Thomson's laboratory. They report a number of cells in embryoid bodies that have contractile activity and express genetic markers consistent commonly found in cardiac myocytes [16] (see Chapter 9. Can Stem Cells Repair a Damaged Heart?). Karl Skorecki and his collaborators have had success in directing the differentiation of human ES cell lines (originating from the Thomson laboratory derivation) into pancreatic islet-like cells that secrete insulin. They have also reported the expression of insulin genes found in islet-like cells of the pancreas [6] (see Chapter 7. Stem Cells and Diabetes).

A new report indicates that it may be possible to direct the differentiation of human EG cells into neuronal cells that may play a role in restoring some function to paralyzed animals. The SDEC human cell line in this study was generated from embryoid bodies that formed in culture by the aggregation of human EG cells, and is referred to as an embryoid-derived cell line. SDEC cells express a panel of neuronal markers that include nestin, neurofilament, tau protein, neuron-specific enolase; the cells also express the glial cells markers glial fibrillary acidic protein, galactocerebroside, and CNPase. No *in vitro* assays that indicate cell function have been reported

for SDEC cell assays. However, when SDEC cells were injected into the central canal of the spinal cord of rats—whose hind limbs were paralyzed by an induced form of amytrophic lateral sclerosis (ALS, also known as Lou Gehrig's disease)—the majority of animals showed some functional recovery. It is not clear whether the human embryoid body-derived cells replaced some of the spinal motor neurons damaged by the experimental ALS, or whether the injected cells triggered neurons in the recipient animals to recover lost function [17] (see Chapter 8. Rebuilding the Nervous System with Stem Cells).

Several groups of investigators are trying to direct the differentiation of human ES cell lines, but their work is not yet published. They reported their findings in interviews with the NIH or during presentations at scientific meetings. They include, but are not limited to, the following:

- Martin Pera, Alan Trounson, and their coworkers are trying to direct the differentiation of human ES cells along a neural lineage using the BMP antagonist noggin. They generate an apparently homogenous population of cells, but have not yet characterized it [23].

- Brenda Kahan, Jon Odorico, and their coworkers are trying to direct the differentiation of the human ES lines H1 and H9 into pancreatic islet cells, which are endodermal derivatives. They induce the formation of embryoid bodies in medium lacking bFGF and assay cultures for the expression of transcripts for the endodermal markers *hnf3, Ifabp, Ifabp,* and *villin 1.* Differentiated progeny from these cells express the genes for insulin, glucagon, and somatostatin, which are normally expressed in pancreatic islet cells [15].

- Micha Drukker, Nissim Benvenisty, and their colleagues are trying to direct the differentiation of human ES cells into neurons by adding retinoic acid or ß-NGF to the growth medium. They report that about 80% of embryoid bodies exposed to these factors contain differentiated neuronal cells, as determined by morphology and the expression of receptors for dopamine or serotonin [8].

- Su-Chang Zhang, James Thomson, and their collaborators are trying to direct the differentiation of human ES cells into neural epithelial cells, by selecting cells from embryoid bodies that express nestin, glial fibrillary acidic protein (GFAP, an astrocyte marker), neural cell adhesion molecule (NCAM), and Musashi-1. The differentiated cell types express (as yet unidentified) markers of neurons and glial cells. After transplantation into the mouse brain, the cells aggregated into clusters and migrate into the brain parenchyma where they express (unidentified) neural and glial markers. By 10 weeks after transplantation, the human embryoid-derived cells had not formed teratomas [38].

- Margaret Inokuma, Melissa Carpenter, and their colleagues are trying to direct the differentiation of human ES cells into neural cells using neurotrophin 3 (NT3) and brain-derived neurotrophic factor (BNDF). Some of the resulting cells stain positive for tyrosine hydroxylase (TH, the rate-limiting enzyme in dopamine synthesis) or gamma-amino butyric acid (GABA), an inhibitory neurotransmitter [13].

- Chunhui Xu, Melissa Carpenter, and their colleagues report preliminary data on growing human ES cells in vitro in serum-free medium without feeder layers. The details of their method have not been published but apparently include Matrigel or laminin as a substrate, basic FGF, and conditioned medium from cultures of mouse embryo fibroblasts [39].

- J.S. Lebkowski and Margaret Inokuma et al. report methods for using genetic modification and changes in culture conditions to direct the differentiation of the human ES cell lines H1 and H7 in vitro. They grow undifferentiated human ES cells in serum-free medium on Matrigel or laminin, and then add 20% serum replacement medium plus DMSO to direct the first stage of differentiation. The second stage is induced by adding sodium butyrate to the medium. Cell maturation occurs in a third medium (not described). To induce differentiation into neural cells, they allow the human ES cells to form embryoid bodies, which are then expanded, and plated in B27 medium (not described), with FGF and EGF. The resulting cells express the neural progenitor markers psNCAM and A2B5.

Some differentiated cells express the glial marker GFAP. Other cells express the neuronal markers ß-tubulin III and synaptophysin, or stain for the neurotransmitters GABA, tyrosine hydroxylase, or glutamate. No quantitative data, electrophysiological data, or responses to neurotransmitter application are reported [18].

HUMAN EMBRYONIC CARCINOMA CELLS

Embryonal carcinoma (EC) cells are the "stem cells" that occur in unusual germ cell tumors, also called teratocarcinomas. As such, they give rise to the differentiated cell types that also occur in the tumors. The tumors probably arise from a malignant form of a primordial germ cell. In humans, germ cell tumors occur most often in the testis of young men; these are always malignant, but usually treatable. Benign germ tumors called ovarian cysts can occur in the ovary; malignant ovarian germ cell tumors are much rarer (malignant ovarian tumors – usually referred to as ovarian cancer – are not germ cell tumors).

Germ cell tumors have been studied extensively in humans and mice. They contain an aberrant mix of differentiated cell types, rather than a single kind of tumor cell. Small groups of the cells may appear organized, but overall, the tissue in the tumor is disorganized. Teratocarcinomas are of particular interest because they contain EC cells, which in many ways resemble normal ES cells [4].

Like human ES cells, human EC cells proliferate extensively in vitro and in teratomas formed in vivo after injection into immunocompromised mice. Because research on human ES cells is so recent, a direct comparison of cultured human EC cells and human ES cells has just begun.[2] Both cell types express a panel of surface markers, including the embryonic stage-specific antigens SSEA-3 and SSEA-4. Neither human ES cells nor human EC cells expresses SSEA-1, as mouse ES and EC cells do [5, 26, 35]. Conversely, mouse EC and ES cells do not express SSEA-3 or SSEA-4. Human EC and ES cells also carry on their surfaces keratin sulfate proteoglycans that can be labeled with specific antibodies, TRA-1-60 and TRA-1-81 [3, 7]. Also, unlike their mouse counterparts,

---

[2] As of May 9, 2001, the comparisons between human ES cells and EC cells have been made only in Peter Andrews' laboratory at the University of Sheffield, United Kingdom. James Thomson, of the University of Wisconsin at Madison, supplied Andrews with four lines of human ES cells [3, 32].

human ES and EC cells express MHC Class I antigens, which are responsible for immunogenicity (see Chapter 6. Autoimmune Diseases and the Promise of Stem Cell-Based Therapies). Like mouse ES and EC cells, undifferentiated human ES and EC cells strongly express the transcription factor Oct-4 [26, 4], which is widely regarded as a hallmark of pluripotent embryonic cells [20, 28, 29] (see Table C.1. Comparison of Mouse, Monkey, and Human Pluripotent Stem Cells).

Human ES and EC cells differ in important ways. Human ES cells are euploid, meaning they carry the normal complement of chromosomes. In contrast, human EC cells are aneuploid; their chromosomes are distinctly abnormal. (Interestingly, the chromosomes in mouse EC cells do not appear as abnormal, although they do carry subtle chromosomal abnormalities.) The ability of both cell types to differentiate into various tissue types has been explored by injecting human ES and EC cells into

Table C.1. Comparison of Mouse, Monkey, and Human Pluripotent Stem Cells

Marker Name	Mouse EC/ ES/EG cells	Monkey ES cells	Human ES cells	Human EG cells	Human EC cells
SSEA-1	+	–	–	+	–
SSEA-3	–	+	+	+	+
SEA-4	–	+	+	+	+
TRA-1-60	–	+	+	+	+
TRA-1-81	–	+	+	+	+
Alkaline phosphatase	+	+	+	+	+
Oct-4	+	+	+	Unknown	+
Telomerase activity	+ ES, EC	Unknown	+	Unknown	+
Feeder-cell dependent	ES, EG, some EC	Yes	Yes	Yes	Some; relatively low clonal efficiency
Factors which aid in stem cell self-renewal	LIF and other factors that act through gp130 receptor and can substitute for feeder layer	Co-culture with feeder cells; other promoting factors have not been identified	Feeder cells + serum; feeder layer + serum-free medium + bFGF	LIF, bFGF, forskolin	Unknown; low proliferative capacity
Growth characteristics in vitro	Form tight, rounded, multi-layer clumps; can form EBs	Form flat, loose aggregates; can form EBs	Form flat, loose aggregates; can form EBs	Form rounded, multi-layer clumps; can form EBs	Form flat, loose aggregates; can form EBs
Teratoma formation in vivo	+	+	+	–	+
Chimera formation	+	Unknown	+		+

KEY

ES cell	=	Embryonic stem cell	TRA	=	Tumor rejection antigen-1
EG cell	=	Embryonic germ cell	LIF	=	Leukemia inhibitory factor
EC cell	=	Embryonal carcinoma cell	bFGF	=	Basic fibroblast growth factor
SSEA	=	Stage-specific embryonic antigen	EB	=	Embryoid bodies

immunocompromised mice. Injected human ES cells will form embryonic stem cell teratomas in mice, and the tumors consist of cells derived from all three primary germ layers [36]. In contrast, human EC cell lines vary in their ability to differentiate *in vivo*, but in general are more limited than are ES cells. For example, NTERA2 cl.D1 cells (which are derived from human TERA2 EC cells) generate only a few kinds of tissues, including primitive gut-like structures, and neural tissue after injection into immunocompromised mice [2].

The *in vitro* growth characteristics of human ES and EC cells are also being compared. Both cell types grow well in serum-containing medium on feeder layers of mouse embryonic fibroblasts that have been treated to block their proliferation. It is difficult to induce human ES cells to proliferate in the absence of feeder layers, unless conditioned medium from feeder cells cultures is added. However, many human EC cells lines, such as the NTERA2 line, are not dependent on feeder layers [2].

If human ES cells are removed from their feeder layers, they differentiate spontaneously into many cell types. Mouse ES cells, after removal from feeder layers, can be stimulated to divide and prevented from differentiating by adding LIF (leukemia inhibitory factor); neither human ES nor EC cells show this response to LIF. Instead, if human ES cells grow to confluence (where the cells grow to completely cover the culture plates), the cells aggregate and begin to differentiate spontaneously [26, 35]. Also, human ES cells grown in suspension cultures at high density will form embryoid bodies. Embryoid bodies are clumps or groupings of cells that form when cultured in plates or media and do not occur in nature. Embryoid bodies contain undifferentiated and partially differentiated cells [14]. However, human EC cells remain undifferentiated when grown at high density [4]. Whether these apparent differences in the *in vitro* growth characteristics of human ES and EC cells are meaningful or real is subject to debate [5].

The pluripotency of human EC cells does not equal that of human ES cells. Human ES cells can differentiate into a wide range of cell types *in vitro*, and can form teratomas with many cell types after injection into immune-deficient mice. The differentiation potential of most lines of human EC cells is more limited, both *in vitro* and *in vivo*. One human EC cell line, however, TERA2, differentiates easily *in vitro*. The

well-studied morphogen, retinoic acid, induces TERA2 cells (and the subline NTERA2) to differentiate into neural precursors, which can then become mature neurons [4]. But when human ES cells are exposed to retinoic acid, they differentiate into a wider array of cell types than do human EC cells. As yet, it is not clear how the mechanism of action of retinoic acid differs in human ES cells versus human EC cells. It may be that, because of their tumor origin, human EC cells carry genetic variations linked to tumorigenesis that restrict their capacity for differentiation [5].

Thus, the *in vitro* and *in vivo* characteristics of human EC cells resembles that of human ES cells in certain respects, but not in others. Although ES cells will likely prove to be a better model for understanding human development than will EC cells [27], there may be some aspects of development that EC cells will reveal that ES cells will not [5].

REFERENCES

1. Amit, M., Carpenter, M.K., Inokuma, M.S., Chiu, C.P., Harris, C.P., Waknitz, M.A., Itskovitz-Eldor, J., and Thomson, J.A. (2000). Clonally derived human embryonic stem cell lines maintain pluripotency and proliferative potential for prolonged periods of culture. Dev. Biol. *227*, 271-278.

2. Andrews, P.W., Damjanov, I., Simon, D., Banting, G.S., Carlin, C., Dracopoli, N.C., and Fogh, J. (1984). Pluripotent embryonal carcinoma clones derived from the human teratocarcinoma cell line Tera-2. Differentiation *in vivo* and *in vitro*. Lab. Invest. *50*, 147-162.

3. Andrews, P.W., Casper, J., Damjanov, I., Duggan-Keen, M., Giwercman, A., Hata, J., von Keitz, A., Looijenga, L.H., Millan, J.L., Oosterhuis, J.W., Pera, M., Sawada, M., Schmoll, H.J., Skakkebaek, N.E., van Putten, W., and Stern, P. (1996). Comparative analysis of cell surface antigens expressed by cell lines derived from human germ cell tumours. Int. J. Cancer. 66, 806-816.

4. Andrews, P.W. (1998). Teratocarcinomas and human embryology: pluripotent human EC cell lines. Review article. APMIS. *106*, 158-167.

5. Andrews, P.W., personal communication.

6. Assady, S., Maor, G., Amit, M., Itskovitz-Eldor, J., Skorecki, K.L., and Tzukerman, M. (2001). Insulin production by human embryonic stem cells. Diabetes. *50*.

7. Badcock, G., Pigott, C., Goepel, J., and Andrews, P.W. (1999). The human embryonal carcinoma marker antigen TRA-1-60 is a sialylated keratan sulfate proteoglycan. Cancer Res. *59*, 4715-4719.

8. Drukker, M., Schuldiner, M., Eiges, R., Eden, A., Yanuka, O., Itskovitz-Eldor, J., and Benvenisty, N. Keystone symposia. Pluripotent stem cells: biology and applications. Induced neuronal differentiation of human embryonic stem cells. Poster abstracts. *207*.

9. Eiges, R., Schuldiner, M., Drukker, M., Yanuka, O., Itskovitz-Eldor, J., and Benvenisty, N. (2001). Establishment of human embryonic stem cell-transduced clones carrying a marker of undifferentiated cells. Curr. Biol. *11*, 514-518.

10. Firpo, M., personal communication.

11. Gearhart, J., personal communication.

12. Hanley, N., personal communication.

13. Inokuma, M.S., Denham, J., Mujtaba, T., Rao, M., and Carpenter, M.K. Keystone symposia. Pluripotent stem cells: biology and applications. Human embryonic stem cells differentiate into neural cells *in vitro*. Poster abstracts. 312.

14. Itskovitz-Eldor, J., Schuldiner, M., Karsenti, D., Eden, A., Yanuka, O., Amit, M., Soreq, H., and Benvenisty, N. (2000). Differentiation of human embryonic stem cells into embryoid bodies comprising the three embryonic germ layers. Mol. Med. *6*, 88-95.

15. Kahan, B.W., Jacobson, L.M., Hullett, D.A., Thomson, J., and Odorico, J.S. Keystone symposia. Pluripotent stem cells: biology and applications. *In vitro* differentiation of human embryonic stem (ES) cell lines: expression of endoderm- and pancreatic islet-specific genes. Poster abstract. 117.

16. Kehat, I., Kenyagin-Karsenti, D., Druckmann, M., Segev, H., Amit, M., Gepstein, A., Livne, E., Binah, O., Itskovitz-Eldor, J., and Gepstein, L. (2001). Human embryonic stem cells can differentiate into myocytes portraying cardiomyocytic structural and functional properties. J. Clin. Invest. (In press)

17. Kerr, D.A., Llado, J., Shamblott, M., Maragakis, N., Irani, D.N., Dike, S., Sappington, A., Gearhart, J., and Rothstein, J. (2001). Human embryonic germ cell derivatives facilitate motor recovery of rats with diffuse motor neuron injury.

18. Lebkowski, J.S., Gold, J., Chiu, C.P., Xu, C., Inokuma, M., Hassanipour, M., Denham, J., Piderit, A., Rosler, E., Golds, K., and Carpenter, M. ASGT Meeting. Targeted Gene Expression I. Human Embryonic Stem Cells: Genetic Modification and Differentiation into Cell Types for Potential Transplantation Applications. Poster Abstract. 205.

19. Odorico, J.S., Kaufman, D.S., and Thomson, J.A. (2001). Multilineage Differentiation from Human Embryonic Stem Cell Lines. Stem Cells. *19*, 193-204.

20. Okamoto, K., Okazawa, H., Okuda, A., Sakai, M., Muramatsu, M., and Hamada, H. (1990). A novel octamer binding transcription factor is differentially expressed in mouse embryonic cells. Cell. *60*, 461-472.

21. Panicker, M., personal communication.

22. Pera, M., personal communication.

23. Rao, M., personal communication.

24. Reubinoff BE, Pera, M., Fong, C.Y., and Trounson, A. (2000). Research Errata. Nat. Biotechnol. *18*, 559.

25. Reubinoff, B.E., Pera, M.F., Fong, C.Y., Trounson, A., and Bongso, A. (2000). Embryonic stem cell lines from human blastocysts: somatic differentiation in vitro. Nat. Biotechnol. *18*, 399-404.

26. Roach, S., Cooper, S., Bennett, W., and Pera, M.F. (1993). Cultured cell lines from human teratomas: windows into tumour growth and differentiation and early human development. Eur. Urol. *23*, 82-87.

27. Rosner, J.L. (1990). Reflections of science as a product. Nature. *345*, 108.

28. Schöler, H.R., Ruppert, S., Suzuki, N., Chowdhury, K., and Gruss, P. (1990). New type of POU domain in germ line-specific protein Oct-4. Nature. *344*, 435-439.

29. Schuldiner, M., Yanuka, O., Itskovitz-Eldor, J., Melton, D., and Benvenisty, N. (2000). Effects of eight growth factors on the differentiation of cells derived from human embryonic stem cells. Proc. Natl. Acad. Sci. U.S.A. *97*, 11307-11312.

30. Shamblott, M.J., Axelman, J., Wang, S., Bugg, E.M., Littlefield, J.W., Donovan, P.J., Blumenthal, P.D., Huggins, G.R., and Gearhart, J.D. (1998). Derivation of pluripotent stem cells from cultured human primordial germ cells. Proc. Natl. Acad. Sci. U.S.A. *95*, 13726-13731.

31. Shamblott, M.J., Axelman, J., Littlefield, J.W., Blumenthal, P.D., Huggins, G.R., Cui, Y., Cheng, L., and Gearhart, J.D. (2001). Human embryonic germ cell derivatives express a broad range of developmentally distinct markers and proliferate extensively *in vitro*. Proc. Natl. Acad. Sci. U.S.A. *98*, 113-118.

32. Thomson, J., personal communication.

33. Thomson, J.A., Kalishman, J., Golos, T.G., Durning, M., Harris, C.P., Becker, R.A., and Hearn, J.P. (1995). Isolation of a primate embryonic stem cell line. Proc. Natl. Acad. Sci. U.S.A. *92*, 7844-7848.

34. Thomson, J.A., Itskovitz-Eldor, J., Shapiro, S.S., Waknitz, M.A., Swiergiel, J.J., Marshall, V.S., and Jones, J.M. (1998). Embryonic stem cell lines derived from human blastocysts. Science. *282*, 1145-1147.

35. Thomson, J.A. and Odorico, J.S. (2000). Human embryonic stem cell and embryonic germ cell lines. Trends. Biotechnol. *18*, 53-57.

36. Totey, S., personal communication.

37. Xu, C., Inokuma, M.S., Denham, J., Golds, K., Kundu, P., Gold, J.D., and Carpenter, M.K. Keystone symposia. Pluripotent stem cells: biology and applications. Growth of undifferentiated human embryonic stem cells on defined matrices with conditioned medium. Poster abstract. 133.

38. Zhang, S.U., Wernig, M., Duncan, I.D., Brüstle, O., and Thomson, J. Keystone symposia. Pluripotent stem cells: biology and applications. Directed differentiation of human ES cells to neural epithelia. Poster abstracts. 235.

APPENDIX D:

STEM CELL TABLES

COMPENDIUM OF SCIENTIFIC PUBLICATIONS REGARDING THE ISOLATION AND CHARACTERIZATION OF STEM CELLS

The following tables provide an overview of information about stem cells that have been derived from mice and humans. The tables summarize published research that characterizes cells that are capable of developing into cells of multiple germ layers (i.e., multipotent or pluripotent) or that can generate the differentiated cell types of another tissue (i.e., plasticity) such as a bone marrow cell becoming a neuronal cell. The tables do not include information about cells

considered progenitor ore precursor cells or those that can proliferate without the demonstrated ability to generate cell types of other tissues.

The tables list the tissue from which the cells were derived, the types of cells that developed, the conditions under which differentiation occurred, the methods by which the cells were characterized, and the primary references for the information.

Appendix D.i.
Published Reports on Isolation and Differentiation of Mouse Stem Cells

Origin Tissue	Cell Type	Cell Types Developed	Differentiation Conditions	Methods of Characterization	Reference
Bone marrow	Hematopoietic stem cell (HSC)	Cardiac muscle	Cardiac injury induced in mice Injected labeled HSCs into injured heart	Measurement of green fluorescent protein (GFP) in regenerating cardiac cells Measurement of cardiac-specific protein and gene expression Cardiac-function tests	Orlic et al., 2001
	HSC	Epithelial cells of the liver, skin, lung, esophagus, stomach, small and large intestine	Transplantation of HSCs into lethally irradiated female mice	Detection of antibodies to cellular and cell-surface proteins Cell staining Probing for Y chromosome-positive cells	Krause et al., 2001
	HSC	Cholangiocyte Hepatocyte	Purification of HSCs from bone marrow Transplantation of HSCs into mice with liver-enzyme deficiency	Observation of normalized liver function and regenerating hepatocytes Measurement of expression of hematopoietic and hepatic cell-surface proteins	Lagasse et al., 2000
	HSC	Platelet Red blood cell White blood cell	Hematopoietic growth factors: interleukin-3, interleukin-6, granulocyte-colony stimulating factor, erythropoietin, and thrombopoietin	Detection of antibodies to cell-surface proteins Colony-forming assays Immunophenotyping	Spangrude et al., 1991 Morrison et al., 1995
	HSC Side population (SP)	Skeletal muscle	Lethal irradiation of female mice Induced muscle injury Purified bone marrow transplanted into mice	Measurement of dystrophin expression in regenerating muscle cells Fluorescence-activated cell sorting (FACS) Probing for Y chromosome-positive cells	Gussoni et al., 1999
	Mesenchymal stem cell (MSC)	Adipocyte Chondrocyte Osteoblast Tenocyte	Dexamethasone Vitamin D_3 Bone morphogenetic protein-2 (BMP-2)	Detection of antibody binding to cell-surface proteins Immunofluorescence	Friedenstein et al., 1976 Pereira et al., 1995 Prockop, 1997

Appendix D.i. (cont.)

Origin		Cell Types Developed	Differentiation Conditions	Methods of Characterization	Reference
Tissue	Cell Type				
Bone marrow (cont.)	MSC	Astrocyte Neuron	Injection of MSC into brain of immunocompromised neonatal mice	Detection of cell-surface markers by using antibodies and immunofluorescence	Kopen et al., 1999
	MSC	Astrocyte Neuron	Epidermal growth factor Brain-derived neurotrophic factor β-mercaptoethanol Retinoic acid	Immunofluorescence Cell sorting	Sanchez-Ramos et al., 2000
	MSC	Neuron	Stromal cells expanded as undifferentiated cells β-mercaptoethanol Butylated hydroxyanisole	Detection of numerous neuron-specific proteins via staining	Woodbury et al., 2000
	MSC	Skeletal muscle	5-azacytidine and amphotericin B	Observation of myotubes Staining for myocytes	Wakitani et al., 1995
	MSC and/or HSC	Astrocyte Microglia Oligodendrocyte	Induced injury to neural tissue Bone marrow transplantation	Detection of antibodies to cell-surface proteins	Eglitis and Mezey, 1997
	MSC and/or HSC	Cardiac muscle	Bone marrow transplantation of 5-azacytidine-treated cells into mice with induced cardiac muscle injury	Cell staining for cardiac muscle proteins Measurement of blood pressure Electron microscopy Observation of beating cells *in vitro* Measurement of atrial natriuretic peptide Staining cells for muscle proteins	Tomita et al., 1999 Makino et al., 1999
	MSC and/or HSC	Hepatocyte	Suppression of liver cell proliferation Induced injury to liver Bone marrow transplantation	Staining cells Antibody labeling of cell-surface markers	Taniguchi et al., 1996 Petersen et al., 1999 Theise et al., 2000

Appendix D.i. (cont.)

Origin Tissue	Cell Type	Cell Types Developed	Differentiation Conditions	Methods of Characterization	Reference
Bone marrow *(cont.)*	MSC and/or HSC	Neuron	Induced neural tissue injury Bone marrow transplantation into female mice	Detection of antibodies to cell-surface proteins Probing for Y chromosome-containing neurons	Mezey et al., 2000 Brazelton et al., 2000
	MSC, HSC, or side population (SP)	Cardiac muscle Skeletal muscle	Lethal irradiation of mice Bone marrow transplantation from normal male donor mice into mice with induced muscle degeneration	Probing for Y chromosome-containing muscle cells Detection of expression of myoregulatory proteins	Bittner et al., 1999
	MSC, HSC, or SP	Skeletal muscle	Induced muscle tissue injury Transplantation of genetically marked bone marrow into immunodeficient mice	Histologic observation of muscle regeneration Detection of antibodies to cell-surface proteins Myogenic differentiation factor transcript expression	Ferrari et al., 1998
	SP	Cardiomyocyte Vascular endothelia	Transplanted into lethally irradiated mice with ischemic damage to cardiac tissue	Immunohistochemistry Staining for cardiomyocte marker (alpha-actin) and endothelial marker (flt-1)	Jackson et al., 2001
Brain	Neural stem cell (NSC)	Astrocyte Neuron Oligodendrocyte	Basic fibroblast growth factor Epidermal growth factor	Detection of antibodies to neural cell-specific proteins	Reynolds et al., 1996 Doetsch et al., 1999 Johansson et al., 1999
	NSC	Red blood cell White blood cell	Transplantation of NSC into irradiated mice	Flow cytometry analysis Genetic labeling assay Detection of antibodies to cell surface proteins	Bjornson et al., 1999

Appendix D.i. *(cont.)*

Origin		Cell Types Developed	Differentiation Conditions	Methods of Characterization	Reference
Tissue	Cell Type				
Brain *(cont.)*	NSC	Skeletal muscle	Transplantation of NSCs into mice *In vitro* co-culture with myogenic cells	Observation of differentiated skeletal muscle cells Analysis of muscle cell-specific proteins and gene expression	Galli et al., 2000
Embryo-blastocyst inner-cell mass	Embryonic stem (ES)	Adipocyte	Retinoic acid Insulin, T3 (thyroid hormone), and Leukemia inhibitory factor (LIF)	Observation of adipocyte differentiation Measurement of adipocyte enzyme activity Measurement of adipocyte-specific gene expression	Dani et al., 1997
	ES	Astrocyte Glial precursor Oligodendrocyte	Cells cultured in neurogenic medium with basic fibroblast growth factor Epidermal growth factor Platelet-derived growth factor Transplanted glial precursor cells into myelin-deficient mice	Observation of spinal cord remyelination Electron microscopy Antibodies to neural cell-specific proteins	Brustle et al., 1999
	ES	Astrocyte Midbrain neuron Neural precursor Neuron Oligodendrocyte	Retinoic acid Cell selection through transgene conferring drug resistance Co-culture with stromal cells	Examination of cell morphology and neuron-specific markers Cell-specific markers Detection of dopamine production	Bain et al., 1995 Strubing et al., 1995 Li et al., 1998 Lee et al., 2000 Kawasaki et al., 2000
	ES	Astrocyte Neuron Oligodendro-cyte	Retinoic acid	Observation of functional synapses Measurement of neurotransmitters	Slager, et al., 1993 Gottlieb, et al., 1999
	ES	Astrocyte Oligodendrocyte	Retinoic acid Fetal calf serum (10%) ß-mercaptoethanol	Antibodies to neural cell-specific proteins Cytochemistry	Fraichard et al., 1995

Appendix D.i. *(cont.)*

Origin		Cell Types Developed	Differentiation Conditions	Methods of Characterization	Reference
Tissue	Cell Type				
Embryo-blastocyst inner-cell mass *(cont.)*	ES	Cardiac muscle Skeletal muscle Smooth muscle	Retinoic acid Dimethyl sulfoxide Transplantation of muscle cells into mice	Histology Detection of cell-specific proteins Cytochemistry	Dinsmore et al., 1996
	ES	Cardiomyocyte	LIF, retinoic acid Fibroblast feeder cells	Histology and observation of beating cardiomyocyte Detection of specific cardiac cell-gene expression and cardiomyocyte surface proteins	Doetschman et al., 1985 Maltsev et al., 1993 Wobus et al., 1995
	ES	Cardiomyocyte	LIF Cell selection through genetic labeling of ES Injection of ES into mouse heart	Detection of genetically labeled cardiomyocytes Electrophysiological studies	Bader et al., 2000
	ES	Cardiomyocyte	LIF Purification of cardiomyocytes from ES culture by genetic labeling and selection	Observation of functional cardiomyocyte grafts in heart Immunohistology	Klug et al., 1996
	ES	Cardiomyocyte	Culture of ES with LIF Selection of cardiomyocytes through genetic labeling Injection of cardiomyocytes into mouse heart	Microscopy and cell-receptor studies Observation of cardiomyocyte differentiation and contractility Analysis of cardiomyocyte gene expression	Westfall et al., 1997
	ES	Chondrocyte (cartilage-forming cell)	BMP-2 and BMP-4	Staining of mature chondrocytes Measurement of chondrocyte-specific gene expression and proteins	Kramer et al., 2000

Appendix D.i. *(cont.)*

Origin		Cell Types	Differentiation	Methods of	
Tissue	Cell Type	Developed	Conditions	Characterization	Reference
Embryo-blastocyst inner-cell mass *(cont.)*	ES	Dendritic (immune cell)	Culture on stromal cell layer Interleukin-3 Granulocyte-macrophage stimulating factor	Immune-function assays Immunophenotyping	Fairchild et al., 2000
	ES	Embryoid bodies (EBs) consisting of structures that contain tissues of the three embryonic germ layers: endoderm, mesoderm, and ectoderm Teratocarcinoma	ES cultured in suspension without feeder cell layer Absence of LIF Injection of ESs into mice	Observation of differentiation into multiple tissue types of the germ layers of blood, skeletal and cardiac muscle, primitive gastro-intestinal and neural tissue Growth of tumor containing tissues from embryonic germ layer	Evans and Kaufman, 1981
	ES	ES self-renewal	LIF Culture on feeder cell layer	Observation of extensive ES proliferation and self-renewal	Evans and Kaufman, 1981
	ES	Endothelial	Culture on collagen substrate Hematopoietic growth factors Semisolid media EB implanted peritoneal cavity	Observation of capillary formation	Risau et al., 1988
	ES	Endothelial Smooth muscle Vascular progenitor	Culture over collagen-IV matrix Absence of LIF Vascular endothelial growth factor	Electron microscopy: observation of endothelial and smooth muscle vascular structures Detection of endothelial cell marker by immunochemistry Detection of smooth muscle markers by immunochemistry	Yamashita et al., 2000

Appendix D.i. (cont.)

Origin		Cell Types Developed	Differentiation Conditions	Methods of Characterization	Reference
Tissue	Cell Type				
Embryo-blastocyst inner-cell mass (cont.)	ES	HSC and erythroid	Interleukin-6 Absence of LIF and cell feeder layer Culture on collagen substrate Hematopoietic growth factors Semisolid media BMP-4	Antibodies against surface markers FACS Immunophenotyping	Wiles and Keller, 1991 Johansson and Wiles, 1995 Perkins et al., 1998
	ES	Keratinocyte (skin)	ß-mercaptoethanol Implantation of ES cells in mice	Microscopy Immunofluorescence Observation of skin tissue differentiation Measurement of keratin	Bagutti et al., 1996
	ES	Lymphoid precursor Lymphocyte	Culture of ES in low oxygen concentration (5%) without hematopoietic growth factors	Antibodies to lymphoid cell-surface proteins Analysis of antibody production and lymphocyte receptors	Potocnik et al., 1994
	ES	Macrophage	Interleukin-3 and macrophage colony stimulating factor	Immunophenotyping Immune-function assays	Lieschke and Dunn, 1995
	ES	Mast	Lethal mutations in ES cells Culture of EBs in media containing interleukin-3, stem cell factor	Transplantation of cells into mast cell-deficient mice Immunologic- and inflammation-function tests Analysis of gene expression	Johansson and Wiles, 1995 Tsai et al., 2000
	ES	Melanocyte	Dexamethasone Stromal cell layer Steel factor	Morphology studies Reactivity to growth factors Expression of melanogenic markers	Yamane et al., 1999

Appendix D.i. (cont.)

Origin		Cell Types Developed	Differentiation Conditions	Methods of Characterization	Reference
Tissue	Cell Type				
Embryo-blastocyst inner-cell mass (cont.)	ES	Neuron	Expression of noggin cDNA in ES Expression of neuronal determination gene EB exposed to retinoic acid	Detection of antibodies to neuronal proteins	O'Shea, 1999
	ES	Oligodendrocyte	Retinoic acid Induced spinal cord injury Transplantation of ES-derived cells into spinal cord of mice	Detection of remyelination in spinal cord Antibodies to oligodendrocyte-specific proteins	Liu et al., 2000
	ES	Osteoblast (bone cell)	Co-cultured with fetal mouse osteoblasts Dexamethasone, retinoic acid, ascorbic acid, β-glycerophosphate	Microscopy; observation of mineralized bone nodules Histochemistry	Buttery et al., 2001
	ES	Pancreatic	Insertion of insulin-gene promoter into ES	Antibodies to cellular proteins Measurement of insulin, glucagon, somatostatin Observation of islet-like organization of cells Transplantation of cells into diabetic mice with resultant lowering of blood glucose	Soria et al., 2000
	ES	Pancreatic islet-like	Serum-free media Absence of feeder-cell layer Basic fibroblast growth factor Nicotinamide	Detection of antibodies to cellular and cell-surface proteins	Lumelsky et al., 2001
	ES	Skeletal muscle	Overexpression of insulin-like growth factor-2 in ES through gene insertion Dimethyl sulfoxide	Observation of myocyte differentiation Measurement of myocyte-specific gene expression and proteins	Prelle et al., 2000

Appendix D.i. *(cont.)*

Origin		Cell Types Developed	Differentiation Conditions	Methods of Characterization	Reference
Tissue	Cell Type				
Embryo-blastocyst inner-cell mass *(cont.)*	ES	Skeletal muscle	Transforming growth factor-beta and retinoic acid ES co-culture with stromal cells Fetal calf serum ß-mercaptoethanol	Observation of myocyte differentiation Detection of functional muscle cell receptors Measurement of myocyte-specific gene expression	Slager et al., 1993 Rohwedel et al., 1994
	ES	Smooth muscle	Retinoic acid and db-cAMP Culture over collagen IV matrix Vascular endothelial growth factor Platelet-derived growth factor-BB	Electron microscopy observation of vascular structures Detection of smooth muscle markers: SMA, CGA7	Drab et al., 1997 Yamashita et al., 2000
	ES	Smooth muscle	Platelet-derived growth factor	FACS Detection of smooth muscle cell proteins	Hirashima et al., 1999
	ES	White blood cell	Interleukin-3 Transplantation of ESs into lymphocyte-deficient mice	Measurement of lymphocyte-specific gene expression Radioimmunoassay	Wiles and Keller, 1991
	ES	White blood cell	Transplantation of ES cells into lymphocyte-deficient mice	Histology Immunophenotyping Antibodies to cell-specific proteins	Rathjen et al., 1998
Gonadal ridge (fetal)	Embryonic primordial germ cell	Endoderm Mesoderm Ectoderm	"Reprogramming" primordial germ cells: culture of primordial germ cell with LIF, basic fibroblast growth factor and Steel factor	Histology Immunocytochemistry	Matsui et al., 1992

Appendix D.i. (cont.)

| Origin | | | | | |
Tissue	Cell Type	Cell Types Developed	Differentiation Conditions	Methods of Characterization	Reference
Liver	HSC	HSC All blood cell lineages	Enrichment of cell populations through immunoselection Purification of CD45+ liver cells Selection of cells with HSC markers Transplantation of HSCs into lethally irradiated mice	Colony-forming assays Detection of *in vitro* growth of hematopoietic colonies by flow cytometry and cell sorting Liver-derived cells reconstituted from bone marrow of transplanted mice FACS	Taniguchi et al., 199
Pancreas	Pancreatic ductal epithelial cell	Alpha, beta, and delta pancreatic islet	Stem cells isolated from prediabetic adult, nonobese mice Cells cultured for an extensive period Pancreatic cells transplanted into diabetic mice	Analysis of pancreatic cell gene expression and differentiation markers Glucose challenge test *in vitro* Observation of reversal of insulin-dependent diabetes in mice with transplants	Ramiya et al., 2000
	Unselected pancreatic cells	Hepatocyte	Pancreatic cells transplanted into mice with liver-enzyme deficiency	Detection of normalized liver function in mice Histological evidence of donor-derived hepatocytes	Wang et al., 2001
Skeletal muscle	Muscle	Adipocyte	Long-chain fatty acids Thiazolidinediones	Assays of adipocyte enzyme function Observation of adipocyte differentiation Detection of adipocyte-specific gene expression	Grimaldi et al., 1997
	Muscle	Osteoclast and osteocyte Osteoprogenitor	Exposure of donor cells to BMP-2 Retroviral transfection of cells with vector and transplantation into severe combined immunodeficient mice (SCID)	Detection of ectopic bone formation Detection of muscle-derived cells Co-localization with osteocalcin-producing cells in newly formed bone matrix	Bosch et al., 2000

Appendix D.i. *(cont.)*

Origin		Cell Types Developed	Differentiation Conditions	Methods of Characterization	Reference
Tissue	Cell Type				
Skeletal muscle *(cont.)*	Muscle Satellite	HSC Myocyte precursor	Isolation of transcription factor Pax7 as a gene expressed specifically in satellite cell-derived myoblasts	Detection of Pax7-/- and Pax7+ muscle cells in hematopoietic and myogenic cells	Seale et al., 2000
	Muscle Satellite or SP	All blood cell lineages HSC	Transplant of muscle-derived cells into lethally irradiated mice	Observation of engraftment of muscle cells in bone marrow Antibodies to hematopoietic cell markers FACS	Jackson et al., 1999 Gussoni et al., 1999
	Satellite	Myocyte Myocyte precursor	Induced tissue injury; mechanical and denervation stress Transcription factor expression	Detection of myocyte progenitor and myocyte-specific proteins and mRNA transcripts	Megeney et al., 199
Spinal cord	NSC	Astrocyte Neuron Oligodendrocyte	Basic fibroblast growth factor Epidermal growth factor	Detection of antibodies to neural cell proteins	Weiss et al., 1996

Appendix D.ii.
Published Reports on Isolation and Differentiation of Human Fetal Tissue Germ Cells

Origin Tissue	Cell Type	Cell Types Developed	Differentiation Conditions	Methods of Characterization	Reference
Gonadal ridge	Primordial germ cell	Embryoid bodies	SDEC line of embryoid body derived cells transplanted into rats paralyzed with a virus induced motor neuron degeneration	Functional assessment of rat locomotion and righting ability (turning from supine to prone) Histopathologic examination of motor axons Immunohistochemistry of mature neurons: NeuN+ and 68-kilodalton neurofilament	Kerr et al., 2001
	Primordial germ cell	Embryoid bodies with neural cells, vascular endothelium, muscle cells, endodermal derivatives	Leukemia inhibitory factor, Basic fibroblast growth factor	Clonal expression, polymerase chain reaction Ethidium bromide fluorescence detection Surface markers: 68-kilodalton neurofilament, neuron-specific enolase, tau, vimentin, human nestin, galactocerebroside, O4, SMI32	Shamblott et al., 2001
	Primordial germ cell	Embryoid bodies with three germ layers: endoderm, mesoderm, ectoderm	Leukemia inhibitory factor, Basic fibroblast growth factor	Detection of surface markers: SSEA-1, SSEA-3, SSEA-4, TRA-1-60, TRA-1-81	Shamblott et al., 1998

Appendix D.iii.
Published Reports on Isolation and Differentiation of Human Embryonic Stem Cells

Origin Tissue	Cell Type	Cell Types Developed	Differentiation Conditions	Methods of Characterization	Reference
Human embryo (from *in vitro* fertilization (IVF))	Blastocyst inner-cell mass	Ectoderm Endoderm Mesoderm Neuronal progenitor cell	Leukemia inhibitory factor Injection into severe combined immunodeficient (SCID) mice	Developed two lines (HES-1, HES-2) Clonal expression Polymerase chain reaction Surface markers: SSEA-1, SSEA-4, TRA-1-60, GTCM-2	Reubinoff et al., 2000
	Blastocyst inner-cell mass (H9 clone line from Thomson et al., 1998)	Cardiomyocyte	Embryoid body formation (See Itskovitz-Eldor et al., 2000)	Visualization of contracting areas in embryoid bodies Immunohistochemistry for cardiac myosin heavy chain, alpha-actinin, desmin, cardiac troponin I, and antinaturetic protein.	Assady et al., 2001
	Blastocyst inner-cell mass (H9 clone line from Thomson et al., 1998)	Cardiomyocyte	Embryoid body formation	Polymerase chain reaction for cardiac-specific genes and transcription factors	Kehat et al., 2001
	Blastocyst inner-cell mass (H9 clone line from Thomson et al., 1998)	Cardiomyocyte Endoderm Hematopoietic Neuron	Leukemia inhibitory factor Basic fibroblast growth factor Collagenase or trypsin/EDTA to induce embryoid body	Clonal expression Polymerase chain reaction Surface markers: gamma-globin, 68-kilodalton neurofilament, alpha-fetoprotein, albumin	Itskovitz-Eldor et al., 2000
	Blastocyst inner-cell mass (H9 clone line from Thomson et al., 1998)	Ectoderm: brain, skin, adrenal Endoderm: liver, pancreas Mesoderm: muscle, bone, kidney, urogenital, heart, hematopoietic, hematopoietic	Basic fibroblast growth factor, transforming growth factor beta 1, activin-A, bone morphogenic protein 4 hepatocyte growth factor, epidermal growth factor, beta nerve growth factor, retinoic acid	Clonal expression Polymerase chain reaction Surface markers	Schuldiner et al., 2000

Appendix D.iii. *(cont.)*

Origin		Cell Types Developed	Differentiation Conditions	Methods of Characterization	Reference
Tissue	**Cell Type**				
Human embryo (from *in vitro* fertilization (IVF) *(cont.)*	Blastocyst inner-cell mass (H9 clone line from Thomson et al., 1998)	Ectoderm: neural epithelium, embryonic ganglia, stratified squamous epithelium Endoderm: gut epithelium Mesoderm: cartilage, bone, smooth muscle, striated muscle	Injection of cell lines into severe combined immunodeficient mice Leukemia inhibitory factor Type IV collagenase	Surface markers: SSEA-3, SSEA-4, TRA-160, TRA-181, alkaline phosphatase Radioimmunoassay detection: alpha-fetoprotein and human chorionic gonadotropin	Thomson et al., 1998
	Blastocyst inner-cell mass (H9 clone line from Thomson et al., 1998)	Pancreatic beta cell	Embryoid body formation (See Itskovitz-Eldor et al., 2000) No leukemia inhibitory factor or basic fibroblast growth factor	Immunohistochemistry for insulin Polymerase chain reaction for insulin, IPF1/PDX1, Ngn3, beta-actin, Glut-1, Glut-2, glucokinase, and Oct 4	Assady et al., 2001

Appendix D.iv.
Published Reports on Isolation and Differentiation of Human Embryonic Carcinoma Stem Cells

Origin		Cell Types Developed	Differentiation Conditions	Methods of Characterization	Reference
Tissue	Cell Type				
Terato-carci-noma	Embryonic carcinoma (EC)	Endodermal progenitor cell	Absence of feeder cell layer Bone morphogenetic protein-2 Retinoic acid	Analysis of stem cell marker-gene transcription Immunochemistry Immunofluorescence	Roach et al., 1994 Pera and Herszfeld, 1998
	EC	Neuron	EC transplanted into mouse brain	Observation of functional synapses Immunochemistry	Trojanowski et al., 1993
	EC	Glial Neuron	Retinoic acid	Measurement of mRNA for GABA(A) receptor-chloride complex Recording of whole-cell voltage-clamp measurements in differentiated cells in the presence of GABA(A) receptor antagonists and activators (bicuculline and flurazepam, respectively)	Reynolds et al., 1994
	EC	Glial Neuron	Retinoic acid	Detection of neurons with HNK-1 antibody Measurement of acetylcholine synthesis and detection of high-affinity uptake sites for GABA	McBurney et al., 1988
	EC	Neuron	Retinoic acid	Morphology and histology Analysis of neuron-specific proteins	Andrews, 1984

Appendix D.iv. (cont.)

Origin		Cell Types Developed	Differentiation Conditions	Methods of Characterization	Reference
Tissue	Cell Type				
Terato-carci-noma or teratoma	EC	Tumors containing tissue types from endoderm, mesoderm, and ectoderm	Bone morphogenetic protein-7 EC cells cultured without feeder cell layer Transplantation of EC cells into mice	Morphology, histology, and cell staining Observation of tissue types from endoderm, mesoderm, and ectoderm Observation of extended self-renewal of EC cells Analysis of chromosomes and specific genes Detection of cell-specific proteins Cytochemical assay	Andrews et al., 1984 Thompson et al., 1984 Pera, 1989

Appendix D.v.
Published Reports on Isolation and Differentiation of Human Adult Stem Cells

Origin Tissue	Origin Cell Type	Cell Types Developed	Differentiation Conditions	Methods of Characterization	Reference
Blood	Circulatory Skeletal	Adipocyte Osteocyte	Leukemia inhibitory factor (LIF) Transplantation of stem cells into bg-nu-xid immunocompromised mice	Antibody labeling Polymerase chain reaction	Kuznetsov, 2001
Bone marrow	Angioblast (endothelial precursor)	Mature endothelia and newly formed blood vessels	Angioblasts isolated by mobilizing peripheral blood with granulocyte-colony stimulating factor Angioblasts injected into rats with experimental myocardial infarction	Observation of neovascularization within myocardium from transplanted cells Detection of improved cardiac function in experimental animals	Kocher et al., 2001
	Hematopoietic stem cell (HSC)	Hepatocyte Cholangiocyte	Bone marrow transplantation	Probed for presence and function of Y chromosome-containing liver cells Measured expression of liver-specific proteins Immunochemistry	Alison et al., 2000 Theise et al., 2000
	Human marrow stromal	Stromal-derived cell engrafted in rat brain	Isolation of marrow stromal cell from human volunteers; injection of stromal cell into rat brain	Observation of engraftment, migration, and survival of stromal-derived cell in rat brain Observation of loss of stromal cell functions Antibodies to cell-surface proteins	Azizi et al., 1998
	Mesenchymal stem cell (MSC)	Adipocyte Chondrocyte Osteocyte	Fetal bovine serum, dexamethasone, isobutylxanthine, insulin, ascorbate, indomethacin, transforming growth factor-B3, and glycerol phosphate	Histology and immunofluorescence Detection of lipids and specific enzyme activity of adipocytes and osteocytes Specific staining for chondrocytes	Pittenger et al., 1999

Appendix D.v. *(cont.)*

Origin		Cell Types Developed	Differentiation Conditions	Methods of Characterization	Reference
Tissue	Cell Type				
Bone marrow *(cont.)*	MSC	Neuron	Prolonged expansion of MSCs as undifferentiated cells β-mercaptoethanol (BME) Butylated hydroxyanisole (BHA)	Histology Detection of numerous neuron-specific proteins via staining and antibody binding	Woodbury et al., 2000
	MSC	Neuron	MSCs cultured with fetal rat brain cells Epidermal growth factor Brain-derived neurotrophic factor	Detection of nestin and nestin-gene expression Detection of neuron-specific proteins	Sanchez-Ramos et al., 2000
	MSC	Adipocyte Bone marrow stromal cell Cardiomyocyte Chondrocyte Myocyte Thymic stromal cell	MSCs isolated from bone marrow Transplantation of MSCs into fetal sheep	Analysis of human gene expression in sheep tissues Confirmed presence of human cells by immunohistochemistry	Liechty et al., 2000
Bone marrow (fetal)	HSC	HSC Red blood cell lineages White blood cell lineages	Enrichment of hematopoietic cell populations by cell selection Transplantation of bone marrow and thymus cells into mice	Establishment of long-term multilineage cultures of hematopoietic colonies Fluorescence-activated cell sorting (FACS) Engraftment of hematopoietic cells in mice	Baum et al., 1992
Brain	Neural stem cell (NSC)	Muscle cell	Exposure of NSCs to myoblasts Dissociation of NSC clusters Transplantation of human NSCs into mice with induced muscle injury	Observation of differentiated skeletal muscle cells from primary and culture-derived NSCs Demonstration of NSC engraftment in mice by detection of expression of specific genes	Galli et al., 2000

Appendix D.v. *(cont.)*

Origin		Cell Types Developed	Differentiation Conditions	Methods of Characterization	Reference
Tissue	**Cell Type**				
Brain (adult and neonatal)	Neural progenitor cell (NPC)	Astrocyte Neuron Oligodendrocyte	NPCs cultured in medium containing glutamine, amphotericin-B, antibiotics, fetal calf serum, basic fibroblast growth factor, epidermal growth factor, and platelet-derived growth factor AB Transplantation of human central nervous system stem cells (hCNS-SCs) into mice	Observation of functional engraftment of NPCs into mouse brain Antibody labeling of neuronal cell-surface proteins	Palmer et al., 2001
Brain (fetal)	Human central nervous system stem cell (hCNS-SC)	Astrocyte Neuron Oligodendrocyte	Fibroblast growth factor-2, epidermal growth factor, lymphocyte inhibitory factor, neural survival factor-1, brain-derived and glial-derived neurotrophic factors	Observation of neurosphere formation and self-renewal of hCNS-SCs Demonstration of engraftment, proliferation, migration, and neural differentiation of hCNS-SCs FACS	Uchida et al., 2000
Fat	Stromal vascular cell fraction of processed lipoaspirate	Adipocyte precursor Osteocyte precursor Chondrocyte precursor Myocyte precursor	Co-cultured with mouse adipocytes, isobutylmethylxanthine, dexamethasone Co-cultured with human osteoblasts, insulin, indomethacin, antibiotic/antimycotic dexamethasone, ascorbate, b-glycerophosphate, antibiotic/antimycotic Co-cultured with human skeletal myocytes, insulin, transforming growth factor-B, ascorbate, antibiotic/antimycotic dexamethasone, hydrocortisone, antibiotic/antimycotic	Staining for lipid accumulation Staining for alkaline phosphatase activity Staining for bone formation Staining for proteoglycan-rich matrix Antibody binding to collagen II Visualization of multinucleation Staining for muscle protein: myosin Antibody binding to MyoD1	Zuk et al., 2001

Appendix D.v. (cont.)

Origin Tissue	Cell Type	Cell Types Developed	Differentiation Conditions	Methods of Characterization	Reference
Liver (fetal)	HSC	Hematopoietic progenitor cell (HPC) Red blood cell lineages White blood cell lineages	Co-culture of HSCs with mouse stromal cells Implantation of fetal hematopoietic liver cells into immunocompromised mice	Demonstration of differentiation into red and white blood cell lineages through colony-forming assays and detection of surface markers characteristic of the hematopoietic system	McCune et al., 1988 Namikawa et al., 1990
Pancreas	Nestin-positive islet-derived progenitor cell (NIP)	Pancreatic Hepatic	NIPs obtained from pancreatic islets and cultured for extended periods	Observation of extended proliferative, self-renewing, and multipotent capacity Expression of hepatic and exocrine pancreatic markers Demonstration of ductal and endocrine pancreatic features Production of insulin and glucagons	Zulewski et al., 2000
Umbilical cord blood	HPC	Most red and white blood cell lineages	Collection and sorting Stimulation with colony-stimulating factors and interleukin-3	Demonstration of multipotent progenitor, granulocyte-macrophage, and erythroid cell lines	Broxmeyer et al., 1989
	HSC Mesenchymal progenitor cell (MPC)	Most red and white blood cell lineages Osteoblasts Adipocytes	Mixtures of dexamethasone, ß-glycerol, ascorbate, insulin, isobutyl-methylxanthine, and indomethacin	Cell morphology Cytochemical analysis of osteoblast and adipocyte products Immunophenotyping	Erices et al., 1999

Appendix D.vi.

REFERENCES

1. Alison, M.R., Poulsom, R., Jeffery, R., Dhillon, A.P., Quaglia, A., Jacob, J., Novelli, M., Prentice, G., Williamson, J., and Wright, N.A. (2000). Hepatocytes from non-hepatic adult stem cells. Nature. *406*, 257.

2. Andrews, P.W., Damjanov, I., Simon, D., Banting, G.S., Carlin, C., Dracopoli, N.C., and Fogh, J. (1984). Pluripotent embryonal carcinoma clones derived from the human teratocarcinoma cell line Tera-2. Differentiation *in vivo* and *in vitro*. Lab. Invest. *50*, 147-162.

3. Assady, S., Maor, G., Amit, M., Itskovitz-Eldor, J., Skorecki, K.L., and Tzukerman, M. (2001). Insulin production by human embryonic stem cells. Diabetes, *50*, http://www.diabetes.org/Diabetes_Rapids/Suheir_Assady_06282001.pdf.

4. Azizi, S.A., Stokes, D., Augelli, B.J., DiGirolamo, C., and Prockop, D.J. (1998). Engraftment and migration of human bone marrow stromal cells implanted in the brains of albino rats—similarities to astrocyte grafts. Proc. Natl. Acad. Sci. U. S. A. *95*, 3908-3913.

5. Bader, A., Al Dubai, H., and Weitzer, G. (2000). Leukemia inhibitory factor modulates cardiogenesis in embryoid bodies in opposite fashions. Circ. Res. *86*, 787-794.

6. Bagutti, C., Wobus, A.M., Fassler, R., and Watt, F.M. (1996). Differentiation of embryonal stem cells into keratinocytes: comparison of wild-type and ß(1) integrin-deficient cells. Dev. Biol. *179*, 184-196.

7. Bain, G., Kitchens, D., Yao, M., Huettner, J.E., and Gottlieb, D.I. (1995). Embryonic stem cells express neuronal properties *in vitro*. Dev. Biol. *168*, 342-357.

8. Baum, C.M., Weissman, I.L., Tsukamoto, A.S., Buckle, A.M., and Peault, B. (1992). Isolation of a candidate human hematopoietic stem-cell population. Proc. Natl. Acad. Sci. U. S. A. *89*, 2804-2808.

9. Bittner, R.E., Schofer, C., Weipoltshammer, K., Ivanova, S., Streubel, B., Hauser, E., Freilinger, M., Hoger, H., Elbe-Burger, A., and Wachtler, F. (1999). Recruitment of bone-marrow-derived cells by skeletal and cardiac muscle in adult dystrophic mdx mice. Anat. Embryol. (Berl) *199*, 391-396.

10. Bjornson, C.R., Rietze, R.L., Reynolds, B.A., Magli, M.C., and Vescovi, A.L. (1999). Turning brain into blood: a hematopoietic fate adopted by adult neural stem cells *in vivo*. Science. *283*, 534-537.

11. Bosch, P., Musgrave, D.S., Lee, J.Y., Cummins, J., Shuler, F., Ghivizzani, S.C., Evans, C., Robbins, P.D., and Huard, J. (2000). Osteoprogenitor cells within skeletal muscle. J. Orthop. Res. *18*, 933-944.

12. Brazelton, T.R., Rossi, F.M., Keshet, G.I., and Blau, H.M. (2000). From marrow to brain: expression of neuronal phenotypes in adult mice. Science. *290*, 1775-1779.

13. Broxmeyer, H.E., Douglas, G.W., Hangoc, G., Cooper, S., Bard, J., English, D., Arny, M., Thomas, L., and Boyse, E.A. (1989). Human umbilical cord blood as a potential source of transplantable hematopoietic stem/progenitor cells. Proc. Natl. Acad. Sci. U. S. A. *86*, 3828-3832.

14. Brustle, O., Jones, K.N., Learish, R.D., Karram, K., Choudhary, K., Wiestler, O.D., Duncan, I.D., and McKay, R.D. (1999). Embryonic stem cell-derived glial precursors: a source of myelinating transplants. Science. *285*, 754-756.

15. Buttery, L.D., Bourne, S., Xynos, J.D., Wood, H., Hughes, F.J., Hughes, S.P., Episkopou, V., and Polak, J.M. (2001). Differentiation of osteoblasts and *in vitro* bone formation from murine embryonic stem cells. Tissue Eng. *7*, 89-99.

16. Dani, C., Smith, A.G., Dessolin, S., Leroy, P., Staccini, L., Villageois, P., Darimont, C., and Ailhaud, G. (1997). Differentiation of embryonic stem cells into adipocytes *in vitro*. J. Cell Sci. *110*, 1279-1285.

17. Dinsmore, J., Ratliff, J., Deacon, T., Pakzaban, P., Jacoby, D., Galpern, W., and Isacson, O. (1996). Embryonic stem cells differentiated *in vitro* as a novel source of cells for transplantation. Cell Transplant. *5*, 131-143.

18. Doetsch, F., Caille, I., Lim, D.A., Garcia-Verdugo, J.M., and Alvarez-Buylla, A. (1999). Subventricular zone astrocytes are neural stem cells in the adult mammalian brain. Cell. *97*, 703-716.

19. Doetschman, T., Eistetter, H., Katz, M., Schmit, W., and Kemler, R. (1985). The *in vitro* development of blastocyst-derived embryonic stem cell lines: formation of visceral yolk sac, blood islands and myocardium. J. Embryol. Exp. Morph. *87*, 27-45.

20. Drab, M., Haller, H., Bychkov, R., Erdmann, B., Lindschau, C., Haase, H., Morano, I., Luft, F.C., and Wobus, A.M. (1997). From totipotent embryonic stem cells to spontaneously contracting smooth muscle cells: a retinoic acid and db-cAMP *in vitro* differentiation model. FASEB J. *11*, 905-915.

21. Eglitis, M.A. and Mezey, E. (1997). Hematopoietic cells differentiate into both microglia and macroglia in the brains of adult mice. Proc. Natl. Acad. Sci. U. S. A. *94*, 4080-4085.

22. Erices, A., Conget, P., and Minguell, J.J. (1999). Mesenchymal progenitor cells in human umbilical cord blood. Br. J. Haematol. *109*, 235-242.

23. Evans, M.J. and Kaufman, M.H. (1981). Establishment in culture of pluripotential cells from mouse embryos. Nature. *292*, 154-156.

24. Fairchild, P.J., Brook, F.A., Gardner, R.L., Graca, L., Strong, V., Tone, Y., Tone, M., Nolan, K.F., and Waldmann, H. (2000). Directed differentiation of dendritic cells from mouse embryonic stem cells. Curr. Biol. *10*, 1515-1518.

25. Ferrari, G., Cusella-De Angelis, G., Coletta, M., Paolucci, E., Stornaiuolo, A., Cossu, G., and Mavilio, F. (1998). Muscle regeneration by bone marrow-derived myogenic progenitors. Science. *279*, 1528-1530.

26. Fraichard, A., Chassande, O., Bilbaut, G., Dehay, C., Savatier, P., and Samarut, J. (1995). *In vitro* differentiation of embryonic stem cells into glial cells and functional neurons. J. Cell Sci. *108*, 3181-3188.

27. Friedenstein, A.J., Gorskaja, U.F., and Kulagina, N.N. (1976). Fibroblast precursors in normal and irradiated mouse hematopoietic organs. Exp. Hematol. *4*, 267-274.

28. Galli, R., Borello, U., Gritti, A., Minasi, M.G., Bjornson, C., Coletta, M., Mora, M., De Angelis, M.G., Fiocco, R., Cossu, G., and Vescovi, A.L. (2000). Skeletal myogenic potential of human and mouse neural stem cells. Nat. Neurosci. *3*, 986-991.

29. Gottlieb, D.I. and Huettner, J.E. (1999). An *in vitro* pathway from embryonic stem cells to neurons and glia. Cells Tissues Organs. *165*, 165-172.

30. Grimaldi, P.A., Teboul, L., Inadera, H., Gaillard, D., and Amri, E.Z. (1997). Trans-differentiation of myoblasts to adipoblasts: triggering effects of fatty acids and thiazolidinediones. Prostaglandins. Leukot. Essent. Fatty. Acids. *57*, 71-75.

31. Gussoni, E., Soneoka, Y., Strickland, C.D., Buzney, E.A., Khan, M.K., Flint, A.F., Kunkel, L.M., and Mulligan, R.C. (1999). Dystrophin expression in the mdx mouse restored by stem cell transplantation. Nature. *401*, 390-394.

32. Hirashima, M., Kataoka, H., Nishikawa, S., Matsuyoshi, N., and Nishikawa, S. (1999). Maturation of embryonic stem cells into endothelial cells in an *in vitro* model of vasculogenesis. Blood. *93*, 1253-1263.

33. Itskovitz-Eldor, J., Schuldiner, M., Karsenti, D., Eden, A., Yanuka, O., Amit, M., Soreq, H., and Benvenisty, N. (2000). Differentiation of human embryonic stem cells into embryoid bodies comprising the three embryonic germ layers. Mol. Med. *6*, 88-95.

34. Jackson, K.A., Mi, T., and Goodell, M.A. (1999). Hematopoietic potential of stem cells isolated from murine skeletal muscle. Proc. Natl. Acad. Sci. U. S. A. *96*, 14482-14486.

35. Jackson, K., Majka SM, Wang H, Pocius J, Hartley CJ, Majesky MW, Entman ML, Michael LH, Hirschi KK, and and Goodell MA (2001). Regeneration of ischemic cardiac muscle and vascular endothelium by adult stem cells. J. Clin. Invest. *107*, 1-8.

36. Johansson, B.M. and Wiles, M.V. (1995). Evidence for involvement of activin A and bone morphogenetic protein 4 in mammalian mesoderm and hematopoietic development. Mol. Cell Biol. *15*, 141-151.

37. Johansson, C.B., Momma, S., Clarke, D.L., Risling, M., Lendahl, U., and Frisen, J. (1999). Identification of a neural stem cell in the adult mammalian central nervous system. Cell. *96*, 25-34.

38. Kawasaki, H., Mizuseki, K., Nishikawa, S., Kaneko, S., Kuwana, Y., Nakanishi, S., Nishikawa, S.I., and Sasai, Y. (2000). Induction of midbrain dopaminergic neurons from ES cells by stromal cell-derived inducing activity. Neuron. *28*, 31-40.

39. Kehat, I., Kenyagin-Karsenti, D., Druckmann, M., Segev, H., Amit, M., Gepstein, A., Livne, E., Binah, O., Itskovitz-Eldor, J., and Gepstein, L. (2001). Human embryonic stem cells can differentiate into myocytes portraying cardiomyocytic structural and functional properties. J. Clin. Invest. *(in press)*.

40. Kerr, D.A., Llado, J., Shamblott, M., Maragakis, N., Irani, D.N., Dike, S., Sappington, A., Gearhart, J., and Rothstein, J. (2001). Human embryonic germ cell derivatives facilitate motor recovery of rats with diffuse motor neuron injury.

41. Klug, M.G., Soonpaa, M.H., Koh, G.Y., and Field, L.J. (1996). Genetically selected cardiomyocytes from differentiating embryonic stem cells form stable intracardiac grafts. J. Clin. Invest. *98*, 216-224.

42. Kocher, A.A., Schuster, M.D., Szabolcs, M.J., Takuma, S., Burkhoff, D., Wang, J., Homma, S., Edwards, N.M., and Itescu, S. (2001). Neovascularization of ischemic myocardium by human bone-marrow-derived angioblasts prevents cardiomyocyte apoptosis, reduces remodeling and improves cardiac function. Nat. Med. *7*, 430-436.

43. Kopen, G.C., Prockop, D.J., and Phinney, D.G. (1999). Marrow stromal cells migrate throughout forebrain and cerebellum, and they differentiate into astrocytes after injection into neonatal mouse brains. Proc. Natl. Acad. Sci. U. S. A. *96*, 10711-10716.

44. Kramer, J., Hegert, C., Guan, K., Wobus, A.M., Muller, P.K., and Rohwedel, J. (2000). Embryonic stem cell-derived chondrogenic differentiation *in vitro*: activation by BMP-2 and BMP-4. Mech. Dev. *92*, 193-205.

45. Krause, D.S., Theise, N.D., Collector, M.I., Henegariu, O., Hwang, S., Gardner, R., Neutzel, S., and Sharkis, S.J. (2001). Multi-organ, multi-lineage engraftment by a single bone marrow-derived stem cell. Cell. *105*, 369-377.

46. Kuznetsov, S.A., Mankani, M.H., Gronthos, S., Satomura, K., Bianco, P., and Robey P.G. (2001). Circulating skeletal stem cells. J. Cell Biol. *153*, 1133-40.

47. Lagasse, E., Connors, H., Al Dhalimy, M., Reitsma, M., Dohse, M., Osborne, L., Wang, X., Finegold, M., Weissman, I.L., and Grompe, M. (2000). Purified hematopoietic stem cells can differentiate into hepatocytes *in vivo*. Nat. Med. *6*, 1229-1234.

48. Lee, S.H., Lumelsky, N., Studer, L., Auerbach, J.M., and McKay, R.D. (2000). Efficient generation of midbrain and hindbrain neurons from mouse embryonic stem cells. Nat. Biotechnol. *18*, 675-679.

49. Li, M., Pevny, L., Lovell-Badge, R., and Smith, A. (1998). Generation of purified neural precursors from embryonic stem cells by lineage selection. Curr. Biol. *8*, 971-974.

50. Liechty, K.W., MacKenzie, T.C., Shaaban, A.F., Radu, A., Moseley, A.B., Deans, R., Marshak, D.R., and Flake, A.W. (2000). Human mesenchymal stem cells engraft and demonstrate site-specific differentiation after in utero transplantation in sheep. Nat. Med. *6*, 1282-1286.

51. Lieschke, G.J. and Dunn, A.R. (1995). Development of functional macrophages from embryonal stem cells in vitro. Exp. Hematol. 23, 328-334.

52. Liu, S., Qu, Y., Stewart, T.J., Howard, M.J., Chakrabortty, S., Holekamp, T.F., and McDonald, J.W. (2000). Embryonic stem cells differentiate into oligodendrocytes and myelinate in culture and after spinal cord transplantation. Proc. Natl. Acad. Sci. U. S. A. 97, 6126-6131.

53. Lumelsky, N., Blondel, O., Laeng, P., Velasco, I., Ravin, R., and McKay, R. (2001). Differentiation of Embryonic Stem Cells to Insulin-Secreting Structures Similiar to Pancreatic Islets. Science. 292, 1389-1394.

54. Makino, S., Fukuda, K., Miyoshi, S., Konishi, F., Kodama, H., Pan, J., Sano, M., Takahashi, T., Hori, S., Abe, H., Hata, J., Umezawa, A., and Ogawa, S. (1999). Cardiomyocytes can be generated from marrow stromal cells in vitro. J. Clin. Invest. 103, 697-705.

55. Maltsev, V.A., Rohwedel, J., Hescheler, J., and Wobus, A.M. (1993). Embryonic stem cells differentiate in vitro into cardiomyocytes representing sinusnodal, atrial and ventricular cell types. Mech. Dev. 44, 41-50.

56. Matsui, Y., Zsebo, K., and Hogan, B.L. (1992). Derivation of pluripotential embryonic stem cells from murine primordial germ cells in culture. Cell. 70, 841-847.

57. McBurney, M.W., Reuhl, K.R., Ally, A.I., Nasipuri, S., Bell, J.C., and Craig, J. (1988). Differentiation and maturation of embryonal carcinoma-derived neurons in cell culture. J. Neurosci. 8, 1063-1073.

58. McCune, J.M., Namikawa, R., Kaneshima, H., Shultz, L.D., Lieberman, M., and Weissman, I.L. (1988). The SCID-hu mouse: murine model for the analysis of human hematolymphoid differentiation and function. Science. 241, 1632-1639.

59. Megeney, L.A., Kablar, B., Garrett, K., Anderson, J.E., and Rudnicki, M.A. (1996). MyoD is required for myogenic stem cell function in adult skeletal muscle. Genes Dev. 10, 1173-1183.

60. Mezey, E., Chandross, K.J., Harta, G., Maki, R.A., and McKercher, S.R. (2000). Turning blood into brain: cells bearing neuronal antigens generated in vivo from bone marrow. Science. 290, 1779-1782.

61. Morrison, S.J., Uchida, N., and Weissman, I.L. (1995). The biology of hematopoietic stem cells. Annu. Rev. Cell. Dev. Biol. 11, 35-71.

62 Namikawa, R., Weilbaecher, K.N., Kaneshima, H., Yee, E.J., and McCune, J.M. (1990). Long-term human hematopoiesis in the SCID-hu mouse. J. Exp. Med. 172, 1055-1063.

63. O'Shea, K.S. (1999). Embryonic stem cell models of development. Anat. Rec. 257, 32-41.

64. Orlic, D., Kajstura, J., Chimenti, S., Jakoniuk, I., Anderson, S.M., Li, B., Pickel, J., McKay, R., Nadal-Ginard, B., Bodine, D.M., Leri, A., and Anversa, P. (2001). Bone marrow cells regenerate infarcted myocardium. Nature. 410, 701-705.

65. Palmer, T.D., Schwartz, P.H., Taupin, P., Kaspar, B., Stein, S.A., and Gage, F.H. (2001). Progenitor cells from human brain after death. Nature. 411, 42-43.

66. Pera, M.F., Cooper, S., Mills, J., and Parrington, J.M. (1989). Isolation and characterization of a multipotent clone of human embryonal carcinoma cells. Differentiation. 42, 10-23.

67. Pera, M.F. and Herszfeld, D. (1998). Differentiation of human pluripotent teratocarcinoma stem cells induced by bone morphogenetic protein-2. Reprod. Fertil. Dev. 10, 551-555.

68. Pereira, R.F., Halford, K.W., O'Hara, M.D., Leeper, D.B., Sokolov, B.P., Pollard, M.D., Bagasra, O., and Prockop, D.J. (1995). Cultured adherent cells from marrow can serve as long-lasting precursor cells for bone, cartilage, and lung in irradiated mice. Proc. Natl. Acad. Sci. U. S. A. 92, 4857-4861.

69. Perkins, A.C. (1998). Enrichment of blood from embryonic stem cells in vitro. Reprod. Fertil. Dev. 10, 563-572.

70. Petersen, B.E., Bowen, W.C., Patrene, K.D., Mars, W.M., Sullivan, A.K., Murase, N., Boggs, S.S., Greenberger, J.S., and Goff, J.P. (1999). Bone marrow as a potential source of hepatic oval cells. Science. 284, 1168-1170.

71. Pittenger, M.F., Mackay, A.M., Beck, S.C., Jaiswal, R.K., Douglas, R., Mosca, J.D., Moorman, M.A., Simonetti, D.W., Craig, S., and Marshak, D.R. (1999). Multilineage potential of adult human mesenchymal stem cells. Science. 284, 143-147.

72. Potocnik, A.J., Nielsen, P.J., and Eichmann, K. (1994). In vitro generation of lymphoid precursors from embryonic stem cells. EMBO J. 13, 5274-5283.

73. Prelle, K., Wobus, A.M., Krebs, O., Blum, W.F., and Wolf, E. (2000). Overexpression of insulin-like growth factor-II in mouse embryonic stem cells promotes myogenic differentiation. Biochem. Biophys. Res. Commun. 277, 631-638.

74. Prockop, D.J. (1997). Marrow stromal cells as stem cells for nonhematopoietic tissues. Science. 276, 71-74.

75. Ramiya, V.K., Maraist, M., Arfors, K.E., Schatz, D.A., Peck, A.B., and Cornelius, J.G. (2000). Reversal of insulin-dependent diabetes using islets generated in vitro from pancreatic stem cells. Nat. Med. 6, 278-282.

76. Rathjen, P.D., Lake, J., Whyatt, L.M., Bettess, M.D., and Rathjen, J. (1998). Properties and uses of embryonic stem cells: prospects for application to human biology and gene therapy. Reprod. Fertil. Dev. 10, 31-47.

77. Reubinoff, B.E., Pera, M.F., Fong, C.Y., Trounson, A., and Bongso, A. (2000). Embryonic stem cell lines from human blastocysts: somatic differentiation in vitro. Nat. Biotechnol. 18, 399-404.

78. Reynolds, B.A. and Weiss, S. (1996). Clonal and population analyses demonstrate that an EGF-responsive mammalian embryonic CNS precursor is a stem cell. Dev. Biol. 175, 1-13.

79. Reynolds, J.N., Ryan, P.J., Prasad, A., and Paterno, G.D. (1994). Neurons derived from embryonal carcinoma (P19) cells express multiple GABA(A) receptor subunits and fully functional GABA(A) receptors. Neurosci. Lett. 165, 129-132.

80. Risau, W., Sariola, H., Zerwes, H.G., Sasse, J., Ekblom, P., Kemler, R., and Doetschman, T. (1988). Vasculogenesis and angiogenesis in embryonic-stem-cell-derived embryoid bodies. Development. 102, 471-478.

81. Roach, S., Schmid, W., and Pera, M.F. (1994). Hepatocytic transcription factor expression in human embryonal carcinoma and yolk sac carcinoma cell lines: expression of HNF-3α in models of early endodermal cell differentiation. Exp. Cell. Res. 215, 189-198.

82. Rohwedel, J., Maltsev, V., Bober, E., Arnold, H.H., Hescheler, J., and Wobus, A.M. (1994). Muscle cell differentiation of embryonic stem cells reflects myogenesis in vivo: developmentally regulated expression of myogenic determination genes and functional expression of ionic currents. Dev. Biol. 164, 87-101.

83. Sanchez-Ramos, J., Song, S., Cardozo-Pelaez, F., Hazzi, C., Stedeford, T., Willing, A., Freeman, T.B., Saporta, S., Janssen, W., Patel, N., Cooper, D.R., and Sanberg, P.R. (2000). Adult bone marrow stromal cells differentiate into neural cells in vitro. Exp. Neurol. 164, 247-256.

84. Schuldiner, M., Yanuka, O., Itskovitz-Eldor, J., Melton, D., and Benvenisty, N. (2000). Effects of eight growth factors on the differentiation of cells derived from human embryonic stem cells. Proc. Natl. Acad. Sci. U. S. A. 97, 11307-11312.

85. Seale, P., Sabourin, L.A., Girgis-Gabardo, A., Mansouri, A., Gruss, P., and Rudnicki, M.A. (2000). Pax7 is required for the specification of myogenic satellite cells. Cell. 102, 777-786.

86. Shamblott, M.J., Axelman, J., Littlefield, J.W., Blumenthal, P.D., Huggins, G.R., Cui, Y., Cheng, L., and Gearhart, J.D. (2001). Human embryonic germ cell derivatives express a broad range of developmentally distinct markers and proliferate extensively in vitro. Proc. Natl. Acad. Sci. U. S. A. 98, 13-118.

87. Shamblott, M.J., Axelman, J., Wang, S., Bugg, E.M., Littlefield, J.W., Donovan, P.J., Blumenthal, P.D., Huggins, G.R., and Gearhart, J.D. (1998). Derivation of pluripotent stem cells from cultured human primordial germ cells. Proc. Natl. Acad. Sci. U. S. A. 95, 13726-13731.

88. Slager, H.G., Van Inzen, W., Freund, E., Van den Eijnden-Van Raaij A.J.M., and Mummery, C.L. (1993). Transforming growth factor-beta in the early mouse embryo: implications for the regulation of muscle formation and implantation. Dev. Genet. 14, 212-224.

89. Soria, B., Roche, E., Berna, G., Leon-Quinto, T., Reig, J.A., and Martin, F. (2000). Insulin-secreting cells derived from embryonic stem cells normalize glycemia in streptozotocin-induced diabetic mice. Diabetes. 49, 157-162.

90. Spangrude, G.J., Smith, L., Uchida, N., Ikuta, K., Heimfeld, S., Friedman, J., and Weissman, I.L. (1991). Mouse hematopoietic stem cells. Blood. 78, 1395-1402.

91. Strubing, C., Ahnert-Hilger, G., Shan, J., Wiedenmann, B., Hescheler, J., and Wobus, A.M. (1995). Differentiation of pluripotent embryonic stem cells into the neuronal lineage in vitro gives rise to mature inhibitory and excitatory neurons. Mech. Dev. 53, 275-287.

92. Taniguchi, H., Toyoshima, T., Fukao, K., and Nakauchi, H. (1996). Presence of hematopoietic stem cells in the adult liver. Nat. Med. 2, 198-203.

93. Theise, N.D., Nimmakayalu, M., Gardner, R., Illei, P.B., Morgan, G., Teperman, L., Henegariu, O., and Krause, D.S. (2000). Liver from bone marrow in humans. Hepatology. 32, 11-16.

94. Thompson, S., Stern, P.L., Webb, M., Walsh, F.S., Engstrom, W., Evans, E.P., Shi, W.K., Hopkins, B., and Graham, C.F. (1984). Cloned human teratoma cells differentiate into neuron-like cells and other cell types in retinoic acid. J. Cell. Sci. 72, 37-64.

95. Thomson, J.A., Itskovitz-Eldor, J., Shapiro, S.S., Waknitz, M.A., Swiergiel, J.J., Marshall, V.S., and Jones, J.M. (1998). Embryonic stem cell lines derived from human blastocysts. Science. 282, 1145-1147.

96. Tomita, S., Li, R.K., Weisel, R.D., Mickle, D.A., Kim, E.J., Sakai, T., and Jia, Z.Q. (1999). Autologous transplantation of bone marrow cells improves damaged heart function 672. Circulation. 100 (Suppl. II), 11247-11256.

97. Trojanowski, J.Q., Mantione, J.R., Lee, J.H., Seid, D.P., You, T., Inge, L.J., and Lee, V.M. (1993). Neurons derived from a human teratocarcinoma cell line establish molecular and structural polarity following transplantation into the rodent brain. Exp. Neurol. 122, 283-294.

98. Tsai, M., Wedemeyer, J., Ganiatsas, S., Tam, S.Y., Zon, L.I., and Galli, S.J. (2000). In vivo immunological function of mast cells derived from embryonic stem cells: an approach for the rapid analysis of even embryonic lethal mutations in adult mice in vivo. Proc. Natl. Acad. Sci. U. S. A. 97, 9186-9190.

99. Uchida, N., Buck, D.W., He, D., Reitsma, M.J., Masek, M., Phan, T.V., Tsukamoto, A.S., Gage, F.H., and Weissman, I.L. (2000). Direct isolation of human central nervous system stem cells. Proc. Natl. Acad. Sci. U. S. A. 97, 14720-14725.

100. Wakitani, S., Saito, T., and Caplan, A.I. (1995). Myogenic cells derived from rat bone marrow mesenchymal stem cells exposed to 5-azacytidine 754. Muscle. Nerve. 18, 1417-1426.

101. Wang, X., Al-Dhalimy, M., Lagasse, E., Finegold, M., and Grompe, M. (2001). Liver repopulation and correction of metabolic liver disease by transplanted adult mouse pancreatic cells. Am. J. Pathol. 158, 571-579.

102. Weiss, S., Dunne, C., Hewson, J., Wohl, C., Wheatley, M., Peterson, A.C., and Reynolds, B.A. (1996). Multipotent CNS stem cells are present in the adult mammalian spinal cord and ventricular neuroaxis. J. Neurosci. 16, 7599-7609.

103. Westfall, M.V., Pasyk, K.A., Yule, D.I., Samuelson, L.C., and Metzger, J.M. (1997). Ultrastructure and cell-cell coupling of cardiac myocytes differentiating in embryonic stem cell cultures. Cell. Motil. Cytoskeleton. *36*, 43-54.

104. Wiles, M.V. and Keller, G. (1991). Multiple hematopoietic lineages develop from embryonic stem (ES) cells in culture. Development. *111*, 259-267.

105. Wobus, A.M., Rohwedel, J., Maltsev, V., and Hescheler, J. (1995). Development of cardiomyocytes expressing cardiac-specific genes, action potentials, and ionic channels during embryonic stem cell-derived cardiogenesis. Ann. N. Y. Acad. Sci. *752*, 460-469.

106. Woodbury, D., Schwarz, E.J., Prockop, D.J., and Black, I.B. (2000). Adult rat and human bone marrow stromal cells differentiate into neurons. J. Neurosci. Res. *61*, 364-370.

107. Yamane, T., Hayashi, H., Mizoguchi, M., Yamazaki, H., and Kunisada, T. (1999). Derivation of melanocytes from embryonic stem cells in culture. Dev. Dyn. *216*, 450-458.

108. Yamashita, J., Itoh, H., Hirashima, M., Ogawa, M., Nishikawa, S., Yurugi, T., Naito, M., Nakao, K., and Nishikawa, S. (2000). Flk1-positive cells derived from embryonic stem cells serve as vascular progenitors. Nature. *408*, 92-96.

109. Zuk, P.A., Zhu, M., Mizuno, H., Huang, J., Futrell, J.W., Katz, A.J., Benhaim, P., Lorenz, H.P., and Hedrick, M.H. (2001). Multilineage cells from human adipose tissue: implications for cell- based therapies. Tissue Eng. *7*, 211-228.

110. Zulewski, H., Abraham, E.J., Gerlach, M.J., Daniel, P.B., Moritz, W., Muller, B., Vallejo, M., Thomas, M.K., and Habener, J.F. (2001). Multipotential nestin-positive stem cells isolated from adult pancreatic islets differentiate ex vivo into pancreatic endocrine, exocrine, and hepatic phenotypes. Diabetes. *50*, 521-533.

APPENDIX E:

STEM CELL MARKERS

Appendix E.i.

HOW DO RESEARCHERS USE MARKERS TO IDENTIFY STEM CELLS?

In recent years, scientists have discovered a wide array of stem cells that have unique capabilities to self-renew, grow indefinitely, and differentiate or develop into multiple types of cells and tissues. Researchers now know that many different types of stem cells exist but they all are found in very small populations in the human body, in some cases 1 stem cell in 100,000 cells in circulating blood. And, when scientists examine these cells under a microscope, they look just like any other cell in the tissue where they are found. So, how do scientists identify these rare type of cells found in many different cells and tissues—a process that is much akin to finding a needle in a haystack? The answer is rather simple thanks to stem cell "markers." This feature describes stem cell marker technology and how it is used in the research laboratory. Following this is a listing of some of the commonly used stem cell markers (see Appendix E.ii. Markers Commonly Used to Identify Stem Cells and to Characterize Differentiated Cell Types).

What are stem cell markers? Coating the surface of every cell in the body are specialized proteins, called receptors, that have the capability of selectively binding or adhering to other "signaling" molecules. There are many different types of receptors that differ in their structure and affinity for the signaling molecules. Normally, cells use these receptors and the molecules that bind to them as a way of communicating with other cells and to carry out their proper functions in the body. These same cell surface receptors are the stem cell markers. Each cell type, for example a liver cell, has a certain combination of receptors on their surface that makes them distinguishable from

other kinds of cells. Scientists have taken advantage of the biological uniqueness of stem cell receptors and chemical properties of certain compounds to tag or "mark" cells. Researchers owe much of the past success in finding and characterizing stem cells to the use of markers.

Stem cell markers are given short-hand names based on the molecules that bind to the stem cell surface receptors. For example, a cell that has the receptor stem cell antigen – 1, on its surface, is identified as Sca-1. In many cases, a combination of multiple markers is used to identify a particular stem cell type. So now, researchers often identify stem cells in short-hand by a combination of marker names reflecting the presence (+) or absence (–) of them. For example, a special type of hematopoietic stem cell from blood and bone marrow called "side population" or "SP" is described as ($CD34^{-/low}$, c-Kit$^+$, Sca-1$^+$) [4].

Researchers use the signaling molecules that selectively adhere to the receptors on the surface of the cell as a tool that allows them to identify stem cells. Many years ago, a technique was developed to attach to the signaling molecule another molecule (or the tag) that has the ability to fluoresce or emit light energy when activated by an energy source such as an ultraviolet light or laser beam (see Figure E.i.1. Identifying Cell Surface Markers Using Fluorescent Tags). At the researchers' disposal are multiple fluorescent tags with emitted light that differ in color and intensity.

Described here are two approaches of how researchers use the combination of the chemical properties of fluorescence and unique receptor patterns on cell surfaces to identify specific populations of stem cells. One approach for using markers as a research tool is with a technique known as fluorescence-activated cell sorting (FACS) (see Figure E.i.2.

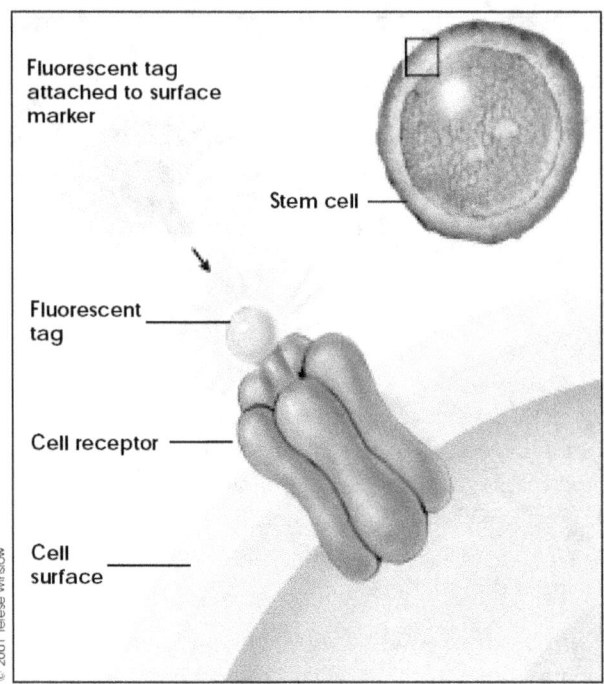

© 2001 Terese Winslow

Figure E.i.1. Identifying Cell Surface Markers Using Fluorescent Tags.

Looking for a Needle in a Haystack: How Researchers Find Stem Cells) [1, 3, 5]. Researchers often use a FACS instrument to sort out the rare stem cells from the millions of other cells. With this technique, a suspension of tagged cells (i.e., bound to the cell surface markers are fluorescent tags) is sent under pressure through a very narrow nozzle—so narrow that cells must pass through one at a time. Upon exiting the nozzle, cells then pass, one-by-one, through a light source, usually a laser, and then through an electric field. The fluorescent cells become negatively charged, while nonfluorescent cells become positively charged. The charge difference allows stem cells to be separated from other cells. The researchers now have a population of cells that have all of the same marker characteristics, and with these cells they can conduct their research.

A second method uses stem cell markers and their fluorescent tags to visually assess cells as they exist in tissues. Often researchers want to assess how stem cells appear in tissues and in doing so they use a microscope to evaluate them rather than the FACS instrument. In this case, a thin slice of tissue is prepared, and the stem cell markers are tagged by the signaling molecule that has the fluorescent tag attached. The fluorescent tags are then activated either by special light energy or a chemical reaction.

The stem cells will emit a fluorescent light that can easily be seen under the microscope.

Genetic and molecular biology techniques are extensively used to study how cells become specialized in the organism's development. In doing so, researchers have identified genes and transcription factors (proteins found within cells that regulate a gene's activity) that are unique in stem cells. Scientists use techniques such as polymerase chain reaction (PCR) to detect the presence of genes that are "active" and play a role guiding the specialization of a cell. This technique has is helpful to researchers to identify "genetic markers" that are characteristic of stem cells. For example, a gene marker called PDX-1 is specific for a transcription factor protein that initiates activation of the insulin gene. Researchers use this marker to identify cells that are able to develop islet cells in the pancreas.

Recently, researchers have applied a genetic engineering approach that uses fluorescence, but isn't dependent on cell surface markers. The importance of this new technique is that it allows the tracking of stem cells as they differentiate or become specialized. Scientists have inserted into a stem cell a "reporter gene" called green fluorescent protein or GFP [2]. The gene is only activated or "reports" when cells are undifferentiated and is turned off once they become specialized. Once activated, the gene directs the stem cells to produce a protein that fluoresces in a brilliant green color (see Figure Ei.3. Microscopic Image of Fluorescent-Labeled Stem Cell). Researchers are now coupling this reporting method with the FACS and microscopic methods described earlier to sort cells, identify them in tissues, and now, track them as they differentiate or become specialized.

These discovery tools are commonly used in research laboratories and clinics today, and will likely play important roles in advancing stem cell research. There are limitations, however. One of them is that a single marker identifying pluripotent stem cells, those stem cells that can make any other cell, has yet to be found. As new types of stem cells are identified and research applications of them become increasingly complex, more sophisticated tools will be developed to meet investigators' needs. For the foreseeable future, markers will continue to play a major role in the rapidly evolving world of stem cell biology.

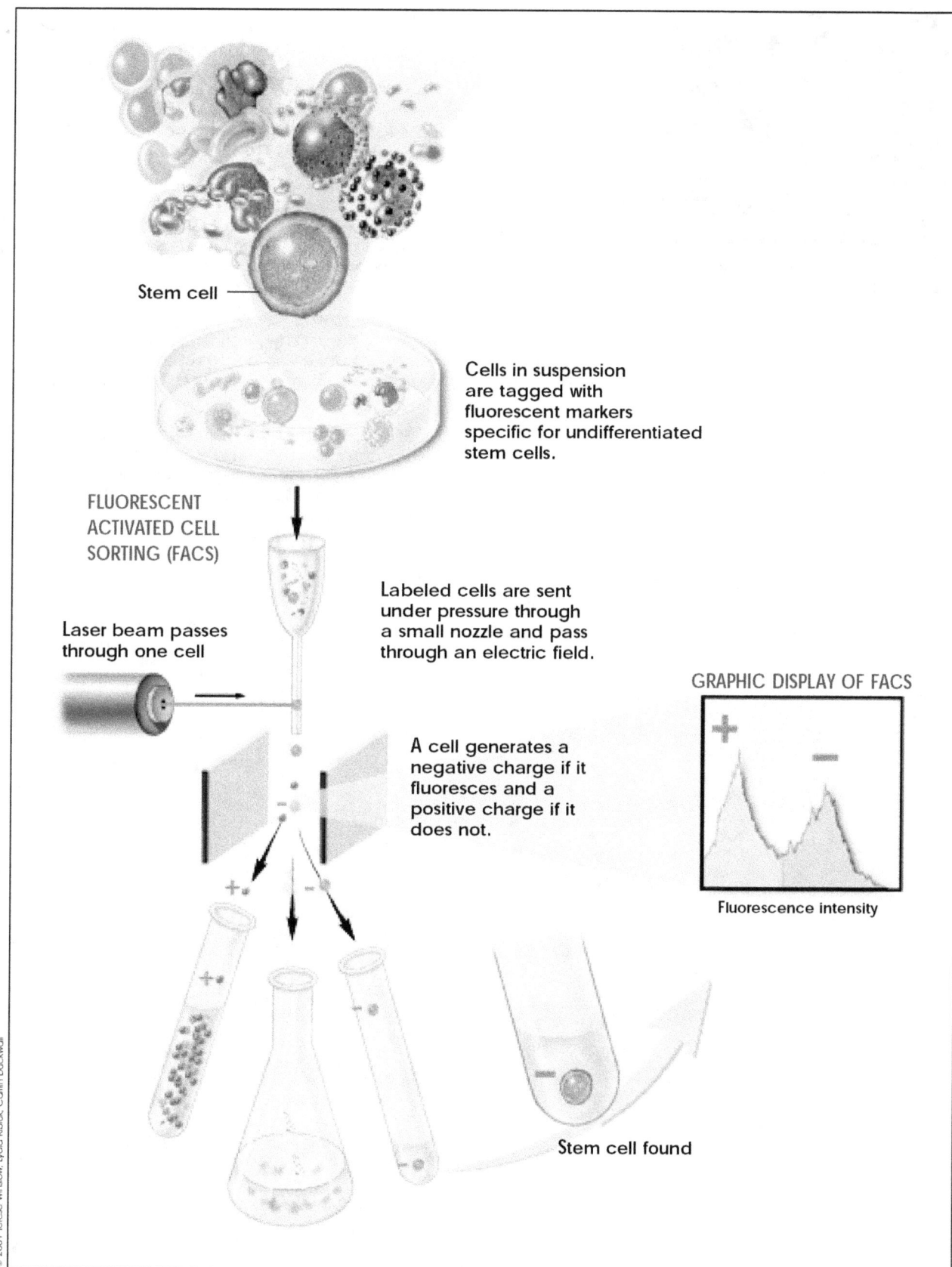

Stem cell

Cells in suspension
are tagged with
fluorescent markers
specific for undifferentiated
stem cells.

FLUORESCENT
ACTIVATED CELL
SORTING (FACS)

Labeled cells are sent
under pressure through
a small nozzle and pass
through an electric field.

Laser beam passes
through one cell

A cell generates a
negative charge if it
fluoresces and a
positive charge if it
does not.

GRAPHIC DISPLAY OF FACS

+

—

Fluorescence intensity

Stem cell found

Figure E.i.2. Looking for a Needle in a Haystack: How Researchers Find Stem Cells.

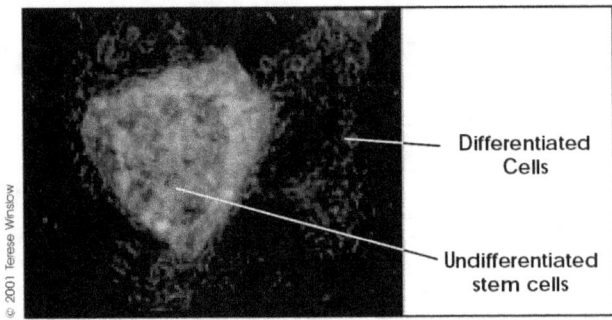

© 2001 Terese Winslow

Differentiated Cells

Undifferentiated stem cells

Figure E.i.3. Microscopic Image of Fluorescent-Labeled Stem Cell.

REFERENCES

1. Bonner, W.A., Hulett, H.R., Sweet, R.G., and Herzenberg, L.A. (1972). Fluorescence activated cell sorting. Rev. Sci. Instrum. *43*, 404-409.

2. Eiges, R., Schuldiner, M., Drukker, M., Yanuka, O., Itskovitz-Eldor, J., and Benvenisty, N. (2001). Establishment of human embryonic sten cell-transduced clones carrying a marker of undifferentiated cells. Curr. Biol. *11*, 514-518.

3. Herzenberg, L.A. and De Rosa, S.C. (2000). Monoclonal antibodies and the FACS: complementary tools for immunobiology and medicine. Immunol. Today. *21*, 383-390.

4. Jackson, K., Majka SM, Wang H, Pocius J, Hartley CJ, Majesky MW, Entman ML, Michael LH, Hirschi KK, and Goodell MA (2001). Regeneration of ischemic cardiac muscle and vascular endothelium by adult stem cells. J. Clin. Invest. *107*, 1-8.

5. Julius, M.H., Masuda, T., and Herzenberg, L.A. (1972). Demonstration that antigen-binding cells are precursors of antibody- producing cells after purification with a fluorescence-activated cell sorter. Proc. Natl. Acad. Sci. U. S. A. *69*, 1934-1938.

Appendix E.ii.
Markers Commonly Used to Identify Stem Cells
and to Characterize Differentiated Cell Types

Marker Name	Cell Type	Significance
Blood Vessel		
Fetal liver kinase-1 (Flk1)	Endothelial	Cell-surface receptor protein that identifies endothelial cell progenitor; marker of cell-cell contacts
Smooth muscle cell-specific myosin heavy chain	Smooth muscle	Identifies smooth muscle cells in the wall of blood vessels
Vascular endothelial cell cadherin	Smooth muscle	Identifies smooth muscle cells in the wall of blood vessels
Bone		
Bone-specific alkaline phosphatase (BAP)	Osteoblast	Enzyme expressed in osteoblast; activity indicates bone formation
Hydroxyapatite	Osteoblast	Minerlized bone matrix that provides structural integrity; marker of bone formation
Osteocalcin (OC)	Osteoblast	Mineral-binding protein uniquely synthesized by osteoblast; marker of bone formation
Bone Marrow and Blood		
Bone morphogenetic protein receptor (BMPR)	Mesenchymal stem and progenitor cells	Important for the differentiation of committed mesenchymal cell types from mesenchymal stem and progenitor cells; BMPR identifies early mesenchymal lineages (stem and progenitor cells)
CD4 and CD8	White blood cell (WBC)	Cell-surface protein markers specific for mature T lymphocyte (WBC subtype)
CD34	Hematopoietic stem cell (HSC), satellite, endothelial progenitor	Cell-surface protein on bone marrow cell, indicative of a HSC and endothelial progenitor; CD34 also identifies muscle satellite, a muscle stem cell
CD34$^+$Sca1$^+$ Lin$^-$ profile	Mesencyhmal stem cell (MSC)	Identifies MSCs, which can differentiate into adipocyte, osteocyte, chondrocyte, and myocyte

Appendix E.ii. *(cont.)*

Marker Name	Cell Type	Significance
	Bone Marrow and Blood cont.	
CD38	Absent on HSC Present on WBC lineages	Cell-surface molecule that identifies WBC lineages. Selection of CD34+/CD38- cells allows for purification of HSC populations
CD44	Mesenchymal	A type of cell-adhesion molecule used to identify specific types of mesenchymal cells
c-Kit	HSC, MSC	Cell-surface receptor on BM cell types that identifies HSC and MSC; binding by fetal calf serum (FCS) enhances proliferation of ES cells, HSCs, MSCs, and hematopoietic progenitor cells
Colony-forming unit (CFU)	HSC, MSC progenitor	CFU assay detects the ability of a single stem cell or progenitor cell to give rise to one or more cell lineages, such as red blood cell (RBC) and/or white blood cell (WBC) lineages
Fibroblast colony-forming unit (CFU-F)	Bone marrow fibroblast	An individual bone marrow cell that has given rise to a colony of multipotent fibroblastic cells; such identified cells are precursors of differentiated mesenchymal lineages
Hoechst dye	Absent on HSC	Fluorescent dye that binds DNA; HSC extrudes the dye and stains lightly compared with other cell types
Leukocyte common antigen (CD45)	WBC	Cell-surface protein on WBC progenitor
Lineage surface antigen (Lin)	HSC, MSC Differentiated RBC and WBC lineages	Thirteen to 14 different cell-surface proteins that are markers of mature blood cell lineages; detection of Lin-negative cells assists in the purification of HSC and hematopoietic progenitor populations
Mac-1	WBC	Cell-surface protein specific for mature granulocyte and macrophage (WBC subtypes)
Muc-18 (CD146)	Bone marrow fibroblasts, endothelial	Cell-surface protein (immunoglobulin superfamily) found on bone marrow fibroblasts, which may be important in hematopoiesis; a subpopulation of Muc-18+ cells are mesenchymal precursors

Appendix E.ii. (cont.)

Marker Name	Cell Type	Significance
	Bone Marrow and Blood cont.	
Stem cell antigen (Sca-1)	HSC, MSC	Cell-surface protein on bone marrow (BM) cell, indicative of HSC and MSC
Stro-1 antigen	Stromal (mesenchymal) precursor cells, hematopoietic cells	Cell-surface glycoprotein on subsets of bone marrow stromal (mesenchymal) cells; selection of Stro-1+ cells assists in isolating mesenchymal precursor cells, which are multipotent cells that give rise to adipocytes, osteocytes, smooth myocytes, fibroblasts, chondrocytes, and blood cells
Thy-1	HSC, MSC	Cell-surface protein; negative or low detection is suggestive of HSC
	Cartilage	
Collagen types II and IV	Chondrocyte	Structural proteins produced specifically by chondrocyte
Keratin	Keratinocyte	Principal protein of skin; identifies differentiated keratinocyte
Sulfated proteoglycan	Chondrocyte	Molecule found in connective tissues; synthesized by chondrocyte
	Fat	
Adipocyte lipid-binding protein (ALBP)	Adipocyte	Lipid-binding protein located specifically in adipocyte
Fatty acid transporter (FAT)	Adipocyte	Transport molecule located specifically in adipocyte
Adipocyte lipid-binding protein (ALBP)	Adipocyte	Lipid-binding protein located specifically in adipocyte
	General	
Y chromosome	Male cells	Male-specific chromosome used in labeling and detecting donor cells in female transplant recipients
Karyotype	Most cell types	Analysis of chromosome structure and number in a cell

Appendix E.ii. *(cont.)*

Marker Name	Cell Type	Significance
		Liver
Albumin	Hepatocyte	Principal protein produced by the liver; indicates functioning of maturing and fully differentiated hepatocytes
B-1 integrin	Hepatocyte	Cell-adhesion molecule important in cell-cell interactions; marker expressed during development of liver
		Nervous System
CD133	Neural stem cell, HSC	Cell-surface protein that identifies neural stem cells, which give rise to neurons and glial cells
Glial fibrillary acidic protein (GFAP)	Astrocyte	Protein specifically produced by astrocyte
Microtubule-associated protein-2 (MAP-2)	Neuron	Dendrite-specific MAP; protein found specifically in dendritic branching of neuron
Myelin basic protein (MPB)	Oligodendrocyte	Protein produced by mature oligodendrocytes; located in the myelin sheath surrounding neuronal structures
Nestin	Neural progenitor	Intermediate filament structural protein expressed in primitive neural tissue
Neural tubulin	Neuron	Important structural protein for neuron; identifies differentiated neuron
Neurofilament (NF)	Neuron	Important structural protein for neuron; identifies differentiated neuron
Neurosphere	Embryoid body (EB), ES	Cluster of primitive neural cells in culture of differentiating ES cells; indicates presence of early neurons and glia
Noggin	Neuron	A neuron-specific gene expressed during the development of neurons
O4	Oligodendrocyte	Cell-surface marker on immature, developing oligodendrocyte
O1	Oligodendrocyte	Cell-surface marker that characterizes mature oligodendrocyte

Appendix E.ii. *(cont.)*

Marker Name	Cell Type	Significance
	Nervous System cont.	
Synaptophysin	Neuron	Neuronal protein located in synapses; indicates connections between neurons
Tau	Neuron	Type of MAP; helps maintain structure of the axon
	Pancreas	
Cytokeratin 19 (CK19)	Pancreatic epithelium	CK19 identifies specific pancreatic epithelial cells that are progenitors for islet cells and ductal cells
Glucagon	Pancreatic islet	Expressed by alpha-islet cell of pancreas
Insulin	Pancreatic islet	Expressed by beta-islet cell of pancreas
Insulin-promoting factor-1 (PDX-1)	Pancreatic islet	Transcription factor expressed by beta-islet cell of pancreas
Nestin	Pancreatic progenitor	Structural filament protein indicative of progenitor cell lines including pancreatic
Pancreatic polypeptide	Pancreatic islet	Expressed by gamma-islet cell of pancreas
Somatostatin	Pancreatic islet	Expressed by delta-islet cell of pancreas
	Pluripotent Stem Cells	
Alkaline phosphatase	Embryonic stem (ES), embryonal carcinoma (EC)	Elevated expression of this enzyme is associated with undifferentiated pluripotent stem cell (PSC)
Alpha-fetoprotein (AFP)	Endoderm	Protein expressed during development of primitive endoderm; reflects endodermal differentiation
Bone morphogenetic protein-4	Mesoderm	Growth and differentiation factor expressed during early mesoderm formation and differentiation
Brachyury	Mesoderm	Transcription factor important in the earliest phases of mesoderm formation and differentiation; used as the earliest indicator of mesoderm formation

Appendix E.ii. *(cont.)*

Marker Name	Cell Type	Significance
Pluripotent Stem Cells cont.		
Cluster designation 30 (CD30)	ES, EC	Surface receptor molecule found specifically on PSC
Cripto (TDGF-1)	ES, cardiomyocyte	Gene for growth factor expressed by ES cells, primitive ectoderm, and developing cardiomyocyte
GATA-4 gene	Endoderm	Expression increases as ES differentiates into endoderm
GCTM-2	ES, EC	Antibody to a specific extracellular-matrix molecule that is synthesized by undifferentiated PSCs
Genesis	ES, EC	Transcription factor uniquely expressed by ES cells either in or during the undifferentiated state of PSCs
Germ cell nuclear factor	ES, EC	Transcription factor expressed by PSCs
Hepatocyte nuclear factor-4 (HNF-4)	Endoderm	Transcription factor expressed early in endoderm formation
Nestin	Ectoderm, neural and pancreatic progenitor	Intermediate filaments within cells; characteristic of primitive neuroectoderm formation
Neuronal cell-adhesion molecule (N-CAM)	Ectoderm	Cell-surface molecule that promotes cell-cell interaction; indicates primitive neuroectoderm formation
Oct-4	ES, EC	Transcription factor unique to PSCs; essential for establishment and maintenance of undifferentiated PSCs
Pax6	Ectoderm	Transcription factor expressed as ES cell differentiates into neuroepithelium
Stage-specific embryonic antigen-3 (SSEA-3)	ES, EC	Glycoprotein specifically expressed in early embryonic development and by undifferentiated PSCs
Stage-specific embryonic antigen-4 (SSEA-4)	ES, EC	Glycoprotein specifically expressed in early embryonic development and by undifferentiated PSCs

Appendix E.ii. *(cont.)*

Marker Name	Cell Type	Significance
Pluripotent Stem Cells cont.		
Stem cell factor (SCF or c-Kit ligand)	ES, EC, HSC, MSC	Membrane protein that enhances proliferation of ES and EC cells, hematopoietic stem cell (HSCs), and mesenchymal stem cells (MSCs); binds the receptor c-Kit
Telomerase	ES, EC	An enzyme uniquely associated with immortal cell lines; useful for identifying undifferentiated PSCs
TRA-1-60	ES, EC	Antibody to a specific extracellular matrix molecule is synthesized by undifferentiated PSCs
TRA-1-81	ES, EC	Antibody to a specific extracellular matrix molecule normally synthesized by undifferentiated PSCs
Vimentin	Ectoderm, neural and pancreatic progenitor	Intermediate filaments within cells; characteristic of primitive neuroectoderm formation
Skeletal Muscle/Cardiac/Smooth Muscle		
MyoD and Pax7	Myoblast, myocyte	Transcription factors that direct differentiation of myoblasts into mature myocytes
Myogenin and MR4	Skeletal myocyte	Secondary transcription factors required for differentiation of myoblasts from muscle stem cells
Myosin heavy chain	Cardiomyocyte	A component of structural and contractile protein found in cardiomyocyte
Myosin light chain	Skeletal myocyte	A component of structural and contractile protein found in skeletal myocyte

This page intentionally left blank

APPENDIX F:

GLOSSARY AND TERMS

Appendix F.i.

GLOSSARY

Adipocyte – Fat cell.

Adult stem cell – An undifferentiated cell found in a differentiated tissue that can renew itself and (with certain limitations) differentiate to yield all the specialized cell types of the tissue from which it originated.

Allogenic – Two or more individuals (or cell lines) are stated to be allogeneic to one another when the genes at one or more loci are not identical in sequence in each organism.

Amnion – The innermost intrauterine membrane around the fetus and the amniotic fluid.

Anterior visceral endoderm (AVE) – Specific tissue structure arising in the early embryo that helps establish the anterior-posterior axis of the organism.

Antibody – A Y-shaped protein secreted by B cells in response to an antigen. An antibody binds specifically to the antigen that induced its production. Antibodies directed against antigens on the surface of infectious organisms help eliminate those organisms from the body.

Antigen – A substance (often a protein) that induces the formation of an antibody. Antigens are commonly found on the surface of infectious organisms, transfused blood cells, and transplanted organs.

Antigen presenting cells (APCs) – One of a variety of cells within the body that can process antigens and display them on their surface in a form recognizable by T cells.

Apoptosis – Genetically programmed cell death.

Astrocyte – One of the large neuroglia cells of nervous tissue.

Autoantibody – An antibody that reacts with antigens found on the cells and tissues of an individual's ownbody. Autoantibodies can cause autoimmune diseases.

Autoimmune disease – A condition that results from T cells and/or antibodies that attack the cells or tissues of an individual's own body.

Autologous transplant – Transplanted tissue derived from the intended recipient of the transplant. Such a transplant helps avoid complications of immune rejection.

Axis – A straight line passing through a spherical body between its two poles. The central line of the body or any of its parts. The vertebral column. The central nervous system. An artery that when created, immediately divides into a number of branches.

B cells – Also known as B lymphocytes. Each B cell is capable of making one specific antibody. When stimulated by antigen and helper T cells, B cells mature into plasma cells that secrete large amounts of their specific antibody.

Blastocoel – The cavity in the blastula of the developing embryo.

Blastocyst – A preimplantation embryo of 30-150 cells. The blastocyst consists of a sphere made up of an outer layer of cells (the trophectoderm), a fluid-filled cavity (the blastocoel), and a cluster of cells on the interior (the inner cell mass).

Blastula – An early stage in the development of an ovum consisting of a hollow sphere of cells enclosing a cavity called the blastocoel.

Bone marrow – The soft, living tissue that fills most bone cavities and contains hematopoietic stem cells, from which all red and white blood cells evolve. The bone marrow also contains mesenchymal stem cells that a number of cells types come from, including chondrocytes, which produce cartilage.

Bone marrow (BM) cell – Refers to both hematopoietic and mesenchymal (stromal) cells.

Bone marrow stem cell (BMSC) – One of at least two types of multipotient stem cells: hematopoietic stem cell and mesenchymal stem cell.

Bone marrow transplantation (BMTx) – Trans-plantation of bone marrow from one individual to another. Autologous BMTx is a process in which a patient's healthy bone marrow is withdrawn and preserved, then injected back into the patient to restore the production of healthy blood and immune cells by the bone marrow. This strategy is often used in patients with certain types of cancer who have undergone radiation therapy or chemotherapy that destroys the bone marrow cells.

Bone morphogenetic proteins (BMPs) – Proteins thatare involved in the formation of embryonic bone. BMPs operate at several stages in this formation of bone, beginning with the early stages of morpho-genesis and continuing to late postnatal life. BMPs also play a critical role in the development of the central nervous system.

Brain-derived neurotrophic factor (BDNF) – A growth factor synthesized in the brain that stimulates neurite outgrowth and supports survival of neurons.

Cavitation – A process that occurs during the forma-tion of the blastocyst and establishes the polarity of embryonic cells.

Cell cycle – The orderly sequence of events by which the cell duplicates its contents and divides into two.

Chimera – An organism composed of cells derived from at least two genetically different zygotes. Theoretically, the zygote could be from separate species.

Chondrocytes – Cartilage cells.

Chorion – The multilayered, outermost fetal membrane. As pregnancy progresses, part of the chorion becomes the placenta.

Chromosomes – Nucleic acid-protein structures in the nucleus of a cell. Chromosomes are composed chiefly of DNA, the carrier of hereditary information. Chromosomes contain genes, working subunits of DNA that carry the genetic code for specific proteins, interspersed with large amounts of DNA of unknown function. A normal human body cell contains 46 chromosomes; a normal human gamete, 23 chromosomes.

Cleavage – The process of cell division in the very early embryo before it becomes a blastocyst.

Clonality – A line of cells that is genetically identical to the originating cell; in this case, a stem cell.

Cluster differentiation (CD) – Cell membrane molecules used to classify leukocytes into subsets.

Colony-forming cells – Groups of cells growing on a solid nutrient surface with each group being created from the multiplication of an individual cell.

Colony-stimulating factors – Diffusible proteins that stimulate the proliferation of hematopoietic stem cells.

Cripto – Transcription factor expressed by pluripotent stem cells and early embryos.

Cyclin-dependent kinase (Cdk protein) – Protein kinase that has to be complexed with a cyclin protein in order to act; different Cdk-cyclin complexes are thought to trigger different steps in the cell-division cycle by phosphorylating specific target proteins.

Cytokines – A generic term for a large variety of regulatory proteins produced and secreted by cells and used to communicate with other cells. One class ofcytokines is the interleukins, which act as inter-cellular mediators during the generation of an immune response.

Cytoplasm – The contents of a cell other than the nucleus; cytoplasm consists of a fluid containing numerous structures, known as organelles, that carry out essential cell functions.

Decidual cells – A cellular matrix that first surrounds an implanted embryo and later occupies most of the endometrium.

Dendrite – Extension of a nerve cell, typically branched and relatively short, that receives stimuli from other nerve cells.

Differentiation – The process whereby an unspecialized early embryonic cell acquires the features of a specialized cell such as a heart, liver, or muscle cell.

Diploid – A cell or tissue having two chromosome sets, as opposed to the haploid situation of gametes, which have only one chromosome set.

DNA – Deoxyribonucleic acid, a chemical found primarily in the nucleus of cells. DNA carries the instructions for making all the structures and materials the body needs to function.

DNA methylation – A type of chemical modification of DNA that regulates gene expression.

Ectoderm – The upper, outermost of the three primitive germ layers of the embryo; it gives rise to skin, nerves, and brain.

Egg cylinder – An asymmetric embryonic structure that helps to determine the body plan of the mouse.

Embryo – In humans, the developing organism from the time of fertilization until the end of the eighth week of gestation, when it becomes known as a fetus.

Embryoid bodies (EBs) – Clumps of cellular structures that arise when embryonic stem cells are cultured. Embryoid bodies contain tissue from all three of the germ layers: endoderm, mesoderm, and ectoderm. Embryoid bodies are not part of normal development and occur only in in vitro conditions.

Embryonal carcinoma (EC) cells – A type of pluripotent stem cell derived from teratocarcinoma (usually a testis tumor).

Embryonic disk – A group of cells derived from the inner cell mass of the blastocyst, which later develops into an embryo. The disc consists of three germ layers known as the endoderm, mesoderm, and ectoderm.

Embryonic germ (EG) cells – Cells found in a specific part of the embryo/fetus called the gonadal ridge that normally develop into mature gametes.

Embryonic stem (ES) cells – Primitive (undifferentiated) cells from the embryo that have the potential to become a wide variety of specialized cell types.

Endoderm – Lower layer of a group of cells derived from the inner cell mass of the blastocyst; it later becomes the lungs and digestive organs.

Epiblast – Gives rise to the ectoderm and mesoderm. The mesoderm then displaces the hypoblast cells and forms the entodermal cell layer on its inner surface.

Epidermal growth factor (EGF) – A protein that stimulates epidermal and various other cells to divide.

Epithelium – The layer of cells forming the epidermis of the skin. These cells serve the general functions of protection, absorption, and secretion, and play a specialized role in moving substances through ducts, in the production of germ cells, and in the reception of stimuli. Their ability to regenerate is excellent; the epithelium may replace itself as frequently as every 24 hours.

Erythroid cell – Red blood cells.

Ex vivo – Outside the living body.

Extracellular matrix – The microenvironment next to a cell that allows for structural support, orientation, and connections for cell-to-cell interactions and formation of connective tissues.

Extraembryonic tissues – Intrauterine tissues that support the embryo's placenta, umbilical cord, and amniotic sac.

Feeder cell layer – Cells that are utilized in co-culture to maintain pluripotent stem cells. Cells usually consist of mouse embryonic fibroblasts.

Fertilization – The process whereby male and female gametes unite.

Fetal calf serum – A type of culture medium often used in the culture of stem cells. It provides a number of growth factors.

Fibroblast – Cells that give rise to connective tissue.

Fluorescence-activated cell sorting (FACS) – A technique that can separate and analyze cells, which are labeled with fluorochrome-conjugated antibody, by their fluorescence and light scattering patterns.

Follistatin – An inhibitory factor produced during embryonic development that affects the growth and differentiation of the pancreas.

Gap junctions – Communicating cell-cell junctions that allow ions and small molecules to pass from the cytoplasm of one cell to the cytoplasm of another cell.

Gastrula – Animal embryo at an early stage of development in which cells are enclosed in a sheath to form the beginning of a gut cavity.

Gene – A functional unit of heredity that is a segment of DNA located in a specific site on a chromosome. A gene Directs the formation of an enzyme of other protein.

Genital Ridge – Formation of a genital ridge requires at least two genes, *WT-1*, which is also important in early kidney formation, and *SF-1*, required for the development of both the gonads and adrenal glands.

Genome – The complete genetic material of an organism.

Genomic imprinting – A biochemical phenomenon that determines, for certain specific genes, which one of the pair of identical genes, the motheris or the fatheris, will be active in that individual.

Germ cell – A sperm or egg, or a cell that can become a sperm or egg. All other body cells are called somatic cells.

Gestation – The period of development of an organism from fertilization of the ovum until birth.

Glia – The nonneuronal or supporting tissue (neuroglia) of the brain and spinal cord.

Glial cells – Supporting cells of the nervous system, including oligodendrocytes and astrocytes in the vertebrate central nervous system and Schwann cells in the peripheral nervous system.

Glial fibrillary acidic protein (GFAP) – A structural protein specifically produced by astrocytes. GFAP is often used as a marker of astrocytes.

Glucagon – A hormone consisting of a straight chain of proteins composed of 29 amino acid residues that can be extracted from certain pancreatic cells.

Glycoprotein – A compound consisting of a carbohydrate and a protein.

Gonadal ridge –Anatomic site in the early fetus where primordial germ cells (PGCs) are formed.

Gonads – The embryonic sex gland before it becomes a definitive testis or ovary.

Goosecoid – Gene that encodes a transcription factor that is important for determining craniofacial orientation and features in the vertebrate embryo.

Graft-versus-host disease (GVHD) – A condition that occurs following bone marrow transplantation in which the donor-derived T cells attack the host's tissues.

Granulocyte – A type of white blood cell filled with microscopic granules that are little sacs containing enzymes, compounds that digest microorganisms. Neutrophils, eosinophils and basophils are all types of granulocytes. They are named by the staining features of their granules in the laboratory.

Granulose cells – Cells surrounding and maintaining the ovarian follicle.

Green fluorescent protein (GFP) – Fluorescent-protein dye used to tag and trace particular genes and cells of interest.

Hanging drop method – A technique used to culture embryonic stem cells so that they develop into embryoid bodies.

Haploid – Refers to a gamete having one chromosome set, as opposed to the diploid situation of cells or tissues, where there are two chromosome sets.

hCNS – Human central nervous system stem cell.

Hematopoiesis – Generation of blood cells, mainly in the bone marrow.

Hematopoietic stem cell (HSC)– A stem cell from which all red and white blood cells evolve.

Hepatic – Relating to the liver.

Hepatocyte – Liver cell.

hES cell – Human embryonic stem cell; a type of pluripotent stem cell.

Hoechst dye – A dye used to identify hematopoietic stem cells (HSCs).

Hox genes – Consists of at least 38 encoded nucleotides that contain genes found in four clusters on four different chromosomes. An important function of hox genes in blood is the regulation of cell proliferation.

HSC markers – Cell-surface molecules that are used to identify hematopoietic stem cells.

Hybridoma – A hybrid cell produced by the fusion of an antibody-producing cell and a multiple myeloma cell. The cell has the capability to produce a continuous supply of identical antibodies.

Hydroxyapatite – A natural mineral structure that contains calcium and phosphate ions that provide the power for the formation of bones and teeth.

Hypoblast – The inner cell layer, or endoderm, which develops during the formation of the embryonic germ layers.

Identical twinning – Process in which genetically identical organisms arise from symmetrical division and separation of totipotent cells.

Immune-function assay – A general term for a number of tests based on an immune cell's ability to carry out a particular immune function.

Immune system cells – White blood cells or leukocytes that originate from the bone marrow. They include antigen presenting cells, such as dendritic cells, T and B lymphocytes, and neutrophils, among many others.

Immunocompromised mice – These genetically altered mice are used for transplantation experiments because they usually do not reject the transplanted tissue.

Immunofluorescence – The detection of antibodies by using special proteins labeled with fluorescein. When present, the specific organism or antibody is observed as a fluorescent material when examined microscopically while illuminated with a fluorescent light source.

Immunogenic – Relating to or producing an immune response.

Immunohistology – Examination of tissues through specific immunostaining techniques.

Immunophenotyping – Identification of various types of immune cells by sorting them according to their cell-surface markers.

In utero – In the uterus.

In vitro – Literally, "in glass;" in a laboratory dish or test tube; an artificial environment.

In vitro fertilization (IVF) – An assisted reproduction technique in which fertilization is accomplished outside the body.

In vivo – In the living subject; in a natural environment.

Indomethacin – An anti-inflammatory, antipain, and antifever drug. Its primary use is in rheumatoid arthritis and degenerative joint disease when aspirin-based products are ineffective or cannot be tolerated.

Inner cell mass – The cluster of cells inside the blastocyst. These cells give rise to the embryonic disk of the later embryo and, ultimately, the fetus.

Insulin-promoting factor 1 – A transcription factor expressed in the pancreas and necessary for the production of insulin.

Interleukin – Selected peptide or protein that primarily mediates local interactions between white blood cells.

Irradiate – Application of radiation from a source (heat, light, Xrays) to a structure or organism.

Karyotype – The full set of chromosomes of a cell arranged with respect to size, shape, and number.

Keratin –An extremely tough protein substance found in hair, nails, skin, and cornea.

Keratinocytes – Cells that synthesize keratin and are found in the skin, hair, and nails. A fibrous protein is produced by keratinocytes and may be hard or soft. The hard keratin is found in hair and nails. The soft keratin is found in the epidermis of the skin in the form of flattened non-nucleated scales that slough continually.

Knock-out mouse – A mouse that has had one or both copies of a specific gene deleted or inactivated.

Lacunae – The spaces occupied by cells (e.g., chondrocytes and osteocytes) of calcified tissues.

Lefty – A developmental factor that helps determine right-left asymmetry in vertebrates.

Leptin –A hormone produced by the placenta and fetal tissues that acts as a growth factor and modulator of metabolic and immune functions.

Leukemia inhibitory factor (LIF) – A growth factor necessary for maintaining mouse embryonic stem cells in a proliferative, undifferentiated state.

Leukocyte – A white blood cell or corpuscle. Leukocytes are formed from undifferentiated stem cells that give rise to all blood cells.

Leukocyte common antigen – Cell-surface molecule found on white blood cells and white blood cell progenitors. Also referred to as CD45.

Lineage surface antigen (Lin) – A mixture of monoclonal antibodies that are directed against antigens found on mature hematopoietic cells of different lineages. A usual Lin mix includes eight different antibodies directed against B and T cells, myeloid cells, and erythroid cells.

Lipase – An enzyme produced by many tissues. Lipase is an important regulator of fat in the blood. A deficiency of this enzyme leads to low levels of high-density lipoproteins (HDLs).

Lipid – Any one of a group of fats or fatlike substances characterized by their insolubility in water and solubility in fat solvents such as alcohol, ether, and chloroform.

Lymph nodes – Widely distributed lymphoid organs within the lymphatic system where many immune cells are concentrated.

Lymphatic system – A network of lymph vessels and nodes that drain and filter antigens from tissue fluids before returning lymphocytes to the blood.

Lymphocyte – A cell present in the blood and lymphatic tissue.

Lymphoid – A shape or form that resembles lymph or lymph tissue.

Macrophage – A monocyte that has left the circulation and settled and matured in a tissue. Because of their placement in the lymphoid tissues, macrophages serve as the major scavenger of the blood, clearing it of abnormal or old cells and cellular debris as well as pathogenic organisms.

Major histocompatibility complex (MHC) – A group of genes that code for cell-surface histocompatibility antigens. These antigens are the primary reason why organ and tissue transplants from incompatible donors fail.

Marker – See Surface marker.

Mast cell – A large tissue cell that does not circulate in the blood. They are also important in producing the signs and symptoms of hypersensitivity reaction, such as those of an insect sting, and certain forms of asthma.

Maternal gene product – A product in the male organism of a gene from the X chromosome.

Meiosis – A process where two successive cells divide and produce cells, eggs, or sperm that contain half the number of chromosomes in the somatic cells. During fertilization, the nuclei of the sperm and ovum fuse and produce a zygote with the full chromosome complements.

Melanocyte – A cell that produces the dark pigment melanin; responsible for the pigmentation of skin and hair.

Memory – The ability of antigen-specific T or B cells to "recall" prior exposure to an antigen and respond quickly without the need to be activated again by CD4 helper T cells.

Memory cells – A subset of antigen-specific T or B cells that "recall" prior exposure to an antigen and respond quickly without the need to be activated again by CD4 helper T cells.

Mesenchymal stem cells (MSCs) – Cells from the immature embryonic connective tissue. A number of cell types come from mesenchymal stem cells, including chondrocytes, which produce cartilage.

Mesoderm – The middle layer of the embryonic disk, which consists of a group of cells derived from the inner cell mass of the blastocyst. This middle germ layer is known as gastrulation and is the precursor to bone, muscle, and connective tissue.

Metaphase – A stage of mitosis where chromosomes are firmly attached to the mitotic spindle at its equator but have not yet segregated toward opposite poles.

Microtubule – An elongated, hollow tubular structure present in the cell. Microtubules help certain cells maintain their rigidity, convert chemical energy into work, and provide a means of transportation of substances in different directions within a cell.

Monoclonal – From a single cell.

Monoclonal antibody (MoAb) – An exceptionally pure and specific antibody derived from hybridoma cells. Because each of the clones is derived from a single B cell, all of the antibody molecules it makes are identical.

Monocyte – A white blood cell derived from myeloid stem cells.

Mononucleocyte – A cell containing a single nucleus. Generally refers to a white blood cell.

Morphology – The shape and structural makeup of a cell, tissue, or organism.

Morula – A solid mass of cells that resembles a mulberry and result from the cleavage of an ovum.

Mouse embryonic fibroblast (MEF) – Mouse embryonic fibroblast cells are used as feeder cells when culturing pluripotent stem cells.

Multipotent stem cells – Stem cells that have the capability of developing cells of multiple germ layers.

Myelin – A fatty sheath that covers axons of nerve cells. It is produced by oligodendrocytes and provides an insulation for nerve conduction through the axons.

Myelin basic protein (MPB) – A structural protein within the myelin sheath surrounding neurons.

Myelin sheath – Insulating layer of specialized cell membrane wrapped around vertebrate axons. This sheath is produced by oligodendrocytes in the central nervous system and by Schwann cells in the peripheral nervous system.

Myeloid – Marrow-like, but not necessarily originating from bone marrow.

Myeloid stem cells – Precursors to the other lines of blood cells: erythrocytes, granulocytes, monocytes, and platelets. The second-generation cells are still pluripotent but their developmental potency is limited because neither can form an offspring of the other type.

Myocyte – A muscular tissue cell.

MyoD1 – A group of four basic myogenic regulatory factors (helix-loop-helix transcription) and a newly discovered factor called muscle enhancer factor-2 which appears to work away from the other three factors. However, all four of the factors in this MyoD family have the capacity of converting nonmuscle cells into cells expressing the full range of muscle proteins.

Myosin – A protein in muscle fibers.

Myosin light chain – There are four light chain subunits containing complex molecules that form contractile units in skeletal muscle.

Nestin – An intermediate filament protein found in cells such as neural and pancreatic precursors.

Neural crest – A band of cells that extend lengthwise along the neural tube of an embryo and give rise to cells that form the cranial, spinal, and autonomic ganglia, as well as becoming odontoblasts, which form the calcified part of the teeth.

Neural plate – A thickened band of ectoderm along the dorsal surface of an embryo. The nervous system develops from this tissue.

Neural stem cell (NSC) – A stem cell found in adult neural tissue that can give rise to neurons, astrocytes, and oligodendrocytes.

Neural tube – The embryological forerunner of the central nervous system.

Neuroectoderm – The central region of the early embryonic ectoderm, which later forms the brain and spinal cord, as well as evolving into nerve cells of the peripheral nervous system

Neuroepithelium – A specialized epithelial structure that forms the termination of a nerve of a special sense, i.e., olfactory cells, hair cells of the inner ear, and the rods and cones of the retina. It is the embryonic layer of the epiblast that develops into the cerebrospinal axis.

Neurofilament (NF) – A type of intermediate filament found in nerve cells.

Neuron – A nerve cell, the structural and functional unit of the nervous system. A neuron consists of a cell body and its processes, an axon, and one or more dendrites. Neurons function by the initiation and conduction of impulses and transmit impulses to other neurons or cells by releasing neurotransmitters at synapses.

Neurosphere –A primitive neural tissue that arises when embryonic stem cells are grown in certain culture conditions.

NMDA receptor – (*N*-methyl-d-aspartate receptor). A neurotransmitter receptor for excitatory synapses.

Nodal – A knob-like protrusion.

Node – A knot, knob; a protrusion or swelling; a constricted region; a small, rounded organ or structure.

Notochord – Forms the axial skeleton in embryos of all chordates. In vertebrates, it is replaced partially or completely by vertebrae.

Oligodendrocyte – Cell that provides insulation to nerve cells by forming a myelin sheath around axons.

Oocyte – Developing egg; usually a large and immobile cell.

Osteocalcin (OC) – A cytokine produced by osteoblasts that promotes bone formation.

Osteoclast – A giant multi-nuclear cell formed in the bone marrow of growing bones.

Osteocyte – A cell from the bone tissue.

Osteoprogenitor – A cell-type that differentiates into a mature osteocyte.

Ovarian follicle – An external, fluid-filled portion of the ovary in which oocytes mature before ovulation.

Oviduct – The passage through which the ova travel from the ovary into the uterus.

Pancreatic polypeptide – An endocrine protein produced by islet cells of the pancreas.

Paracrine factors – Cytokines or hormones that act on cells or tissues within an extremely limited area.

Passage – A round of cell growth and proliferation in culture.

Placenta – The oval or discoid spongy structure in the uterus from which the fetus derives its nourishment and oxygen.

Plasticity – The ability of stem cells from one adult tissue to generate the differentiated types of another tissue.

Pluripotent stem cell (PSC) – A single stem cell that has the capability of developing cells of all germ layers (endoderm, ectoderm, and mesoderm).

Polarity – The presence of an axial, non symmetric gradient along a cell or tissue.

Population doublings – A doubling in the number of cells when grown in culture.

Precursor Cells – In fetal or adult tissues, these are partly differentiated cells that divide and give rise to differentiated cells.Also known as progenitor cells.

Pre-implantation embryo – The very early, free-floating Embryo, from the time the egg is fertilized until implantation in the mother's womb is complete.

Primary germ layers – The three initial embryonic germ layers–endoderm, mesoderm, and ectoderm–from which all other somatic tissue-types develop.

Primitive streak – The initial band of cells from which the embryo begins to develop. The primitive streak establishes and reveals the embryo's head-tail and left-right orientations.

Radioimmunoassay – A sensitive method of determining the concentration of a substance, particularly a protein-bound hormone, in blood plasma.

Retinoic acid – A metabolite of vitamin A.

Ribonucleic acid (RNA) – A chemical that is similar in structure to DNA. One of its main functions is to translate the genetic code of DNA into structural proteins.

Ribosome – Any of the RNA- and protein-rich cytoplasmic organelles that are sites of protein synthesis.

Schwann cell – In the embryo, Schwann cells grow around the nerve fiber, forming concentric layers of cell membrane (the myelin sheath).

Side population (SP) stem cell – Two examples of multipotent stem cell populations found in bone marrow and skeletal muscle. SPs are not yet fully characterized. Their significance is their unexpected ability to differentiate into cell types that are distinct from their tissue of origin.

Signal transduction pathways – Relay of a signal by the conversion from one physical or chemical form to another. In cell biology, signal transduction is the process in which a cell converts an extracellular signal into a response.

Somatic cell nuclear transfer – The transfer of a cell nucleus from a somatic cell into an egg from which the nucleus has been removed.

Somatic cells – Any cell of a plant or animal other than a germ cell or germ cell precursor.

Somatostatin – A hormone that inhibits the secretion of insulin and gastrin.

Steel factor – See stem cell factor.

Stem cell – A cell that has the ability to divide for indefinite periods in culture and to give rise to specialized cells.

Stem cell antigen 1 (Sca-1) – Cell-surface protein on bone marrow cell, indicative of hematopoietic stem cells and mesenchymal stem cells.

Stem cell factor (SCF) – Relatively undifferentiated cell that can continue dividing indefinitely, throwing off daughter cells that can undergo terminal differentiation into particular cell types. (Also known as steel factor).

Stromal cell – A non-blood cell that is derived from blood organs, such as bone marrow or fetal liver, which is capable of supporting growth of blood cells in vitro. Stromal cells that make this matrix within the bone marrow are also derived from mesenchymal stem cells.

Sulfated proteoglycan – Molecules found primarily in connective tissues and joint fluids and that provide lubrication.

Surface marker – Surface proteins that are unique to certain cell types capable of detection by antibodies or other detection methods.

Syncytiotrophoblast – A multinucleated cell formed from the cells of the trophoblast. Only a small area of the syncytiotrophoblast is evident at the start of the formation of the embryo, but this cell tissue is highly invasive, quickly expands and soon surrounds the entire embryo.

Syncytium – A mass of cytoplasm containing many nuclei that are enclosed by a single plasma membrane. This is usually the result of either cell fusion or a series of incomplete division cycles in which the nuclei divide but the cell does not.

T cells – A type of white blood cell that is of crucial importance to the immune system. Immature T cells migrate to the thymus gland in the upper chest cavity, where they mature and differentiate into various types of mature T cells and become active in the immune system in response to a hormone called thymosin and other factors. T-cells that are potentially activated against the body's own tissues are normally killed or changed ("down-regulated") during this maturation process.

Telomerase – An enzyme that is composed of a catalytic protein component and an RNA template and that synthesizes DNA at the ends of chromosomes and confers replicative immortality to cells.

Telomere – The end of a chromosome, associated with a characteristic DNA sequence that is replicated in a special way. A telomere counteracts the tendency of the chromosome to shorten with each round of replication.

Tenocyte – Tendon-producing cell.

Teratocarcinoma – A tumor that occurs mostly in the testis.

Teratogen – A drug or other agent that raises the incidence of congenital malformations.

Teratoma – A tumor composed of tissues from the three embryonic germ layers. Usually found in ovary and testis. Produced experimentally in animals by injecting pluripotent stem cells, in order to determine the stem cells' abilities to differentiate into various types of tissues.

Thiazolidinediones – A class of antidiabetes drugs that enhances the activity of insulin.

Thrombopoietin – Growth factor for the proliferation and differentiation of platelet forming cells called megakaryocytes.

Thymus – A lymphoid organ located in the upper chest cavity. Maturing T cells go directly to the thymus, where they are "educated" to discriminate between self and foreign proteins. (See tolerance induction.)

Tissue culture – Growth of tissue in vitro on an artificial medium for experimental research.

Tolerance – A state of specific immunologic unre-ponsiveness. Individuals are normally tolerant to their own cells and tissues. Autoimmune diseases occur when tolerance fails.

Tolerance induction – The "education" process that T cells undergo to discriminate between self and foreign proteins. This process takes place primarily in the thymus. In addition to inactivating or deleting self-reactive T cells, those T cells that can recognize the body's MHC proteins, but not be activated solely by this recognition, are also selected to leave the thymus (circulate through the body).

Totipotent – Having unlimited capability. The totipotent cells of the very early embryo have the capacity to differentiate into extra embryonic membranes and tissues, the embryo, and all postembryonic tissues and organs.

Transaminase – An enzyme that catalyzes chemical reactions in the body in which an amino group is transferred from a donor molecule to a recipient molecule.

Transcription – Making an RNA copy from a sequence of DNA (a gene). Transcription is the first step in gene expression.

Transcription factor – Molecules that bind to RNA polymerase III and aid in transcription.

Transgene – A gene that has been incorporated from one cell or organism and passed on to successive generations.

Translation – The process of forming a protein molecule at a ribosomal site of protein synthesis from information contained in messenger RNA.

Trophectoderm – The outer layer of the developing blastocyst that will ultimately form the embryonic side of the placenta.

Trophoblast – The extraembryonic tissue responsible for negotiating implantation, developing into the placenta, and controlling the exchange of oxygen and metabolites between mother and embryo.

Trypsin – An enzyme that digests proteins. Often used to separate cells.

Undifferentiated – Not having changed to become a specialized cell type.

Unipotent – Refers to a cell that can only develop in a specific way to produce a certain end result.

Vascular – Composed of, or having to do with, blood vessels.

Villi – Projections from the surface, especially of a mucous membrane. If the projection is minute, as in a cell surface, it is called a microvillus.

Vimentin – The major polypeptide that joins with other subunits to form the intermediate filament cytoskeleton of mesenchymal cells. Vimentin may also have a role in maintaining the internal organization of certain cells.

White blood cell (WBC) – The primary effector cells against infection and tissue damage. WBCs are formed from the undifferentiated stem cell that can give rise to all blood cells. Also known as a leukocyte.

X inactivation – The normal inactivation of one of the two X chromosomes in females.

Y chromosome – The chromosome which determines male gender.

Yolk sac – Vital to the embryo for the formation of primordial and other cells that form the embryo. In mammals, it is small and devoid of a yolk.

Zona pellucida – A thick, transparent noncellular layer that surrounds and protects the oocyte.

Zygote – A cell formed by the union of male and female germ cells (sperm and egg, respectively).

Appendix F.ii.

TERMS

AGM – The region where the aorta, gonads, and fetal kidney mesh.

ALS – A myotrophic lateral sclerosis. Also known as Lou Gehrig's disease.

BME – Beta-mercaptoethanol.

BMP-1 to BMP-9 – Bone morphogenetic proteins that are signaling molecules.

BRCA1 – Breast Cancer Gene 1.

BRCA2 – Breast Cancer Gene 2.

C/EBC – CCAAT/Enhancer binding protein.

CD4 – Helper T cells that are instrumental in initiating an immune response by supplying help in the form of special cytokines to both CD 8 cytotoxic T cells and B cells.

CD8 – Cytotoxic (killer) T cells that are capable of killing infected cells once activated by cytokines secreted by antigen-specific CD4 helper T cells.

CMV – Cytomegalovirus.

EBs – Embryoid bodies.

EG – Embryonic germ cell.

ES – Embryonic stem cell.

FACS – Fluorescence-activated cell sorting.

Fas receptor (CD95) – Fatty acid synthase.

FGF-1 to FGF-10 – Fibroblast growth factor 1 to 10. A growth factor molecule.

GATA4 – Transcription factor. Important in embryonic stem differentiation into yolk sac endoderm.

GATA6 – Important for embryonic stem cell differentiation into heart smooth muscle.

GCSF – Granulocyte-colony stimulating factor.

Gdf-5 – Growth/differentiation factor – 5. A growth factor molecule.

GDNF – Glial cell-derived neurotrophic factor. A growth factor molecule.

GFP – Green fluorescent protein.

Gp130 – Glycoprotein. Signal transducing receptor of Cytokines.

Gsc – Goosecoid. A signaling molecule.

hCNS-SC – Human central nervous system stem cell.

Hesx1 – Pituitary transcription factor.

Hex – Hexosaminidase. Enzyme for processing lipid (fat).

HGF – Hepatic growth factor molecule. Also a scatter factor.

HLAs – Human leukocyte antigens.

Hoxa-d – Homeobox-containing a to d. A transcription factor.

HPC – Hematopoietic progenitor cell.

HSC – Hematopoietic stem cell.

ICM – Inner Cell Mass.

IVF – In vitro fertilization.

LIF – Leukemia inhibitory factor. A growth factor molecule.

Lim1 – A transcription factor molecule.

Mac-1 (CD11b) – Antigen found in blood cells. Indicative of murine and progenitor cells.

MPC – Mesenchymal progenitor cell.

MR4 – Metabolic regulator. Important for electron transport and ATP synthesis.

MSC – Mesenchymal stem cell.

Myf-5 – Myogenic regulatory factor molecule.

NK – Natural killer lymphocytes.

NSC – Neural stem cell.

Oct4 – Octamer binding gene. Important for germ cell generation.

Otx2 – A transcription factor molecule.

Pax-1 to Pax-9 – Paired box 1-9. A transcription factor molecule.

PDGF – Platelet-derived growth factor.

PDX-1 – A transcription factor molecule.

PECAM 1 – Platelet. Endothelial cell adhesion molecule.

SDF-1/CXCR4 – Stromal-derived factor and its receptor.

SHH – Sonic hedgehog.

SMA – Alpha-smooth muscle actin.

SP – Side population stem cell.

Stat 3 – Signal Transducers and Activators of Transcription 3.

T3 – Triiodothyronine. A thyroid hormone important for hematopietic cells.

TGF-β1 to TGF-β5 – Transforming growth factors.

TPO/mpl – Thrombopoietin and receptor.

VEGF – Vascular endothelial growth factor.

Wnt1 – A signaling molecule.

XIST – X-inactive specific transcript. Uncertain function.

APPENDIX G:

INFORMATIONAL RESOURCES

Appendix G.i.

PERSONS INTERVIEWED

Peter Andrews
University of Sheffield
Sheffield, UK

Piero Anversa
New York Medical College
Valhalla, NY

Nissim Benvenisty
Hebrew University
Tel Aviv, Israel

Christopher Bjornson
University of Washington
Seattle, WA

Helen Blau
Stanford University
Palo Alto, CA

David Bodine
National Human Genome
   Research Institute
Bethesda, MD

Ariff Bongso
National University Hospital
Singapore

Susan Bonner-Weir
Harvard University
Cambridge, MA

Richard Burt
Northwestern Medical Center
Chicago, IL

Karen Chandross
Aventis Pharmaceuticals Inc.
Bridgewater, NJ

Richard Childs
National Heart, Lung, and Blood
   Institute
Bethesda, MD

Dennis Choi
Washington University School of
   Medicine
St. Louis, MO

Alan Colman
PPL, Ltd
Blacksburg, VA

Jonathan Dinsmore
Diacrin, Inc.
Charlestown, MA

Cynthia Dunbar
National Heart, Lung, and Blood
   Institute
Bethesda, MD

Stephen Dunnett
Cardiff University
Cardiff, Wales

Elaine Dzierzak
Erasmus University
Rotterdam, Holland

Connie Eaves
University of British Columbia
Vancouver, BC Canada

Chris Evans
Harvard University
Cambridge, MA

James Fallon
University of California, Irvine
Irvine, CA

Gary Fathman
Stanford University
Palo Alto, CA

Meri Firpo
University of California at
   San Francisco
San Francisco, CA

Itzhak Fischer
MCP Hahnemann University
Philadelphia, PA

Curt Freed
University of Colorado
Denver, CO

Fred Gage
Salk Institute
La Jolla, CA

Richard Gardner
University of Oxford
Oxford, UK

John Gearhart
Johns Hopkins University
Baltimore, MD

Steven Goldman
Cornell University
New York, NY

Margaret Goodell
Baylor College of Medicine
Houston, TX

Joel Habener
Harvard University
Cambridge, MA

Neil Hanley
University of Southampton
Southampton, UK

Alberto Hayek
University of California, San Diego
San Diego, CA

Robert Hawley
American Red Cross
Rockville, MD

Thomas Ho
Neuronyx Corporation
Malvern, PA

Ronald Hoffman
University of Illinois Cancer Center
Chicago, IL

Ole Isacson
Harvard Medical School
Boston, MA

Silviu Itescu
Columbia University
New York, NY

Josef Itskovitz-Eldor
Technion-Israel Institute of
   Technology
Haifa, Israel

Douglas Kerr
Johns Hopkins University
Baltimore, MD

Jeffrey Kordower
Rush Presbyterian Medical Center
Chicago, IL

Kristy Kraemer
National Institute of Allergy and
Infectious Diseases
Bethesda, MD

William Langston
Parkinson's Institute
Sunnyvale, CA

Robert Lanza
Advanced Cell Technologies
Cambridge, MA

Ihor Lemischka
Princeton University
Princeton, NJ

Fred Levine
University of California, San Diego
San Diego, CA

John McDonald
Washington University School of
   Medicine
St. Louis, MO

Ron D. McKay
National Institute of Neurological
   Disorders and Stroke
Bethesda, MD

Jeffrey Macklis
Harvard Medical School
Boston, MA

Douglas Melton
Harvard University
Cambridge, MA

Eva Mezey
National Institute of Neurological
   Disorders and Stroke
Bethesda, MD

Shin-Ichi Nishikawa
Kyoto University Medical School
Kyoto, Japan

Jon Odorico
University of Wisconsin
Madison, WI

Warren Olanow
Mt. Sinai School of Medicine
New York, NY

Thomas Okarma
Geron Inc.
Menlo Park, CA

Donald Orlic
National Human Genome
   Research Institute
Bethesda, MD

Mitradas Panicker
National Centre for Biological
   Sciences
Bangalore, India

Ammon Peck
University of Florida
Gainesville, FL

Roger Pedersen
University of California at San
   Francisco
San Francisco, CA

Martin Pera
Monash University
Melbourne, Australia

Vijayakumar Ramiya
Ixion Biotechnology
Alachua, FL

Mahendra Rao
National Institute on Aging
Bethesda, MD

Eugene Redmond
Yale University
New Haven, CT

Juan Reig
Universidad Miguel Hernandez
Alicante, Spain

Camillo Ricordi
University of Miami
Miami, FL

Pamela Gehron Robey
National Institute of Dental and
Craniofacial Research
Bethesda, MD

Janet Rossant
University of Toronto
Ontario, Canada

Jeffrey Rothstein
Johns Hopkins University
Baltimore, MD

Manfred Ruediger
Cardion, Inc.
Erkrath, Germany

Hans R. Schöler
University of Pennsylvania
Kennett Square, PA

James Shapiro
University of Alberta
Edmonton, Canada

Karl Skorecki
Technion ñ Israel Institute of
    Technology
Haifa, Israel

Austin Smith
University of Edinburgh
Edinburgh, Scotland

Evan Snyder
Harvard Medical School
Boston, MA

James Thomson
University of Wisconsin ñ Madison
Madison, WI

Satish Totey
National Institute of Immunology
New Delhi, India

Pantelis Tsoulfas
University of Miami School of
    Medicine
Miami, FL

Ann Tsukamoto
Stem Cells, Inc.
Palo Alto, CA

Gary Van Zant
University of Kentucky Medical
    Center
Lexington, KY

Catherine Verfallie
University of Minnesota
Minneapolis, MN

Inder M. Verma
The Salk Institute
La Jolla, CA

Irving Weissman
Stanford University Medical School
Stanford, CA

Esmail Zanjani
University of Nevada
Reno, NV

Leonard Zon
Harvard Medical School
Boston, MA

G-4

Appendix G.ii.

SPECIAL CONTRIBUTIONS

John Gearhart
Johns Hopkins University
Baltimore, MD

Ron D. McKay
National Institute of Neurological
Disorders and Stroke
Bethesda, MD

Pamela Gehron Robey
National Institute of Dental and
Craniofacial Research
Bethesda, MD

Janet Rossant
University of Toronto
Ontario, Canada

James Thomson
University of Wisconsin – Madison
Madison, WI

Appendix G.iii.

SPECIAL ACKNOWLEDGMENTS

Cynthia Allen
Silver Spring, MD

Deborah M. Barnes
Bethesda, MD

Marty Brotemarkle
Office of Science Policy &
  Planning, NIH
Bethesda, MD

Elizabeth Miller Dean
Office of Science Policy &
  Planning, NIH
Bethesda, MD

Gregory J. Downing
Office of Science Policy &
  Planning, NIH
Bethesda, MD

Donald M. Fink, Jr.
U.S. Food and Drug Administration
Bethesda, MD

Bruce Fuchs
Office of Science Education, NIH
Bethesda, MD

Charles Anderson Goldthwaite, Jr.
Charlottesville, VA

Mary Groesch
Office of Biotechnology Activities,
  NIH
Bethesda, MD

Celia Hooper
Office of Intramural Research, NIH
Bethesda, MD

Robin I. Kawazoe
Office of Science Policy &
  Planning, NIH
Bethesda, MD

Kristy Kraemer
National Institute of Allergy and
  Infectious Diseases
Bethesda, MD

Robert Levin
Office of Science Policy &
  Planning, NIH
Bethesda, MD

Marina O'Reilly
Office of Biotechnology Activities,
  NIH
Bethesda, MD

Amy P. Patterson
Office of Biotechnology Activities,
  NIH
Bethesda, MD

Peggy Schnoor
Office of Science Policy &
  Planning, NIH
Bethesda, MD

Robert Taylor
Falls Church, VA

Dat Tran
Office of Science Policy &
  Planning, OSP
Bethesda, MD

Nancy Touchette
Science Designs, inc.
Monkton, MD

Jeff Walker
Sutter Design
Lanham, MD

MEDICAL ILLUSTRATIONS

Terese Winslow
Medical Illustration
Alexandria, VA

Caitlin Duckwall
Duckwall Productions
Baltimore, MD

Lydia Kibiuk
Baltimore, MD

Rob Duckwall
Duckwall Productions
Baltimore, MD

This page intentionally left blank